Functional Electrical Stimulation: Standing and Walking after Spinal Cord Injury

Authors

Alojz R. Kralj, D.Sc.
Professor
Electrical and Biomedical Engineering
and Robotics
Faculty of Electrical Engineering
Edvard Kardelj University
Ljubljana, Yugoslavia

Tadej Bajd, D.Sc.
Associate Professor
Electrical and Biomedical Engineering
and Robotics
Faculty of Electrical Engineering
Edvard Kardelj University
Ljubljana, Yugoslavia

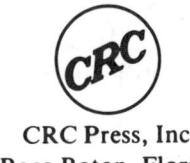

CRC Press, Inc.
Boca Raton, Florida

Library of Congress Cataloging-in-Publication Data

Functional electrical stimulation : standing and walking after spinal
  cord injury / authors, Alojz R. Kralj, Tadej Bajd.
    p.   cm.
  Includes bibliographies and index.
  ISBN 0-8493-4529-4
  1. Spinal cord–Wounds and injuries–Patients–Rehabilitation.
2. Electric stimulation.   I. Kralj, Alojz R., 1937-   II. Bajd,
Tadej, 1949-
   [DNLM: 1. Electric Stimulation. 2. Electrotherapy. 3. Spinal
  Cord Injuries–rehabilitation.   WL 400 F979]
RD594.3.F86 1989
617'.482044—dc19
DNLM/DLC
for Library of Congress   88-14508
                                                                        CIP

This book represents information obtained from authentic and highly regarded sources. Reprinted material is quoted with permission, and sources are indicated. A wide variety of references are listed. Every reasonable effort has been made to give reliable data and information, but the author and the publisher cannot assume responsibility for the validity of all materials or for the consequences of their use.

All rights reserved. This book, or any parts thereof, may not be reproduced in any form without written consent from the publisher.

Direct all inquiries to CRC Press, Inc., 2000 Corporate Blvd., N.W., Boca Raton, Florida, 33431.

© 1989 by CRC Press, Inc.

International Standard Book Number 0-8493-4529-4

Library of Congress Card Number 88-14508
Printed in the United States

To Irina and Barbara

PREFACE

The knowledge displayed in this book represents the present state of the art in functional electrical stimulation (FES) in spinal cord injured (SCI) subjects as developed and practiced in Ljubljana, Yugoslavia. This knowledge is a result of 20 years of systematic FES research and of more than 15 years of research and use of FES in SCI patients. This knowledge was established by clinical practice and by patients' daily use. The text of this book is also based on experiences gained during university classroom teaching to graduate students at the Faculty of Electrical Engineering, Edvard Kardelj University, Ljubljana, Slovenia, Yugoslavia, at University of Southern California, Los Angeles, CA, and at Illinois Institute of Technology, Chicago, IL. It is also based on practical experiences arising from numerous FES seminars conducted regularly by the University Rehabilitation Institute, Edvard Kardelj University Ljubljana, Slovenia, Yugoslavia. The material presented was adapted and shaped according to the experience gained in transferring the FES methodology to other institutions, like the Illinois Institute of Technology, the Michael Resse Hospital, and the Pritzker Institute of Chicago, all in Chicago, IL, and to different institutions in Europe, such as the Bioengineering Unit, University of Strathclyde, Glasgow, U.K. During preparation of this manuscript, our approach has been adopted by several research and clinical institutions, such as Lowenstein Rehabilitation Hospital, Raanana, Israel, Institut für Biokybernetik und Biomedizinische Technik, Universität Karlsruhe, W. Germany, Department of Physical Medicine and Rehabilitation, University of Minnesota, MN, and Department of Electrical Engineering, Bath University, Salisbury, U.K. Dissemination of our research results through journals, conferences, and articles presented at scientific meetings strongly influenced the format of this book.

Our principal goal was to prepare an organized fundamental text stressing the basic principles of the field on a systems knowledge level. The presentation and format was arranged for students and professionals in engineering and medicine, specially in rehabilitation, who are starting or are already engaged in FES utilization. We consider that this book represents a starting effort in regard to unifying the scattered concepts and principles of synthesis, design, development, and utilization of FES as a mean in rehabilitation of SCI subjects. Because of selecting among different methodologies, while presenting an unified approach to the matter, this work is also a reference source. Occasionally, we have sacrified theory in favor of simplicity. We hope the practitioners in the field of rehabilitation and FES will find this book a useful reference for FES in general, because it presents clearly and critically relevant concepts and provides pointers to more detailed literature which they may prefer to read. Our educational objective was the selection of fundamentals and basic principles for presenting in an unified and ordered way the scientifically based matter.

FES of SCI patients is not a scientific discipline by itself, it is rather a combination of engineering and medical disciplines. Recognizing the stated, our aim was to select and present those exclusive topics in the field of FES in SCI patients which can be considered as fundamentals and system science. Because of pedagogical soundness, we have included only a minimal number of examples for illustrating the basic matter covered. Our objective was to teach concepts without balast, enabling the reader to gain new knowledge in regard to fundamentals and formalized basic principles of FES in SCI. We tried not to include too many research reports, results, and statistical evaluations. This matter is included only to the extent necessary for illustrating and presenting the present state of art. Such an approach is favored as basic principles, and fundamentals will remain, while technology dependent solutions and results may change in near future. By intentionally doing so, we hope that the book will remain useful for a longer time.

Here, it is fair to state, that if scientific principles exist in the field of FES in SCI patients gait restoration, we have not yet discovered or proved them. Our knowledge on FES and gait restoration, in particular, is almost empirical and subjective, being the product of nearly 20 years of FES experimental use. FES and the whole rehabilitation field in general have a strong heuristic component and are lacking formalized, scientific, and fundamental knowledge. Theoretical aspects can be introduced to FES and SCI rehabilitation from related fields, but there is little of formal knowledge that can be directly applied to FES in SCI patients. The important product of the 20 years of subjective and empirical FES research is the experience from which we can learn the most relevant issues which may bring us a step closer to scientific fundamentals and formalized knowledge in regard to locomotion restoration in man.

This book is presenting the fundamental aspects of FES in SCI subjects from the Ljubljana research and development point of view. This approach is stressing the attributes such as simplicity, incorporation of patient's preserved mechanisms, and structures in the locomotion restoration scheme, including the dissected spinal cord, reflexes, natural body sensors, biomechanical construction principles, constraints, invariants, bone and joint mechanics, neural control, patient autonomy, etc. all with the aim to enhance function and prevent development of secondary pathologies. This broader understanding of FES and restoration of movement in man forces us to realize how little we know about the human locomotor system. It forces us also to consider innovative ways to utilize the means provided by nature when developing further possibilities of FES utilization. The human system uses redundancy, synergism, reflexes, etc. for improving function, reliability, and efficiency of a graceful movement. We do not yet understand fully the human system synergism and redundancy and how they relate to the neural control of movement.

The future of FES will predominantly depend on the quality of controlled excitation of neural tissue, on selective recording techniques, and also strongly upon innovative FES control approaches, incorporation of preserved structures like sensors and reflex loops, sensory information interpretation, as well as complete system mechanics and neural control. It can be recognized that the task of designing and implementing patient integrated FES locomotion restoration is a complex and difficult one, and we hope and wish that this book will add some new aspects and pieces of knowledge to the emerging formal knowledge base in this very slowly growing FES field. Therefore, it is understandable why our aim was, in spite of many open areas, controversies and disputable problems, to provide a simple textbook with an appropriately organized and up-to-date selection of basic principles and fundamentals presented as formally as possible. As FES in SCI patients is an interdisciplinary field, we limited our interests on engineering issues and, only when necessary, also on rehabilitation problems. For a newcomer to the field, to learn the scattered material from the available literature and to realize the principles and fundamentals of FES application, is a rather difficult task. Therefore, we have tried to put the relevant matter in an ordered and arranged manner enabling easier study. The book was written by engineers with the aim to display basic engineering knowledge in FES, presenting at the same time the major part of system knowledge around which all the FES methodology in SCI patients is integrated. Therefore, it is providing to the nonengineers and professionals with medical and rehabilitation background education, the scientific, formalized, and unified basic knowledge, and fundamentals of FES application in SCI patients. It presents also a starting textbook for engineers, medical students, medical professionals, physical therapists, and orthotists interested in FES and rehabilitation of SCI patients in a broader sense. We hope that this book will provide an effective way of disseminating knowledge and enable many rehabilitation institutions to start effective and successful utilization of FES for the rehabilitation of SCI patients.

Alojz Kralj
and
Tadej Bajd

THE EDITORS

Alojz R. Kralj, D.Sc., was born in 1937 and lived in Maribor until he finished higher gimnazium in 1956. He completed his studies at the Faculty of Electrical Engineering, University of Ljubljana, Slovenia, Yugoslavia. In 1964, he graduated as Diplom. Engineer in Electronics, he obtained his M.Sc. in Automatic Control in 1969, and in 1970, his D.Sc. degree. Since 1965, he has been involved in functional electrical stimulation and biomechanics research. He has performed research in multichannel FES for stroke patients including the development of three- and six-channel electrical stimulators for therapy and early gait initiation. Since 1968, he has been conducting research in FES of spinal cord injured patients and has led the research toward the developments for the Ljubljana methodology for FES-assisted standing and four-channel enabled gait in spinal cord injured patients. Over the years, Professor Kralj has published more than 100 papers and co-authored several books. At the Faculty of Electrical Engineering, Edvard Kardelj University, Ljubljana, he is a professor and teaches courses in Biomedical Engineering, Robotics, and Electronics. Professor Kralj was director of the Rehabilitation Engineering Center, Ljubljana, from 1978 until 1985 and also served as co-president to the Yugoslav Society of Medical and Biological Engineering. In 1973/74, he was visiting professor at the University of Southern California, Los Angeles, CA and research associate with the Rancho Los Amigos Hospital. From 1980 to 1986, Professor Kralj was visiting professor to the Illinois Institute of Technology and Pritzker Institute of Medical Engineering in Chicago, IL where in 1980, he already started introducing FES for spinal cord injured patients. In 1986, he was visiting professor at the Rush Medical College, Rush-Presbyterian-St. Luke's Medical Center, Department of Neurosurgery in Chicago, IL. Dr. Kralj has received several national and international awards for his work in functional electrical stimulation.

Tadej Bajd, D.Sc., was born in Ljubljana, Yugoslavia in 1949. In 1972, he graduated from the Faculty of Electrical Engineering, University of Ljubljana, where in 1976, he obtained his M.Sc. degree and in 1979, his D.Sc. degree.

He has been a research assistant at J. Stefan Institute in Ljubljana and a visiting research fellow at Rancho Los Amigos Hospital, Los Angeles, CA and Strathclyde University, Glasgow, U.K. He is presently an assoicate professor and vice dean of the Faculty of Electrical Engineering in Ljubljana.

Tadej Bajd is the author or co-author of numerous scientific publications from the field of biomedical engineering and industrial robotics. He is also secretary of the Slovene Society of Medical and Biological Engineering which is part of the International Federation of Medical and Biological Engineering. He was twice awarded with the national "Boris Kidrič" award for his scientific achievements in the field of functional electrical stimulation for paralyzed subjects.

ACKNOWLEDGMENTS

Functional electrical stimulation (FES) is a young and growing interdisciplinary field. The foundation of a new field is almost never an accomplishment of a single person. For the progress of FES, many institutions and individuals have to be credited. Many institutions and individuals directly or indirectly, by knowing it or not, contributed also to our research work. First, we would like to acknowledge the funding of our research activities obtained through many years from the Slovenian Research Council, Ljubljana, Slovenia, Yugoslavia, and from the National Institute of Handicapped Research, and at present National Institute for Disability and Rehabilitation Research, Washington, D.C. We also gratefully acknowledge the valuable support from the Faculty of Electrical Engineering, Edvard Kardelj University, Ljubljana, Slovenia, Yugoslavia, and the University Rehabilitation Institute, Ljubljana, Yugoslavia.

We are very grateful to our co-researchers and medical members of the Ljubljana team for FES of spinal cord injured patients. In particular, we would like to thank for their enthusiasm, help, suggestions, and constant support during the many years of our work the following professionals: Principal Rajko Turk, Head of Department of Spinal Cord Injury, Professor Martin Štefančič, and physiotherapists, Helika Benko and Pavla Obreza. We would like to express our gratitude also to Mr. Janez Šega for his devoted technical support through all these years. To all of them, we would like to thank their advisory support, careful work with patients, and professional development of FES equipment.

The outstanding criticism and enthusiasm of our physiotherapists many times made the research work more enjoyable and progressive. In addition, we received many useful suggestions and comments from our teachers and consultants who shared, through all these years with us, the eagerness, enthusiasm, disappointments, and happiness during the development and establishment of FES locomotor principles. Here, we would like to thank first Professor Lojze Vodovnik, a member of Slovenian Academy of Sciences, for his advices, creative support, and for evoking in us the enthusiasm for this very special and challenging field. For constantly supporting our research efforts, we cordially thank to Mr. Joseph E. Traub, Director of Technology Transfer at NIDRR, Washington, D.C. We are extending our special thanks and appreciation for their many contributions to our professors: Principal Slobodan Grobelnik, Anton Širca, Bogdan Brecelj, James Reswick, Jacqueline Perry, Paul Meyer, and Robert Waters.

Our patients and students have substantially contributed many times to our views, our ideas, and reasoning. We are indebted to them for their criticism and enthusiasm.

Particularly, we would like to extend our thanks to those who helped to prepare the manuscript. For expeditive typing and retyping our thanks are expressed to Mrs. Jožica Trobec-Gračanin. Technical drawings were prepared by Mr. Smiljan Dečman, while excellent photographic material by Mr. Marko Tiran.

We would like to extend our most sincere thanks and give the greatest credit to our wives for their support which was and continues to be invaluable.

Therefore, we are dedicating this book to Irina Kralj and Barbara Bajd. Irina also prepared the artist drawings in this book, while Barbara was more than helpful in searching and providing references which are abundant in the present text. Our best thanks are directed also to our children and parents for their continuous support and patience.

We hope that the readers of this book will be inspired enough to continue on their own, discovering the beautiful and challenging world of FES which is bringing medicine and engineering to many patients. We would like to pass this challenge to you to join and continue the battle for improved life quality of so many humans suffering from spinal cord injury.

TABLE OF CONTENTS

Chapter 1
Introduction 1
I. Review of Lower Extremity Functional Electrical Stimulation (FES)
    Research in Paraplegic Subjects 1
II. FES Restoration of Locomotion in Paraplegic Patients and Scope of
    the Present Book 9
References 13

Chapter 2
Muscle Restrengthening and Patient Conditioning 17
I.   The Basics of Muscle Physiology and the State of Skeletal Muscle
     Following Spinal Cord Injury 17
II. The Basics of Muscle Electrophysiology and Parameters of
     Electrical Stimulation 18
III. Electrical Stimulation Exercise in Neurologically Intact Subjects 23
IV. Animal Models 25
V.   The Restrengthening Methodology, Training, and Monitoring 26
     A. Training Modalities 26
     B. Measuring Methods 28
     C. Effects of Exercise on Strength Increase and Fatigue Resistance ... 29
References 33

Chapter 3
Influence of Electrical Stimulation on Spasticity in Spinal Cord Injured Patients .. 37
I.   Characteristics of Spinal Spasticity 37
II. Clinical Assessment of Spasticity 38
III. Treatment of Spasticity and Influence of Electrical Stimulation on
     Agonist and Antagonist Muscle Spasticity 41
IV. Transcutaneous Electrical Stimulation of Dermatomes 44
References 47

Chapter 4
Restoration of Standing 49
I.   Introduction 49
II. Mechanics of Standing 49
     A. Forces and Movements 49
     B. Work, Energy, and Power 53
     C. Fundamentals of Standing 56
     D. Stability and Energy Criteria Related to Standing 57
        1. Solid Objects 57
        2. Segmented Structures 58
     E. Posture Selection and Standing 63
     F. Postural Space 65
     G. Postural Movements and Bone Functions 67
     H. Biomechanics of Standing-Up and Sitting-Down 75
        1. Standing-Up and Sitting-Down Movements: Definition
           of Terms 76
        2. Biomechanical Parameters of Stand/Sit Maneuvers 79
        3. The Stand/Sit Trajectories 85

III. Patients Selection 91
       A. Patients Selection According to Level and Status of Lesion 92
       B. Patients Selection According to Their Neurological Status 94
       C. Patients Selection According to Physiological Status 94
       D. Physical Evaluation and Indications for FES 96
  IV. FES Standing 97
       A. Supporting Frames for FES Standing 101
       B. Posture Dependence of Standing Performance 102
       C. Posture Switching 105
  V. Benefits of FES Standing 109
  VI. Functional Use of FES Standing 114
  References 119

Chapter 5
FES Ambulation Program in Incomplete SCI Patients 123
  I. General Characteristics of Incomplete SCI Lesions 123
  II. Neurophysiological Characteristics of Incomplete SCI Lesions Relevant
       to FES Application 124
  III. FES Therapeutic Program 129
  IV. FES-Assisted Walking 133
  References 137

Chapter 6
FES-Assisted Walking in Complete SCI Patients 139
  I. Patient Selection 139
  II. Fundamentals of FES Gait Restoration 140
  III. Principles of Gait Synthesis and Control 147
       A. Patient Model 150
       B. Control Principles 154
       C. Expansion of Control Information 159
  IV. Gait Training 164
       A. Training of Walker Ambulation 169
       B. Training of Crutch Ambulation 169
  V. Applications and Results 173
       A. Review of Stimulators and Balancing Aids 174
       B. Accomplishments and Results 177
  References 189

Index 193

Chapter 1

INTRODUCTION

I. REVIEW OF LOWER EXTREMITY FUNCTIONAL ELECTRICAL STIMULATION (FES) RESEARCH IN PARAPLEGIC SUBJECTS

Electricity can have various effects on living tissues or cells. The possibility of exciting the action potential in a neural cell appears to be very attractive. The stimulus then propagates along ramified pathways of the nervous system. In this way, almost any organ of the human body can be influenced by electrical pulses.

A theoretical description for propagated action potential was given by the model proposed by Hodgkin and Huxley.[1] A novel practical application of electricity in medicine was presented by the artificial cardiac pacemaker.[2] There was a series of electrical stimulators proposed and patented by different authors already in the 1950s.[3] The development of electronics made it possible for Wladimir Liberson[4] to create the stimulator, preventing foot-drop in hemiplegic patients. It was triggered by a heel switch in the shoe of the affected leg. Stimulation electrodes were positioned above the peroneal nerve in the fossa poplitea area. Each time the patient raised the heel, the heel switch triggered the stimulator, causing dorsal flexion.

This idea has opened the way to a new field of modern rehabilitation known as functional electrical stimulation (FES).[4,5] In 1967, FES was described as "electrical stimulation of muscle deprived of nervous control with a view of providing muscular contraction and producing a functionally useful movement".[6]

Apart from provoking contraction of heart and skeletal muscles, electrical currents can be applied to alleviate pain, help inhibit or void the urinary bladder, reduce epileptic seizures, prevent the progress of scoliosis, improve blood circulation in a certain part of the body, promote bone growth, excite spinal cord neurons, control breathing, and influence the auditory nerve and even the visual cortex. Most of these applications are extensively described in several review papers.[7-12]

FES of peripheral nerves provoking contractions in skeletal muscles can be applied to a patient with a preserved excitability of the lower motor neuron, i.e., to a patient with a paralysis resulting in upper motor neuron lesion (UMNL). It is primarily used with hemiplegic patients, spinal cord injured (SCI) subjects, children with cerebral palsy, and with other patients suffering from an impairment or disease of the central nervous system (CNS), e.g., head injury, multiple sclerosis. Spinal cord injury is one of the most devastating injuries of the nervous system. It results in a frustrating, often irreversible change in the patient's quality of life. The number of SCI patients is not negligible. There are, for example, about 10,000 American patients admitted to hospitals each year.[13] Half of them are younger than 25 years of age. Their life expectancy is today becoming close to that of the normal population. Current mobility rehabilitation of SCI subjects is limited to the use of the wheelchair and, to a much lesser extent, to the use of passive long leg braces, which permit crutch ambulation.

FES may offer a new promising alternative to the present rehabilitation modalities. Excellent research work has been performed in the use of FES in the upper extremities for producing functional hand rehabilitation in quadriplegics.[14,15] Even more attractive appears to be the application of FES in the lower extremities of paraplegic patients, producing the standing and biped gait of completely paralyzed persons. A review of accomplishments utilizing FES for locomotion restoration in complete SCI patients will be given. The first application of FES to a paraplegic patient was reported by Kantrowitz[16] in 1963. The quadriceps and glutei muscles of a T-3 paraplegic subject were stimulated using surface electrodes. The patient's erect standing was achieved for a few minutes. The next similar trial was made by Wilemon et al.[17] and Reswick[18] at Rancho Los Amigos Hospital in California. They implanted stimulators to both femoral and gluteal nerves in an attempt to obtain contraction of knee and hip extensors. A T-5 female paraplegic patient was able to stand and even walk with her knees extended (swing-to or swing-through gait). The ankle joints were stabilized by the help of short leg ankle braces. The stimulation frequency was set between 20 and 25 Hz, while a 0.3-ms pulse duration was chosen. Muscles already atrophied were retrained through an electrical stimulation program lasting 12 h/d over a period of 2 months. The strength of the stimulated muscle was increased, and the fatigue time significantly prolonged from 15 s to 2 h of sustained muscle contraction. Although using crutches, the patient had problems with balance, and ambulation without an accompanying person was not possible. A not very successful trial of FES application in paraplegia was performed by Cooper et al.[19] He used a two-channel bilateral implant for stimulation of femoral and sciatic nerves to obtain the contraction of both hamstrings. It was supposed that knee extensors are too weak to support the body weight of a T-11,12 paraplegic patient. The patient was, therefore, put into a special frame and the reciprocal contractions of knee flexors provided a pushing of the supporting frame. The control over the stimulated muscle groups of the right and left leg was obtained through a mercury switch attached to the patient's sternum and activated by a tilting of the patient's trunk.

It is characteristic for all three investigations described that these achievements were only single trials and no research or clinical activities followed. First, continual research efforts were started by Kralj et al. in 1972.[20] The data were gathered on muscle forces exerted by FES in 50 paraplegic patients with different etiology, time past injury, sex, and age. It was demonstrated that almost all patients with lesions above T-12 have leg muscles which are electrically excitable. The influence of FES training on muscle force and fatigue resistance was documented. It was further shown that the dynamic properties of a paraplegic patient's muscle are close to that of normal muscle. Next, it was demonstrated that almost with no assistance, rising from the sitting to the standing position can be performed with the aid of surface FES.[21] Functional prolonged standing produced by only FES locked knee joints was proposed in 1979.[22] First reciprocal biped walking of a completely paralyzed paraplegic patient was described by the same group of authors 1 year later.[23] The most important characteristic of the walking pattern suggested[24,25] was the use of the preserved withdrawal reflex in order to synthesize swing phase movements. During the stance phase, knee extensors were stimulated providing sufficient support to the body. In this way, the minimal number of stimulation channels required for simple reciprocal ambulation of a completely paralyzed paraplegic subject was defined. It is further characteristic for the simple four-channel gait pattern that the patient himself controls the gait events and no stimulation sequences are prestored in the FES orthotic system. Additional lower extremity muscle groups, such as hip extensors, hip abductors, and ankle plantar flexors, were stimulated with the aim to improve locomotor functions.[23,25] The four-channel electrical stimulator was introduced into the clinical environment and later, walking out of a rehabilitation unit was also made possible. As a consequence, there were, as of 1987, about 70 SCI patients using daily surface FES of the lower extremities. Among them, ten paraplegic patients were able to walk by the help of FES and crutches outside of their homes. Another ten were using FES and a walker and walking regularly at their homes. An additional 30 paraplegic subjects were practicing regular FES standing exercises.[26] In further research, FES standing was prolonged by using intermittent stimulation of several muscle groups, rather than constant muscle activation of a single muscle group. This FES strategy was named posture switching.[27,28] Noticeable improvements also were achieved in the walking ability of incomplete SCI patients when using FES-triggered flexion response.[29]

Interesting research work was performed by Petrofsky and his colleagues when applying surface electrical stimulation to SCI patients. First, an exercise device to train a paraplegic's paralyzed muscle was designed.[30] Electrical stimulation, delivered to the knee extensors, was microcomputer-controlled. The magnitude of electrical pulses was dependent on information obtained from either a strain gauges transducer or precision potentiometer. Isometric, isokinetic, or isotonic exercise could be preprogramed. More efficient training was provided by an indoor bicycle.[31] Here, the paralyzed quadriceps and iliacus muscles were stimulated in order to elicit pedaling by the paraplegic subject. Blood pressure, heart rate, and body temperature monitoring made the training system safer for home use. Even more attractive exercising was conducted by use of the three-wheel outdoor bicycle.[32] The muscles stimulated were the gluteus maximus and quadriceps muscles of both extremities. The following parameters were assessed before and after active physical therapy: blood pressure, heart rate, ventilatory rate, oxygen consumption rate, blood lactate, selected blood gases, and bone density changes.[33] Resting blood pressure, which is often unstable in SCI patients, was found significantly more stable. FES exercise was found to be able to reverse bone demineralization and noticably stress the cardiopulmonary system. Closed-loop computer-controlled walking was proposed by Petrofsky and Phillips.[34] Special shoes with pressure transducers were developed and electrogoniometers attached to the leg joints. Walking was divided into four phases. The first activity was to raise the right heel. The next phase of walking involved lifting the ipsilateral hip. The third phase was represented by the straightening (knee extension) of the right leg. The aim of the final phase of the gait cycle was to bring the extended leg forward. This was accomplished by rotation at the opposite ankle through contracting the gastrocnemius muscle. This walking has only been tested in the laboratory environment.

Walking pattern, based on flexion response triggering, was also applied by Graupe et al.[35,36] In the investigation conducted by Bajd et al.,[24] simple hand switches, built into the handles of a walker or crutches, were used to initiate a step. The advantage of Graupe's approach was the control of stimulation sequences through a patient's electromyogram (EMG) signals. EMG control signals were generated voluntarily at erector spinae and lower back muscles. Surface recording electrodes were used in the experiment. Four different EMG signatures were satisfactorily generated and discriminated by the help of a microprocessor interface circuit. The four corresponding functions were as follows: stand-up command, right leg-up command, left leg-up command, and sit-down command. These functions were performed as a consequence of the following respective voluntary movements: both shoulders back while sitting, right shoulder back and left shoulder forward, left shoulder back and right shoulder forward, and, finally, both shoulders back while standing. The total computation delay was about 0.5 s. The EMG signatures chosen closely relate to natural activities of erector spinae muscles while balancing the trunk during normal standing-up and walking.

Mizrahi et al.[37,38] have also utilized the four-channel gait pattern described by adding the stimulation of gluteus maximus muscles. Six channels of electrical stimulation were delivered through surface electrodes, thus restoring the paraplegic subject's walking. The quadricep and gluteus maximus muscles were stimulated simultaneously in the supporting extremity, while the flexion reflex was triggered to obtain swinging of the contralateral limb. The gait of the patients was evaluated by means of an electrical contact system, assessing the time and distance parameters of walking. Low walking speed and short stride length, accompanied by a rather long stance and swing time, were recorded. The stride parameters were followed throughout the training period. A significant increase of stride length and gait velocity, together with a decrease of stance phase and stride time, were observed in all four paraplegic subjects. Heart rate and oxygen comsumption during FES exercise, standing, and walking were also assessed. Heart rate was increased 20% during FES exercise while the subject was in a sitting position. It was increased 100% during standing and 150% during FES-induced walking. Similarly, the oxygen uptake was doubled during exercise, tripled during standing, and it was about five times higher during walking as compared to the resting values. These results demonstrate the high level of effort during FES-restored walking, which also requires anaerobic sources of energy.

Standing performance with the knees locked by the help of surface FES of paralyzed knee extensors has been extensively studied by Cybulski et al.[39,40] Standing, while using knee-ankle-foot orthoses (KAFOs) was compared to FES standing. FES of the quadricep muscles resulted in standing stability slightly lower than that with KAFOs. It was also observed that visual information was much more important to a paraplegic subject than to a healthy individual during quiet stance. The aim of further research[41] was to develop a closed-loop control system for restoration of quiet standing. It was supposed that the hip joint is stabilized through maximal hyperextension, while the knee joint is fixed by FES. Motion could therefore occur only about the ankle. In this way, a single-link inverted pendulum model was proposed with electrically stimulated ankle joint agonist and antagonist muscles providing balancing at the ankle joint. Implementation of a controller providing stable FES standing would require assessment of ankle angle or the antero-posterior coordinate of reaction force application.

An implanted multichannel FES system providing standing and swing-to or swing-through walking was developed in 1979 by Brindley et al.[42] Passive radio receivers were implanted, together with subcutaneous (s.c.) wires and electrodes to stimulate the femoral nerves and the inferior and superior gluteal nerves. The fatigue of the continuously stimulated muscle was approached in three different ways. First, the stimulation frequency was decreased as low as 13 Hz. Second, the electrodes were placed on three branches of each femoral nerve. By cycling the stimulation between the electrodes, different parts of the quadriceps muscle could rest. It is interesting to note that no improved fatiguing of stimulated muscle was observed by this second approach. Fatigue resistance was mainly improved through an electrical training program. Two paraplegic subjects have received implants. After the training program was established, the first patient was able to stand for 35 min or walk for 15 min, while the second could stand for 75 min or walk for 5 min. During recent years, a 24-channel output implanted stimulator containing a special hybrid circuit was developed by the members of the same research group,[43] indicating that the field of implanted FES is progressing and gaining in interest.

The main advantage of implanted FES is presented by the low stimulation currents or voltages required for muscle activation. In this way, smaller energy sources are needed, providing more specific excitation possibilities and considerably reduced size of stimulators. High electrical stimulation amplitudes applied transcutaneously by surface electrodes can also result in burn injuries to the skin when applied inappropriately. Another disadvantage of surface FES is the positioning of electrodes, which is sometimes inconvenient and time consuming. An implantable 16-channel device for mobilization of paraplegic patients was proposed by Thoma et al.[44,45] The implantable stimulator was the size of a commercially available cardiac pacemaker. Here, epineurium-attached electrodes were introduced. The femoral and gluteal nerves were stimulated to obtain knee and hip joint extension. A stimulation frequency of 30 Hz was used. Fatiguing of the electrically stimulated muscle was approached by so-called "roundabout stimulation". It consists of periodic switching of the electrical current among four electrodes placed radially and equidistantly around the nerve. In this way, different nerve fibers are activated by a rotating electrical field during each stimulation sequence. Swing-through walking over short distances was obtained in two paraplegic patients. Extensive animal studies were conducted in order to determine histopathological changes of nerve and muscle because of implanted FES. The damages observed were caused by mechanical rather than electrical influences. The force of the stimulated muscle has increased up to four times. Biopsy examinations of stimulated paralyzed muscle showed that many of the type II muscle fibers were transformed into type I muscle fibers after the FES training program. The mean diameter of type I fibers decreased by about 20%, whereas the diameter of type II fibers showed a slight increase. The increase in the number of type I fibers demonstrates a transformation toward a slow-contracting muscle. In further research, the authors from the same group also demonstrated a significant increase of the muscle cross-sectional area by using the computer tomography approach.[46] A significant increase of skin and muscle blood flow was already observed after several minutes of electrical stimulation.

Apart from surface and implanted FES, there also exists the third modality of delivering electrical stimuli to the nerves of the paralyzed muscles. This technique is presented by the use of percutaneous intramuscular electrodes. The electrodes are made from extremely thin (76 μm) stainless steel wire.[47] The multistrain wire is coated by Teflon® and it is deinsulated at the end. The bared wire is wound in the shape of a very thin coil, which is ended by an anchoring hook. Implantation of the wire electrode is carried out with the help of a hypodermic needle. The wires pass through the skin and are soldered to small connectors. This arrangement makes percutaneous electrodes somewhat less attractive for patients wishing to use FES on a daily basis. A serious problem is also presented by the limited lifetime of wire electrodes. Cosmetic appearance is poor and there are also difficulties in toileting. The patient must also take care to not damage the electrodes. The electrode penetration site is to be cleansed daily. Percutaneous electrical stimulation is, without doubt, an excellent research electrode and modality for gaining the precious knowledge necessary to design adequate multichannel implanted stimulators.[48]

The main advantage of percutaneous FES applied to the lower extremities of completely paralyzed paraplegic subjects is the possibility of activation of many different muscles which are active during single phases of the gait cycle. The idea of Marsolais and Kobetic[49,50] was, therefore, to synthesize a stimulation pattern individually for each subject, which would be as close as possible to the normal activity of muscles during gait. The fine-wire electrodes were implanted at the motor points of knee extensors (quadriceps, vastus medialis, vastus lateralis, vastus intermedius), hip flexors (sartorius, tensor fasciae latae, gracilis, iliopsoas), hip extensors (semimembranosus, gluteus maximus), hip abductors (gluteus medius), ankle dorsiflexors (tibialis anterior, peroneous longus), and ankle plantar flexors (soleus). An average of 46 2-h sessions were needed to implant each paraplegic subject. It is important to note that only two body entry points were found to provide access to the muscles mentioned. One was on the medial aspect of the thigh, approximately halfway between the hip and the knee to access the hip extensors, flexors, and abductors, and the knee flexors and extensors. The second point was chosen on the medial calf just below the knee, for access to the ankle plantar and dorsiflexors. Electrodes were removed and replaced when they exhibited a breakage or loss of adequate function. The failures usually resulted from electrode movement. Complete withdrawal of those electrodes was in most cases possible. The implanted electrodes delivered biphasic current pulses with an amplitude of 20 mA, frequency from 20 to 50 Hz, and pulse width up to 150 μs. The wire electrode represented the cathode, while the anode was a surface electrode.

The stimulation sequences were accomplished with a 32-channel microprocessor-controlled stimulator. Each step was started by a hand switch, while the pattern of particular muscle action was stored and generated by a microcomputer program. Of the 11 paraplegic subjects participating in the investigation, 9 were able to stand, 7 could walk in parallel bars, and 6 were able to also walk with a walker. They were able to walk maximum distances up to 300 m. The reason for stopping was usually cardiopulmonar fatigue or muscle fatigue of the knee extensors. Gait evaluation was performed by assessing foot-floor contacts, walking speed, foot reaction forces, and joint goniograms. A very satisfactory walking speed of 0.8 m/s was measured with two subjects. An interesting study was also performed when comparing two different gait patterns.[51] The first pattern included stimulation of hip flexors, knee extensors, and ankle dorsiflexors. With the second gait pattern, hip extensors and abductors and ankle plantar flexors were added. With the second pattern, the paraplegic subject was better able to transfer the body weight from one leg to the other. Stride length and speed of walking were significantly increased, while the double-stance phase time was decreased. Less transfer of weight onto the walker was also observed. In detailed force plate studies, it was further demonstrated that the gluteus medius was most effective in mediolateral body weight shift during walking, while gluteus maximus and semimembranosus were taking care of bringing the center of pressure forward. Different locomotion modes were stored into the memory of the FES orthotic system and later selected like menus.

The stimulation pattern stored in the memory of a 32-channel microprocessor-controlled stimulator was also found as an efficient aid in ascending and descending stairs.[52] Three out of eleven subjects were able to climb stairs. Paraplegic subjects used one rail and one crutch for balance. The transfer from a walking aid to the railings of the staircase was found a problem that is not yet adequately solved. Surface stimulation of erector spinae and quadratus lumborum was added for control of trunk extension and sideways movements of the trunk. During the stance phase of walking, the plantar flexion momentum was large enough to lift the subject on his toes. This was found helpful to bring the contralateral extremity to the next higher step. Through the measurements of vertical reaction forces, it was observed that excessive weight was borne by the arms.

After this short review of different approaches to FES restoration of the walking pattern in paraplegic subjects with complete SCI lesions, it is only logical to compare these achievements with current methods of functional mobility. The primary means of mobilization for SCI subjects is a wheelchair. Use of a wheelchair on a level surface proves to be a highly efficient means of locomotion.[53,54] Average speed and rate of oxygen uptake are similar to the values assessed in normal walking. A somewhat elevated heart rate is observed in patients using a wheelchair. It is attributable to the fact that a higher heart rate is associated with upper extremity exercise rather than with lower extremity activity. However, use of a wheelchair is not without problems. Two major limitations are environmental barriers and decubitus ulcers.[55]

The conventional rehabilitation method for standing and walking in paraplegia emphasizes mechanical passive orthoses such as the KAFO. A typical KAFO has a fixed ankle joint. The knee joint is capable of flexion, but during standing and walking is locked in a position of extension. Paraplegic subjects are taught to stand with hips in hyperextension. Patients with paraplegia who require two KAFOs usually do not continue to stand or walk after discharge from a rehabilitation unit.[54] In a study of 98 paraplegic patients who were fitted with KAFOs, 16 used them for functional walking, 25 for exercise walking or standing, and 57 did not use them at all.[56]

It has already been mentioned in the beginning of this chapter that FES can only be applied to patients with a preserved excitability of the lower motoneuron. In more practical clinical terms, it means that only paraplegic subjects displaying spastic paraplegia are candidates for FES-restored ambulation. These are the patients with thoracic levels of SCI. These patients can, because of a lack of pelvic control, walk only with a swing-to or swing-through gait pattern when fitted with long leg braces. It was demonstrated[54] that the average speed for a patient using a swing-through crutch-assisted gait is 64% slower than normal, yet the rate of oxygen uptake is 38% greater, and the heart rate is increased 46%. It was further demonstrated that even able-bodied subjects have a marked elevation in the heart rate and rate of oxygen consumption when walking with a swing-through gait pattern.[57] These findings account for the fact that wheelchair propulsion approximates the energy cost in normal walking, whereas energy expenditure with KAFOs is significantly higher. The energy cost of FES walking in complete paraplegic subjects was compared to that of long leg brace ambulation.[58] Similar energy costs were observed with both walking modalities.

An important difference occurs with increased velocity of walking. As the speed of KAFOs walking increases, so does the energy cost. During FES walking, as speed increases, no significant variation of energy cost is seen. FES has, therefore, the potential to use less energy than KAFOs at speeds approaching those of normal walking.[58] Considering energy cost, FES locomotion does not at present appear to be a realistic functional goal for the patient with complete thoracic paraplegia. Nevertheless, the number of FES ambulating paraplegia subjects is constantly growing in various rehabilitation units all over the world. They are not only exercise or household walkers, some of them reach the level of community ambulation,[26] according to the classification proposed by Stauffer et al.[59] Psychological issues are also among the main reasons for an increased interest in FES walking. In the early period of the FES rehabilitation process, the enthusiasm of the patient when he sees his paralyzed muscles contract again is certainly important. When providing functional movements such as standing-up, this enthusiasm is further increased. In the last stage, when the patient is able to walk with the help of crutches, it appears to be most important that FES walking is much more aesthetic than the unnatural and noisy swing-through gait with KAFOs. In addition, when the goal of FES walking is only exercise ambulation, it brings, because of the efferent and afferent influences of FES walking, several benefits that cannot be attained by passive bracing. These functional benefits of FES ambulation still need to be rigorously confirmed.

It is a quite logical approach to combine the benefits of passive long leg braces intended for the standing and walking of paraplegic patients with the possibilities given by FES. The method was called hybrid orthotics and was proposed as early as 1973.[60] In the beginning, the goals were rather ambitious. A hierarchical control concept was considered for a hybrid actuator. First, voluntary effort of the muscle under consideration is to be exploited to a reasonable maximum. Second, electrical stimulation is added. Third, external power is added if the first two energy sources are inadequate to obtain the movement desired. The basic principle of the hybrid assistive method is, thus, to support FES when biological actuators fail to follow the prescribed trajectory of joint motion or the biological power supply cannot meet the dynamic requirements.

In present hybrid orthotic systems, no active actuators were utilized. The main advantage of hybrid systems is higher patient safety. Hybrid orthoses can also be efficiently applied in some cases of combined lower and upper motor neuron lesions, where FES alone would not yield satisfactory results. Within a hybrid orthosis combining FES and passive bracing, the mechanical component serves to support the subject's body weight, while electrical stimulation is used to provide propulsion. Hybrid orthosis proposed by Schwirtlich and Popović[61] consists of self-fitting modular orthosis, where a patient's control over knee joint locking is provided during walking. Four channels of electrical stimulation are used. The paraplegic subject makes a step-through flexion response triggering. Knee extensors stimulation is needed only to lock the knees. Locking is based on friction of the joint of the passive brace and is activated by a micromotor. Therefore, no electrical stimulation is necessary during the double-support phase. This eliminates the problem of neuromuscular fatigue. Shoe insole switches, inclinometers, and joint angle sensors provide necessary information to a microprocessor controller. Non-numerical (logic) control based on a set of predetermined rules is proposed, rather than the conventional closed-loop concept.

Hybrid orthosis suitable for patients presenting a combination of innervated and denervated muscles was proposed by Andrews and Bajd.[62] In low thoracic or high lumbar lesions, cases are encountered where knee extensors are peripherally denervated and, thus, cannot be electrically excited. Muscles governing ankle joint movement are centrally denervated and respond to electrical stimuli. A mechanical orthosis maintaining the knees in full extension can be used with these patients. Two channels of electrical stimulation are applied to the surface of each leg. One pair of electrodes is positioned over the muscle gastrocnemius and soleus to provide ankle plantar flexion. The second pair of electrodes is placed over the common peroneal nerve to produce a flexion reflex resulting in foot dorsiflexion and hip flexion. This electromechanical arrangement allows a tiptoe type of four-point gait. The subject first shifts his body weight onto one leg. Electrical stimulation is then applied to the plantar flexors of this leg and also to the peroneal nerve of the contralateral leg. During single-support time, the subject is therefore standing on the toes of one leg, which allows the contralateral extremity to swing forward.

Use of reciprocating-brace orthosis is described by Solomonow et al.[63] The orthosis is a long leg brace with the knees locked at extension, ankles fixed at 90°, and hip joints capable of motion. The hip joints are connected with a bowden cable. On movement of one leg forward (hip flexion), the bowden cable assembly forces the contralateral leg backward (hip extension). In this way, a push-off causing a forward shift of the center of gravity of the trunk is provided. It is proposed that a dual-channel implantable electrical stimulator will induce alternate hip flexion by excitation of the iliopsoas muscle group.

A practical solution of a hybrid orthosis appears to be a system based on a short leg-floor reaction orthosis.[64] This below-knee orthosis has the functional advantage of being able to lock the knee joint in hyperextension, provided that the body weight ground-reaction vector passes anterior to the knee joint axis. In such a case, no electrical stimulation of knee extensors is necessary. This state of so-called amuscular standing is characterized by a pressure applied in the region of the patella tendon by the restraining strap. When strap tension assessed by a special transducer drops below a preset threshold level, maximal stimulation of knee extensors is started. The use of this hybrid orthosis minimizes the amount of quadriceps stimulation required to stabilize the leg and thereby avoids fatigue of these muscles. A step is again initiated by triggering the flexion response. An interesting improvement is introduced by using a force transducer built into the handles of crutches or a walker. Whenever a greater degree of flexion is required, the subject presses proportionally harder on the force transducer.

After this short review of the main achievements in the use of FES in paraplegia, the advantages of the electrical stimulation approach over conventional rehabilitation treatment can be listed:

1. Patient's own muscles are used together with functional use of bone support and joints.
2. FES-provoked movements are using the patient's own metabolic energy.
3. Preserved neuromuscular reflexes can be functionally used.
4. Use of FES is accompanied by several therapeutic side effects such as: prevention of muscle atrophy, improvement of muscle and skin blood flow, increase in stimulated muscle bulk and strength, prevention of contractures and joints ossification, improved skin condition, reduction of spasticity, and prevention of bone demineralization.
5. FES orthosis has a favorable appearance, has no attachments to cause pressure spots or decubiti, does not require any external bracing, and need not be custom-made, thus, serial in-stock production is possible, does not depend upon extremity size for fit, thereby eliminating problems caused by change in girth, and costs less than or about the same as mechanical orthosis.

Surface FES, being mostly applied in the clinical environment, has important advantages, but also several disadvantages. For the restrengthening of muscles, patient training, and evaluation of a patient's abilities, surface FES appears to be a practical solution. Positioning of surface electrodes is time consuming and each application is time limited. It is not possible to obtain satisfactory stimulation selectivity because of relatively large surface electrodes. High amplitudes of stimuli are necessary, resulting in bulky stimulators. An improperly used FES orthotic system may produce skin irritations. The force of stimulated muscle is noticeably lower than that of normally innervated muscle.

These problems can, to a large extent, be solved by the multichannel implantable FES systems. Several technological problems need to be solved before introducing implanted FES into a broader clinical practice. The answer to the dilemma is to find whether to use muscle or nerve-implanted electrodes and hermetic or nonhermetic packaging of electronic circuits. Optimal topology of a multichannel implanted FES system for restoration of walking in paraplegia is to be determined. Minor, but important, problems of electrode wires and connectors must be adequately solved before the desired reliability of implants can be attained.

There are, finally, barriers to present-day FES, implanted or surface, imposed by a lack of physiological and engineering knowledge. The problem of fast fatiguing of electrically stimulated muscle remains to be overcome. FES may, through afferent pathways have an effect on the autonomous nervous system. This influence is not yet adequately investigated. The time-variant neuromuscular system is not simply controllable. Sensors providing lacking exteroceptive and proprioceptive information are necessary for an efficient control approach. These sensors can be implanted force or position transducers.[65,66] Natural sensors are preserved in SCI subjects and can also be used if sensory signals are adequately assessed.[67] The myoelectric signal of an electrically stimulated muscle may represent another parameter useful in the design of the FES control system.[68]

In spite of the problems of present FES technology, one can imagine that several tasks of daily living can be successfully accomplished with FES orthosis without using a wheelchair. It is not too ambitious to think about a young paraplegic student coming by car close to the university building and then walking with the help of the FES orthotic system into the lecturing room. Restoration of such activities of daily living is at present the realistic goal of FES application to the lower extremities of paraplegic subjects.

II. FES RESTORATION OF LOCOMOTION IN PARAPLEGIC PATIENTS AND SCOPE OF THE PRESENT BOOK

In the present book, first the FES restrengthening modalities for atrophied spastic paralyzed muscles are described. Next, the influence of electrical stimulation on skeletal muscle spasticity is discussed. A systematic approach to the biomechanical properties of FES-induced standing is given in the fourth chapter. Finally, FES ambulation programs in incomplete SCI and completely paralyzed paraplegic subjects are described. Research achievements and clinical experiences gained in 15 years of FES application to SCI patients in the Ljubljana Rehabilitation Engineering Center (REC), Yugoslavia are presented in the book. This book is first intended for those practitioners who wish to introduce FES into their rehabilitation environment. The authors strongly believe that the present text can also be found useful by all those who would like to put their research efforts into this challenging and promising field. Parts of the book might also be interesting to students of biomedical engineering, physical medicine, and physical therapy. Some basic knowledge of physiology and physics, mechanics and electricity, is necessary for the reader. It was the aim of the authors to describe general principles of FES restoration of standing and walking in paraplegic subjects. These fundamentals are, to a large extent, independent from FES technology, which has rapidly changed in the last 10 years.

The candidates for FES treatment are selected among patients with spastic paraplegia resulting from complete or incomplete spinal cord lesion. The following are the criteria for patient selection: upper motor neuron lesion, adequately preserved skin, intact joints and bones, adequate balance, satisfactory psychosocial condition, motivation, and good cooperation. The contraindications for FES application are the following: peripheral nerve lesions, osteoporosis, heterotropic ossifications, contractures, obesity, and severe spasticity.

When several months or even years have passed after the injury, a paraplegic subject has to undergo the FES restrengthening program of the disuse-atrophied muscles. The exercise program in the Ljubjana REC consists of daily application of cyclic electrical stimulation delivered to the knee extensors through surface electrodes. The stimulation periods of 4 s are followed by a pause of 4 s. The stimulation frequency of 20 Hz, the pulse duration of 0.3 ms and the stimulation amplitude to bring the legs to full extension are used. The electrical stimuli are rectangular and monophasic. During the isotonic training exercise, the patients are positioned supine with both lower extremities semiflexed over a pillow under the knees. Each FES session lasts for 30 min. There are usually two or three FES muscle-strengthening sessions performed every day. As a result of the FES training program, the muscle force is increased while the muscle fatigue is lessened. The effects of FES strengthening are monitored with the help of isometric measurements. In the beginning, the paraplegic subjects can often produce no more than 10 Nm of knee joint torque when stimulated with the highest amplitude of stimuli. With 2 to 3 months of the FES program their paralyzed knee extensors can be restrengthened to functional levels. According to our experiences, 30 to 50 Nm is the minimal knee joint torque required for successful standing-up or walking by FES. It is interesting to note that a healthy subject can voluntarily produce over 200 Nm. When stimulating knee extensors of a normal subject with surface FES of low frequency, not more than 100 to 150 Nm can be obtained. These are the knee torque values that are also often encountered in the paraplegic subjects after they successfully complete the FES training program.

Somewhat improved fatigue resistance can be obtained by applying a lower stimulation frequency, e.g., 10 Hz, during the muscle conditioning program. The FES exercise can also prevent contractures, reduce spasticity, provide better blood flow within the stimulated extremity, and improve skin condition.

The candidates for FES standing and walking are spastic SCI patients. Therefore it is interesting to investigate the influence of electrical stimulation on spinal spasticity. The efficacy of three electrical stimulation modalities was tested in SCI patients: cyclic agonist stimulation, cyclic antagonist stimulation, and continuous dermatome stimulation. The muscle groups governing knee joint movement were treated. The degree of spasticity was assessed with the help of pendulum testing. It was shown that cyclic agonist and antagonist stimulation treatments do not increase the level of spasticity so that they can be safely used for therapeutic exercises or functional activities. The degree of spasticity was reduced to a noticeable extent while applying dermatome stimulation. It was further demonstrated that transcutaneous electrical stimulation delivered to the dermatomes, corresponding to the same spinal segmental level as the spastic muscle group under consideration, produces the greatest reduction of spasticity.

Rising from the sitting to the standing position was first studied in healthy subjects. It was determined with the help of the dynamic measurements that at least 80 Nm of knee joint torque must be provided by knee extensors during the standing-up procedure. Such values of knee joint torque can be produced by electrically stimulated knee extensors in many paraplegic subjects. Arm support is necessary during the standing-up maneuver to maintain balance. When patients assist with arm-lifting, 50 Nm are sufficient for successful rising from a sitting to a standing position. The hip joint torque required to accomplish standing-up can be counterbalanced through the activity of arms and preserved trunk muscles. In this way, bilateral stimulation of knee extensors is sufficient to provide standing-up in a completely paralyzed paraplegic subject. The initial position of lower extremities and upper body are of utmost importance for an efficient standing-up maneuver. Measurement of kinematic joint trajectories and their presentation in the postural space represent a useful approach in an effort to find standing-up procedures that are satisfactory from the point of view of minimal energy expenditure. Continuous FES, causing knee extensors to contract, maintains the knee joints in extension and thus allows standing. The advantages of FES-assisted standing exercise are manifold. It can help prevent decubiti, improve function of the bladder and other internal organs, and provide better blood flow in paralyzed parts of the body. Standing also can be a useful functional activity, e.g., to get an object out of reach from the wheelchair. FES standing at any location is enabled by a special wheelchair-attached folding frame. This supporting frame is lightweight and designed so as to slip into the holders for the arm support of a regular wheelchair. The height of the handles can be adjusted according to the patient's needs. When the frame is folded it does not interfere with the normal use of the wheelchair. Through the use of two stimulation channels and arm support, some patients can stand for only a few minutes, while others can stand-up to 1 h or more. Similar values of maximal knee joint torque were found in all paraplegic subjects tested. Isometric knee joint torque certainly is a necessary condition for successful standing, but is not a sufficient one. Force plate assessment of static biomechanical parameters revealed that well-aligned posture is a prerequisite for adequate FES-induced standing. Such posture results in low knee joint torques, which can be effectively counterbalanced by FES contracted muscles. Contractures or strong abdominal spasticity result in biomechanically inadequate posture and hence large joint torques, which can be counterbalanced by FES for only a few minutes.

Standing by FES-activated knee extensors is not the only possible standing posture. When the body weight line is passing in front of knee joints (when the paraplegic subject is leaned slightly forward) standing can be achieved by stimulating ankle plantar flexors only. Fatiguing of a stimulated muscle is considerably decreased when applying cyclical rather than continuous FES. By switching between the posture with stimulated knee extensors and the posture with activated ankle plantar flexors, the total standing time can be significantly increased. The stimulation sequences during posture switching must be carefully chosen. It is not the aim to copy the muscle activities occurring during the standing of a normal subject. Nevertheless, the selection of an appropriate FES pattern is to be determined on the basis of existing constraints and invariants. These constraints are presented by the human skeletal system.

According to statistical observations, many more incomplete SCI patients have arrived in spinal units during the last 10 years. The first step in the FES program for incomplete cases is again application of therapeutic cyclical electrical stimulation. The training program lasts for about 2 months. After the training program is accomplished, three different groups of incomplete patients are encountered. In the first group, there are patients where both voluntary and electrically stimulated muscle force are improved. In the patients from the second group, only the stimulated muscle force is increased. In the third group of patients, neither voluntary nor stimulated response is augmented. The patients from the second group are candidates for further FES treatment. The final goal of the electrical stimulation program is restoration of ambulation in incomplete SCI patients. In many incomplete paraplegic and tetraplegic patients exaggerated extensor tone was observed in their lower extremities, providing more or less safe standing to some of those patients. Many patients are unable to break this exaggerated extensor tone during standing and hence, they are unable to achieve adequate flexion for gait. It has been shown that in thoracic and cervical SCI patients, electrical stimulation of an afferent nerve augments ankle, knee, and hip flexion in a total lower-limb flexion reflex pattern. In this way, peroneal stimulation can be efficiently used to initiate a step in incomplete SCI patients. Three different groups of patients were encountered with respect to their needs for application of different orthoses based on FES. First, there are incomplete SCI patients who are able to stand, but require unilateral peroneal stimulation to elicit the flexion response and initiate a step. In the second group, there are patients where bilateral peroneal stimulation is found helpful. It was observed that in a great number of incomplete SCI patients, one leg is almost completely paralyzed while the other leg is under voluntary control and sufficiently strong to provide safe standing for short periods with only crutches. Unilateral stimulation of knee extensors and an afferent nerve is helpful in these patients.

It was found that a minimum of four channels of FES are required for synthesis of a simple reciprocal gait pattern in completely paralyzed paraplegic subjects. During reciprocal walking, the stimulator must be controlled through three different phases of walking: double stance, right swing, and left swing. This is achieved by two hand switches. When neither of the switches is pressed, both knee extensors are stimulated. On pressing the switch in the right hand, the right leg is stimulated to flex. The same is true for the left leg. The flexion of the paralyzed limb is accomplished through withdrawal reflex triggering. The electrodes are placed along one of the following mixed sensory nerves: common peroneal nerve, sural nerve, saphenous nerve, or superficial peroneal nerve. Usually, the peroneal nerve is electrically excited. In this way, ankle dorsiflexion is obtained through efferent stimulation. By slightly increasing the amplitude over the value required for ankle dorsiflexion, the flexion reflex is started, resulting in simultaneous knee and hip flexion. The duration of the swing phase based on flexion reflex triggering is equal to the time of pressing the hand switch. When the patient has to overcome an obstacle during walking, the strength of the flexion response must be increased. This can be achieved by increasing either the amplitude of stimuli, or stimulation frequency, or the duration of the train of pulses. Also interesting to note is the build-up phase of the flexion response. During the first few steps the flexion response is, namely, slightly increased from step-to-step. It is then gradually decreased and after some 15 steps, it remains fairly constant. Initial trials of the paraplegic subject's walking are performed in parallel bars or with the help of a special frame with attached wheels. For safety reasons, the patient can be suspended to the frame with leather belts. In the very first walking sessions the hand switches are held and controlled by the physical therapist. Later, the switches are built into the handles of the walker or crutches, and the patient controls them. Kinematic analysis of the walking of paraplegic subjects demonstrated that the speed of their ambulation is about three times lower than the velocity of a normal man. The swing phase is because of the delays provoked by the polysynaptic flexion reflex triggering noticeably longer than in the normal gait pattern. Even more critical is the duration of the double-support phase. During this period, the patient must bring his body forward. With the simple four-channel gait pattern, forward progression is performed solely with the help of arms and preserved trunk muscles.

Stairs represent a major obstacle in the locomotion of wheelchair-confined patients. Stair climbing is therefore the most important advantage of FES-assisted rehabilitation of complete paraplegic patients. The reciprocal gait pattern described also is used while walking on the stairs. The synergistic flexion response in most patients was found strong enough to lift the leg to the next step. The switching control over walking must be given to one hand only, as the patient is holding a handrail with the other hand. A swing-to gait with continuously stimulated knee extensors was found the most appropriate for descending stairs.

The field of FES locomotion restoration is lacking fundamental principles necessary for the successful synthesis of walking. An attempt to provide objective rules for composing multichannel stimulation sequences is proposed, based on constraints imposed by the human musculotendinoskeletal system and pathology itself. The locomotor system, developed during the evolution process, reflects important principles, constraints, and invariants which are essential for appropriate muscle activation synthesis and also an understanding of neural control. Additional constraints inevitable when approaching gait synthesis and control are presented by pathological changes of the locomotor system. Taking into account both types of constraints, new principles for objective mathematical gait synthesis can be obtained. This knowledge will represent the software of future generations of FES locomotion rehabilitation systems.

Although there are already the first signs of encouraging practical clinical results, the research work described in this book is to be understood as a feasibility demonstration. Assisted ambulation of paraplegic patients with complete lesions represents an advanced example of the great effectiveness of FES. It is not difficult to imagine that FES-restored walking represents a new alternative mode of locomotion in some paraplegic patients and a means of overcoming barriers posed to them.

REFERENCES

1. **Hodgkin, A. L. and Huxley, A. F.**, Resting and action potentials in single nerve fibers, *J. Physiol. (London)*, 104, 176, 1945.
2. **Zoll, P. M.**, Resuscitation of the heart in ventricular standstill by external electric stimulation, *N. Engl. J. Med.*, 247, 768, 1952.
3. **Reswick, J. B.**, A brief history of functional electrical stimulation, in *Neural Organization and Its Relevance to Prosthetics*, Fields, W. S. and Leavitt, L. A., Eds., Intercont. Med Book Corp., New York, 1973, 3.
4. **Liberson, W. T., Holmquest, H. J., Scott, D., and Dow, A.**, Functional electrotherapy: stimulation of the peroneal nerve synchronized with the swing phase of the gait in hemiplegic patients, *Arch. Phys. Med. Rehabil.*, 42, 101, 1961.
5. **Vodovnik, L.**, Functional electrical stimulation of extremities, in *Advances in Electronics and Electron Physics*, Vol. 30, Marton, L., Ed., Academic Press, NY, 1971, 282.
6. **Gračanin, F., Prevec, T., and Trontelj, J.**, Evaluation of use of functional electronic peroneal brace in hemiparetic patients, in Proc. Int. Symp. External Control Human Extremities, Dubrovnik, Yugoslavia, August 29 to September 2, 1967, 198.
7. **Vodovnik, L., Bajd, T., Gračanin, F., Kralj, A., and Strojnik, P.**, Functional electrical stimulation for control of locomotor system, *CRC Critical Rev. Bioeng.*, 6, 63, 1981.
8. **Hambrecht, F. T. and Reswick, J. B., Eds.**, *Functional Electrical Stimulation — Applications in Neural Prostheses*, Marcel Dekker, NY, 1977.
9. **Trnkoczy, A.**, Functional electrical stimulation of extremities: its basis, technology and role in rehabilitation, *Automedica*, 2, 59, 1978.
10. **Hambrecht, F. T.**, Neural prostheses, *Annu. Rev. Biophys. Bioeng.*, 8, 239, 1979.
11. **McNeal, D. R. and Reswick, J. B.**, Control of skeletal muscles by electrical stimulation, in *Advances of Biomechanical Engineering*, Vol. 6, Academic Press, NY, 1979, 209.
12. **Kralj, A. and Vodovnik, L.**, Functional electrical stimulation of the extremities: parts 1 and 2, *J. Med. Eng. Tech.*, 12, 75, 1977.
13. **Eccles, J. and Dimitrijević, M. R.**, *Recent Achievements in Restorative Neurology, Upper Motor Neuron Functions and Dysfunctions*, S. Karger, Basel, 1985.
14. **Peckham, P. H., Mortimer, J. T., and Marsolais, E. B.**, Controlled prehension and release in the C5 quadroplegic elicited by functional electrical stimulation of the paralyzed forearm musculature, *Ann. Biomed. Eng.*, 8, 369, 1980.
15. **Peckham, P. H., Marsolais, E. B., and Mortimer, J. T.**, Restoration of key grip and release in the C6 tetraplegic patient through functional electrical stimulation, *J. Hand Surg.*, 5, 462, 1980.
16. **Kantrowitz, A.**, Electronic physiologic aids, Report of the Maimonides Hospital, Brooklyn, NY, 1963.
17. **Wilemon, W. K., Mooney, V., McNeal, D. R., and Reswick, J. B.**, Surgically implanted peripheral neuroelectric stimulation, Internal report of Rancho Los Amigos Hospital, Downey, CA, 1970.
18. **Reswick, J. B.**, Development of feedback control prosthetic and orthotic devices, in *Advances in Biomedical Engineering*, Vol. 2, Brown, J. H. U. and Dickson, J. F., Eds., Academic Press, NY, 1972, 139.
19. **Cooper, E. B., Bunch, W. H., and Campa, J. F.**, Effects of chronic human neuromuscular stimulation, *Surg. Forum*, 14, 477, 1973.
20. **Kralj, A., Grobelnik, S., and Vodovnik, L.**, Electrical stimulation of paraplegic patients — feasibility study, in Proc. Int. Symp. External Control Human Extremities, Dubrovnik, Yugoslavia, August 28 to September 2, 1973, 561.
21. **Kralj, A. and Grobelnik, S.**, Functional electrical stimulation — a new hope for paraplegic patients, *Bull. Prosthet. Res.*, BPR 10-20, 75, 1973.
22. **Kralj, A., Bajd, T., Turk, R., and Benko, H.**, Paraplegic patients standing by functional electrical stimulation, in Digest 12th Int. Conf. Med. Biol. Eng., Jerusalem, Israel, August 19 to 24, 1979, 59.3.
23. **Kralj, A., Bajd, T., and Turk, R.**, Electrical stimulation providing functional use of paraplegic patient muscles, *Med. Prog. Technol.*, 7, 3, 1980.

24. Bajd, T., Kralj, A., Turk, R., Benko, H., and Šega, J., The use of a four-channel electrical stimulator as an ambulatory aid for paraplegic patients, *Phys. Ther.*, 63, 1116, 1983.
25. Kralj, A., Bajd, T., Turk, R., Krajnik, J., and Benko, H., Gait restoration in paraplegic patients: a feasibility demonstration using multichannel surface electrode FES, *J. Rehabil. Res. Dev.*, 20, 3, 1983.
26. Kralj, A., Bajd, T., Turk, R., and Benko, H., Results of FES application to 71 SCI patients, in *Proc. 10th RESNA Annu. Conf.*, RESNA Association for the Advancement of Rehabilitation Technology, Washington, D.C., 1987, 645.
27. Kralj, A., Jaeger, R. J., and Bajd, T., Posture switching enables prolonged standing in paraplegic patients functionally electrically stimulated, in *Proc. 5th RESNA Annu. Conf.*, RESNA Association for the Advancement of Rehabilitation Technology, Washington, D.C., 1982, 60.
28. Kralj, A., Bajd, T., Turk, R., and Benko, H., Posture switching for prolonging functional electrical stimulation standing in paraplegic patients, *Paraplegia*, 24, 221, 1986.
29. Bajd, T., Andrews, B. J., Kralj, A., and Katakis, J., Restoration of walking in incomplete spinal cord injured patients by use of surface electrical stimulation — preliminary results, *Prosthetics Orthotics Int.*, 9, 109, 1985.
30. Petrofsky, J. S., Heaton, H. H., III, and Phillips, C. A., Leg exerciser for training of paralysed muscle by closed-loop control, *Med. Biol. Eng. Comput.*, 22, 298, 1984.
31. Petrofsky, J. S., Phillips, C. A., Almeida, J., Briggs, R., Couch, W., and Colby, W., Aerobic trainer with physiological monitoring for exercise in paraplegic and quadriplegic patients, *J. Clin. Eng.*, 10, 307, 1985.
32. Petrofsky, J. S., Heaton, H. H., III, and Phillips, C. A., Outdoor bicycle for exercise in paraplegics and quadriplegics, *J. Biomed. Eng.*, 5, 292, 1983.
33. Phillips, C. A., Petrofsky, J. S., Hendershot, D. M., and Stafford, D., Functional electrical exercise. A comprehensive approach for physical conditioning of the spinal cord injured patient, *Orthopedics*, 7, 1112, 1984.
34. Petrofsky, J. S. and Phillips, C. A., Closed-loop control of movement of skeletal muscle, *CRC Crit. Rev. in Biomed. Eng.*, 13, 35, 1983.
35. Graupe, D., Kohn, K. H., Kralj, A., and Basseas, S., Patient controlled electrical stimulation via EMG signature discrimination for providing certain paraplegics with primitive walking functions, *J. Biomed. Eng.*, 5, 220, 1983.
36. Graupe, D., Kohn, K. H., Basseas, S., and Naccarato, E., Electromyographic control of functional electrical stimulation in selected patients, *Orthopedics*, 7, 1134, 1984.
37. Mizrahi, J., Braun, Z., Najenson, T., and Graupe, D., Quantitative weightbearing and gait evaluation of paraplegics using functional electrical stimulation, *Med. Biol. Eng. Comput.*, 23, 101, 1985.
38. Isakov, E., Mizrahi, J., and Najenson, T., Biomechanical and physiological evaluation of FES-activated paraplegic patients, *J. Rehabil. Res. Dev.*, 23, 9, 1986.
39. Cybulski, G. R., Penn, R. D., and Jaeger, R. J., Lower extremity functional neuromuscular stimulation in cases of spinal cord injury, *Neurosurgery*, 15, 132, 1984.
40. Cybulski, G. R. and Jaeger, R. J., Standing performance of persons with paraplegia, *Arch. Phys. Med. Rehabil.*, 67, 103, 1986.
41. Jaeger, R. J., Design and simulation of closed-loop electrical stimulation orthoses for restoration of quiet standing in paraplegia, *J. Biomech.*, 19, 825, 1986.
42. Brindley, G. S., Polkey, C. E., and Rushton, D. N., Electrical splinting of the knee in paraplegia, *Paraplegia*, 16, 428, 1979.
43. Donaldson, N. and Donaldson, N., A 24-output implantable stimulator for FES, in Proc. 2nd Vienna Int. Workshop Functional Electrostimulation, Vienna, Austria, September 21 to 24, 1986, 197.
44. Thoma, H., Holle, J., Moritz, E., and Stöhr, H., Walking after paraplegia — a principle concept, in Proc. Int. Symp. External Control Human Extremities, Dubrovnik, Yugoslavia, 1978, 71 (Suppl.).
45. Holle, J., Frey, M., Gruber, H., Kern, H., Stöhr, H., and Thoma, H., Functional electrostimulation of paraplegics — experimental investigations and first clinical experience with an implantable stimulation device, *Orthopedics*, 7, 1145, 1984.
46. Kern, H., Kainz, J., Lechner, F., et al., Morphologic and enzymatic changes of the muscles of paraplegics caused by electrical stimulation, in Proc. 2nd Vienna Int. Workshop Functional Electrostimulation, Vienna, Austria, August 28 to September 1, 1986, 105.
47. Caldwell, C. W. and Reswick, J. B., A percutaneous wire electrode for chronic research use, *IEEE Trans. Biomed. Eng.*, 22, 429, 1975.
48. Peckham, P. H., Ko, W. H., Poon, C. W., and Marsolais, E. B., A multichannel implantable stimulator for control of paralyzed muscle, *IEEE Trans. Biomed. Eng.*, 28, 530, 1981.
49. Marsolais, E. B. and Kobetic, R., Functional walking in paralyzed patients by means of electrical stimulation, *Clin. Orthop.*, 175, 30, 1983.
50. Marsolais, E. B. and Kobetic, R., Implantation techniques and experience with percutaneous intramuscular electrodes in the lower extremities, *J. Rehabil. Res. Dev.*, 23, 1, 1986.

51. **Marsolais, E. B. and Kobetic, R.**, Kinematics of paraplegic gait produced by electrical stimulation, in Proc. of RESNA 8th Annu. Conf., RESNA Association for the Advancement of Rehabilitation Technology, Washington, D.C., 1985, 108.
52. **Kobetic, R., Carroll, S. G., and Marsolais, E. B.**, Paraplegic stair climbing assisted by electrical stimulation, in Proc. 39th Annu. Conf. Eng. Med. Biol., Chevy Chase, MD, 1986, 256.
53. **Waters, R. L. and Lunsford, B. R.**, Energy cost of paraplegic locomotion, *J. Bone Joint Surg.*, 67A, 1245, 1985.
54. **Cerny, K., Waters, R., Hislop, H., and Perry, J.**, Walking and wheelchair energetics in persons with paraplegia, *Phys. Ther.*, 60, 1133, 1980.
55. **Perry, J.**, Rehabilitation of the neurologically disabled patient: principles, practice, and scientific basis, *J. Neurosurg.*, 58, 799, 1983.
56. **Coghlan, J. K., Robinson, C. E., Newmarch, B., and Jackson, G.**, Lower extremity bracing in paraplegia — a follow-up study, *Paraplegia*, 18, 25, 1980.
57. **Chantraine, A., Crielaard, J. M., Oukelinx, A., and Pirnay, F.**, Energy expenditure of ambulation in paraplegics: effects of long term use of bracing, *Paraplegia*, 22, 173, 1984.
58. **Edwards, B. G., Lew, R. D., and Marsolais, E. B.**, Relative energy costs of long-leg-brace and FNS ambulation, in Proc. 9th RESNA Annu. Conf., Minneapolis, MN, August 28 to September 2, 1986.
59. **Stauffer, E. S., Hoffer, M. M., and Nickel, V. A.**, Ambulation in thoracic paraplegia, *J. Bone Joint Surg.*, 60A, 823, 1978.
60. **Tomović, R., Vukobratović, M., and Vodovnik, L.**, Hybrid actuators for orthotic systems — hybrid assistive system, in Proc. Int. Symp. External Control Human Extremities, Dubrovnik, Yugoslavia, 1973, 73.
61. **Schwirtlich, L. and Popović, D.**, Hybrid orthoses for deficient locomotion, in Proc. Int. Symp. External Control of Human Extremities, Dubrovnik, Yugoslavia, September 3 to 7, 1984, 23.
62. **Andrews, B. J. and Bajd, T.**, Hybrid orthoses for paraplegics, in Proc. Int. Symp. External Control Human Extremities, Dubrovnik, Yugoslavia, 1984, 55(Suppl.).
63. **Solomonow, M., Shoji, H., D'Ambrosia, R., and Douglas, R.**, Electromechanical walking system for paraplegics, in *Proc. IEEE 7th Annu. Conf. Engineering in Medicine and Biology Society*, IEEE Service Center, Piscataway, NJ, 1985, 4.
64. **Andrews, B. J.**, A short leg hybrid FES orthosis for assisting locomotion in SCI subjects, in Proc. 2nd Vienna Int. Workshop Functional Electrostimulation, Vienna, Austria, September 21 to 24, 1986, 311.
65. **Crago, P. E., Chizeck, H. J., Neuman, M. R., and Hambrecht, F. T.**, Sensors for use with functional neuromuscular stimulation, *IEEE Trans. Biomed. Eng.*, 33, 256, 1986.
66. **Troyk, P. R., Jaeger, R. J., Haklin, M., Poyezdala, J., and Bajzek, T.**, Design and implementation of an implantable goniometer, *IEEE Trans. Biomed. Eng.*, 33, 215, 1986.
67. **Hoffer, J. A. and Sinkjaer, T.**, A natural "force sensor" suitable for closed-loop control of functional neuromuscular stimulation, in Proc. 2nd Vienna Int. Workshop Functional Electrostimulation, Vienna, Austria, September 21 to 24, 1986, 47.
68. **Solomonow, M., Baratha, R., Shoji, H., and D'Ambrosia, R. D.**, The myoelectric signal of electrically stimulated muscle during recruitment: an inherent feedback parameter for a closed-loop control scheme, *IEEE Trans. Biomed. Eng.*, 33, 735, 1986.

Chapter 2

MUSCLE RESTRENGTHENING AND PATIENT CONDITIONING

I. THE BASICS OF MUSCLE PHYSIOLOGY AND THE STATE OF SKELETAL MUSCLE FOLLOWING SPINAL CORD INJURY

The signals corresponding to the origin of conscious volitional movement can be traced in the brain. The command is then sent over the spinal cord, peripheral nerve, and neuromuscular junction to a skeletal muscle. From the neuromuscular junction the signal spreads in all directions throughout the muscle cell membrane and through the transverse tubular system into the inside of muscle cells. Calcium is then released, and cross-bridges between the actin and myosin filaments are formed. The final task of skeletal muscles, representing some 40% of the body cell mass,[1] is to generate force. According to current concepts of muscle physiology, the amount of force developed within a muscle is determined by the number of bridges formed between the filaments as they slide past each other during a contraction.

The generation of force is also the aim of functionally electrically stimulated paralyzed skeletal muscle. Because of a damage to the spinal cord in the case of paraplegia, an electronic bypass of the neural lesion is necessary.[2] Electrical stimuli are still triggered volitionally by the patient using different control transducers such as hand or foot switches. They are then, through surface or implanted electrodes, delivered to the peripheral nerve, where they are triggering action potentials. From here on, the command chain is the same as described in the case of voluntary contraction of skeletal muscle. This flow of commands was analyzed in a variety of physiological systems ranging from isolated cells to animal preparations. All the different processes and phenomena associated with muscle contraction are described in many physiology textbooks.

It is not too serious an oversimplification to think of human muscle as a combination of slow fibers capable of sustaining low levels of contractile activity without fatigue for prolonged periods and fast fibers capable of developing large forces, but fatiguing so rapidly that they can be used only in intermittent activities.[3] Often in literature, slow twitch or type I fibers are denoted as red, while fast twitch or type II fibers are called white fibers. Red fibers contain myoglobin, which gives them a characteristic color and serves as a reserve of oxygen. Being slower, they have less adenosine triphosphate (ATP)ase activity than white fibers. In histochemical observations, red or type I fibers are, therefore, staining light for myosin ATPase, while white or type II fibers give a dark reaction. Biomechanically, the two fiber types can be distinguished by measuring the duration of the rising and falling phases of the muscle-twitch contraction. The duration of the twitch contraction is prolonged in type I fibers. Slow-twitch oxidative fibers are smaller in the cross-sectional area, have a high capacity for oxidative metabolism, and a low capacity for glycolytic metabolism.[4] In contrast fast-twitch glycolytic fibers are large in cross-section, they have a low capacity for oxidative metabolism, and a high capacity for glycolytic metabolism. Fast-twitch fibers exhibit a twitch contraction of short duration. Some muscles are predominantly made up of white fibers, some predominantly of red, and some of a given mixture of the two. Muscle fiber-type populations were, for example, determined in 32 humans who were autopsied within 25 h of death and histochemically examined.[5] Soleus and vastus intermedius muscles have 70 and 47% of slow-twitch fibers, respectively, while their synergists, gastrocnemius and vastus lateralis, 50 and 32%.

All muscle fibers innervated by the same motoneuron have been found to be of the same histochemical type. Motoneurons innervating predominantly slow muscles discharge at a low frequency (10 to 20 Hz), and those supplying fast muscles at a higher frequency (30 to 60 Hz).[6] Motoneurons activating slow types of muscle are in general called tonic, while phasic types of motoneurons act on fast muscles. Tonic motoneurons have axons of small diameter,[7] and phasic motoneurons have axons with a larger diameter. In a voluntary contraction of normally innervated muscle, the slow-twitch fibers are recruited first, and as increased tension is required, the fast-twitch fibers are recruited.[8] Slow muscle fibers are, therefore, activated frequently, while fast fibers are employed only infrequently, during a burst of intense activity. When applying electrical stimulation, fibers with a greater diameter respond earlier. These are phasic motoneurons innervating fast muscle fibers. When a motoneuron is electrically stimulated, the normal order of recruitment is, therefore, inverted.[3]

Also, it has been demonstrated that the concentration of collagen is higher for a slow than for a fast skeletal muscle.[9] Collagen is the major connective tissue protein, having the main responsibility for mechanical strength of a muscle. More flexible connective tissue of a fast muscle allows faster movements, while slow muscle can store more elastic energy in its collagenous compartments.

When describing the state of skeletal muscle following spinal cord injury, it is important to distinguish between upper and lower motor neuron lesion. Central lesion results in speeding, whereas peripheral denervation results in slowing of contractile properties.[10] The loss of force in electrically stimulated muscles paralyzed with an upper motor neuron lesion is due to disuse atrophy of the involved fibers.[11] The state of the muscle following upper motor neuron lesion is, therefore, to some extent similar to the state occurring after immobilization.[12] Immobilization of healthy human skeletal muscle seems to involve preferentially type I fibers. It causes a remarkable reduction in oxidative enzyme activity, whereas the glycolitic activity seems to be increased. Both immobilization and lesion of the spinal cord result in a decrease in metabolic demand.[13]

It was shown through animal experiments that all limb muscles are slow at birth, and differentation into the fast and slow types occurs during the first few weeks after birth. The differentation of fast muscles is virtually unaffected by spinal cord transection, while the differentation of slow muscles is greatly depressed. A few weeks after spinal cord lesion, predominantly slow muscles become nearly as fast in every respect as normally fast muscles.[13]

The candidates for functional electrical stimulation (FES) locomotion activities are patients with upper motor neuron lesion. Histochemical examination of spastic quadriceps muscle demonstrated type I fiber hypertrophy and type II fiber atrophy (decrease in single fiber area).[14] On the contrary, a marked predominance of type II fibers was observed in patients suffering from spinal cord lesion.[15] Blood circulation also plays an important role when describing muscle properties. It has a direct influence on muscle fatiguing.[16] The nutritional blood flow in the paralyzed tibial muscle of paraplegic patients was found[16] to be significantly lower than in normal biceps muscle of the same patient.

II. THE BASICS OF MUSCLE ELECTROPHYSIOLOGY AND PARAMETERS OF ELECTRICAL STIMULATION

Electrical stimulation is performed in a series of rectangular monophasic or biphasic (symmetrical or asymmetrical) electric pulses described by the following parameters: amplitude or intensity of pulses, frequency or pulse repetition rate, duration of single pulse, and duration of a pulse train. In most cases of surface electrical stimulation applications, periodic monophasic or unidirectional pulses are used. Biphasic or bidirectional pulses prevent a slow deterioration of the electrodes, while the chemical conditions on the skin and in the neuromuscular tissue remain unchanged.

An example of periodic unidirectional pulse current or voltage is presented in Figure 1. With respect to the stimulator output circuit, electric pulses are either voltage- or current-

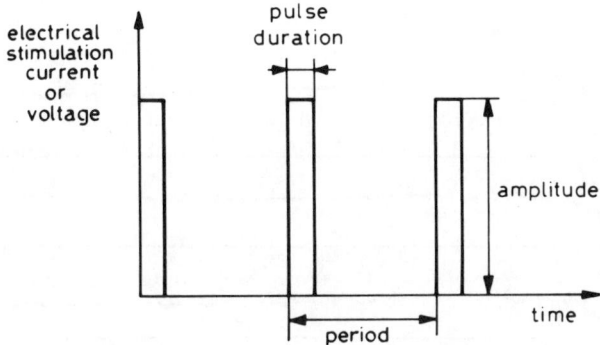

FIGURE 1. Periodic unidirectional stimulation pulse current or voltage.

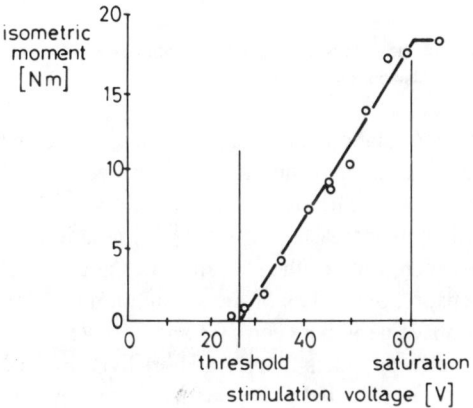

FIGURE 2. Joint torque depending upon the amplitude of stimulation pulses.

controlled pulses. Stimulators providing a constant output voltage can maintain a voltage desired, irrespective of resistance changes in the stimulated muscle tissue. Stimulators with current output stages make possible constant-current pulses. An important difference between the two stimulator types becomes evident in the case of an improper contact between the electrode and the skin. In the case of a constant-current stimulator, a smaller effective electrode surface results in greater current density, which can cause skin burns. At the voltage source the resistance increases, due to an insufficient contact, which results in a decrease of current and, consequently, of the muscle response, causing no skin damage.

Figure 2 yields measurement results in which the amplitude of dorsal flexion stimulation was increased, while the isometric ankle torque was measured. Such measurement is performed at a constant muscle length. The extremity is firmly fixed into a special measuring device and the joint torque is measured. A measurement was performed in a healthy subject. However, similar responses are also obtained in the case of paraplegic patients, as well as other patients with an impairment of the central nervous system (CNS). It can be noticed from Figure 2 that the joint torque is not linearly dependent upon the stimulation intensity. There occurs, above all, two nonlinearities, i.e., threshold and saturation. The increase in joint torque due to an increasing amplitude of electrical stimulation occurs as a result of activating new fibers in a nerve bundle laying in an electric field between the electrodes. The main reason why all nerve fibers do not react to the same stimulation amplitude is found

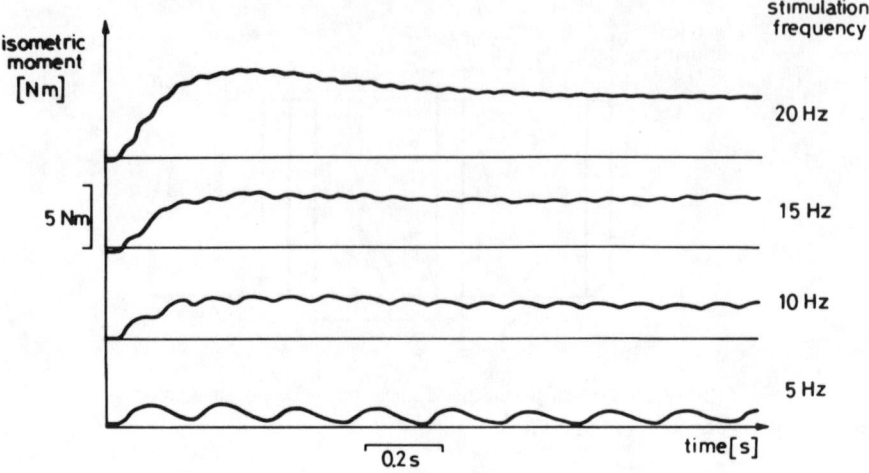

FIGURE 3. Dependency of the contraction of dorsal flexors on the frequency of stimulation pulses (stimulation voltage 60 V, pulse duration 0.3 ms).

in the differences in the stimulation threshold and various distances from the stimulation electrodes. First, the fibers closest to the electrodes are stimulated. In addition, the fibers with a greater diameter respond earlier. As of a certain stimulation intensity onward, the force of contraction no longer increases. At such a stimulation amplitude, all nerve fibers are excited, and a further increasing of the stimulus does not increase contraction. In surface stimulation of knee extensors, the values of the stimulation threshold range between 20 and 60 V, while the saturation value is between 100 and 150 V.

A single stimulation pulse provokes merely a short-lived muscle twitch of no more than 0.2 s. If electrical stimuli are repeated every second, a twitch occurs every second, meanwhile, the muscle relaxes. If the frequency of stimulation pulses increases up to 10 pulses per second (10 Hz), between two twitches there is no time left for muscle relaxation. When measuring isometric contraction, we get twitching responses (Figure 3). This twitching is considerably reduced at stimulation frequencies between 15 and 20 Hz. At higher frequencies, the response is already smooth: this is known as tetanic contraction. The frequency at which tetanic contraction occurs is called fusion frequency; it is not the same for all muscles and depends on properties of muscle fibers. Changes in stimulation frequency also affect the intensity of the response. Figure 4 shows the dependence of the joint torque on the stimulation amplitude at frequencies of 20, 30, and 40 Hz. As regards the response intensity, slight losses are observed at lower stimulation frequencies. On the whole, the changing of frequency between 40 and 100 Hz causes small differences in the isometric torque as measured in the joint. A low stimulation frequency results in a less pronounced fatigue of the neuromuscular system. An electrically stimulated muscle fatigues more quickly than in the case of voluntary contraction. By electrical stimulation, the same nerve fibers are stimulated all the time, whereas with a healthy muscle the work is divided among different motor units of the same muscle. Due to a high stimulation frequency, the transmitter in the neuromuscular junctions is being exhausted, so the muscle stimulated soon shows signs of fatigue. In Figure 5, time courses of the isometric torque during the stimulation of plantar flexors of a paraplegic patient are shown.[17] The measurements were carried out at three different frequencies, namely, 50, 30, and 20 Hz. The smallest decrease of the response can be observed at the lowest frequency used.

In a fashion similar to the amplitude, pulse duration too, exerts a direct effect upon the intensity of contraction. Figure 6 shows an isometric torque in the ankle joint, while changing

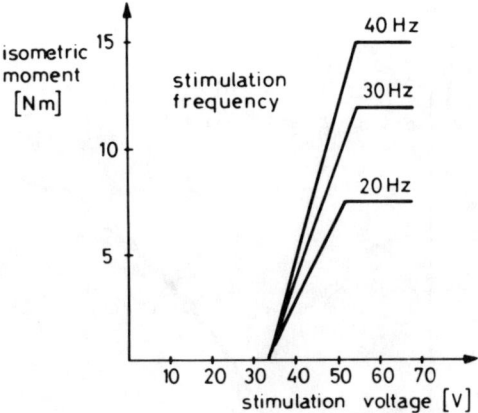

FIGURE 4. Influence of stimulation frequency upon the intensity of the response (dorsal flexors, pulse duration 0.3 ms).

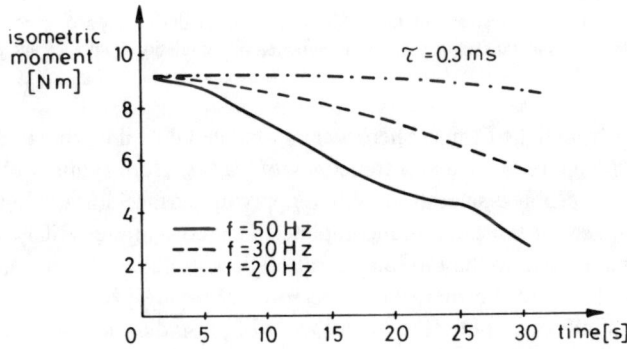

FIGURE 5. Time courses of the isometric torque in the ankle joint at three different stimulation frequencies (pulse duration 0.3 ms).

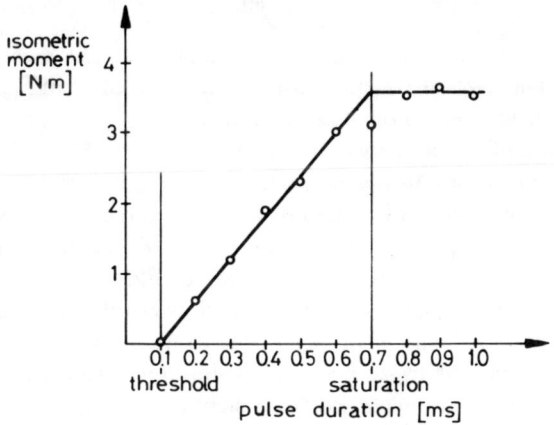

FIGURE 6. Dependence of the intensity of isometric contraction on pulse duration.

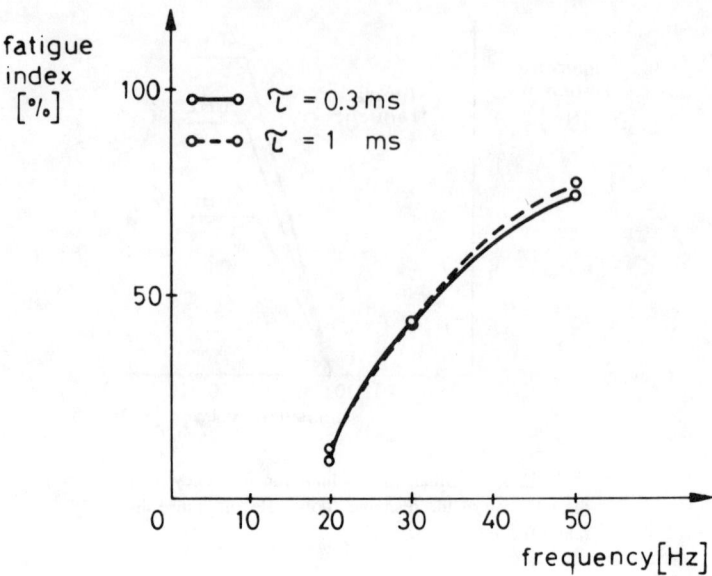

FIGURE 7. The decrease of the ankle joint moment during 30 s of continuous stimulation of plantar flexors plotted as a function of stimulation frequency and pulse duration.

stimulation pulses from 0.1 to 1 ms. There were stimulated dorsal flexors of a healthy person at a stimulation voltage of 50 V and a frequency of 30 Hz. Here again, we have to do with threshold value and response saturation. When applying surface stimulation electrodes, the accompanying unpleasant sensation in incomplete spinal cord injured (SCI) patients, or even skin damage is mainly due to the too long duration of a stimulus, therefore, short durations are preferably used (0.1 to 0.5 ms), while the force of a paralyzed extremity is controlled by increasing the stimulus amplitude. The influence of pulse duration on muscle fatiguability is demonstrated in Figure 7. Here, the following fatigue index was defined:

$$\text{fatigue index} = \frac{\text{initial moment} - \text{moment after 30 s stimulation}}{\text{initial moment}} \cdot 100\%$$

The results shown are average values of ten measurements. The most favorable fatiguing was again found at the lowest frequency. It is further evident from Figure 7 that changing the pulse duration has little effect on stimulated muscle fatigue. Shorter pulse durations are also preferred because of lower energy consumption.

A functional movement of a paralyzed extremity cannot be obtained by a single electric stimulus, but rather, by a series of stimuli of a certain duration, following one another at an appropriate frequency. Such a series of stimuli is called a stimulation pulse train. Figure 8 shows an isometric torque as a response to a train of stimulation pulses. Conclusions on dynamic parameters of a stimulated muscle can be drawn from increase time (t_2), decrease time (t_4), and two delays (t_1 and t_3). In therapeutic stimulation, a stimulation pulse train is followed by a pause, and this by another stimulation train. The relation of train duration and pause is often called the duty cycle and exerts an influence upon the fatigue of a stimulated muscle. In Figure 9, the drop in the knee extension is presented during 20 min of cyclic stimulation applied to knee extensor muscles of a healthy subject. First applying a 50-Hz stimulation frequency, the following on/off duty cycles were used: 4 s/8 s, 4 s/4 s, 8 s/4 s,

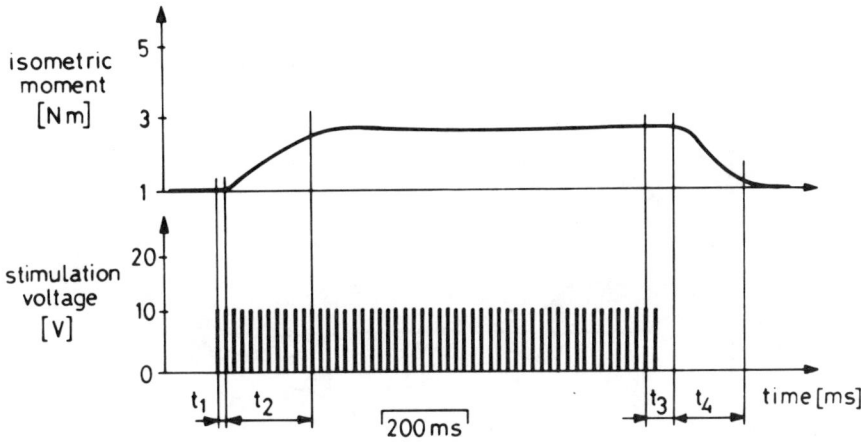

FIGURE 8. Dorsiflexion isometric torque as a response to a stimulation pulse train.

and 8 s/8 s (Figure 9A). The results shown in Figure 9B were obtained in identical experimental conditions, except that the stimulation frequency was decreased to 20 Hz. Muscle fatiguing is considerably more intense with higher stimulation frequency. Less fatiguability can be observed with a 20-Hz stimulation frequency, where only an 8 s/4 s duty cycle results in significant muscle fatigue.

III. ELECTRICAL STIMULATION EXERCISE IN NEUROLOGICALLY INTACT SUBJECTS

Similar characteristic properties of disuse atrophy were found in conditions of joint immobilization and spinal cord lesion. In both cases, a decrease in metabolic demand was found. An increase in metabolic demand and consequently, a restrengthened immobilized or paralyzed muscle can be obtained by physical exercise or by electrical stimulation of the peripheral nerve. Because of the similarity between the state of the skeletal muscle after immobilization and spinal cord injury, some guidelines for planning an electrical stimulation training program can be gained from the experiences gathered from the use of electrical stimulation exercising in neurologically intact patients.

Rather short electrical stimulation sessions were applied in three comparable investigations.[8,18,19] They consisted of only 10 trains of stimuli delivered daily to knee extensor muscles. The duration of the stimulation train was 10 s in all three cases, followed by a 50-s pause. The stimulation frequency used in the three studies[8,18,19] was 50, 60, and 75 Hz, respectively. The objective of the first study[18] performed on healthy subjects was to compare the effectiveness of the electrical stimulation protocol with the isokinetic training. It was found that both isokinetics and electrical stimulation increase the muscle force of the knee extensors. Isokinetics was found superior, when compared with electrical stimulation exercising. In the two other studies, electrical training was compared with isometric exercise. Patients following surgery or injury to the knee were treated by Godfrey et al.,[19] while normal healthy subjects were included in the investigation performed by McMiken et al.[8] In patients, higher improvement was observed when using an electrical stimulation strengthening program. In healthy subjects, there was a marked improvement demonstrated with both treatment regimes, but no significant difference in strength gains was observed. It is interesting to note that no significant differences were found also between the following five conventional training procedures: (1) progressive resistance exercise; (2) bicycle exercise; (3) maximum isometric contractions; (4) isokinetic low-; and (5) isokinetic high-speed train-

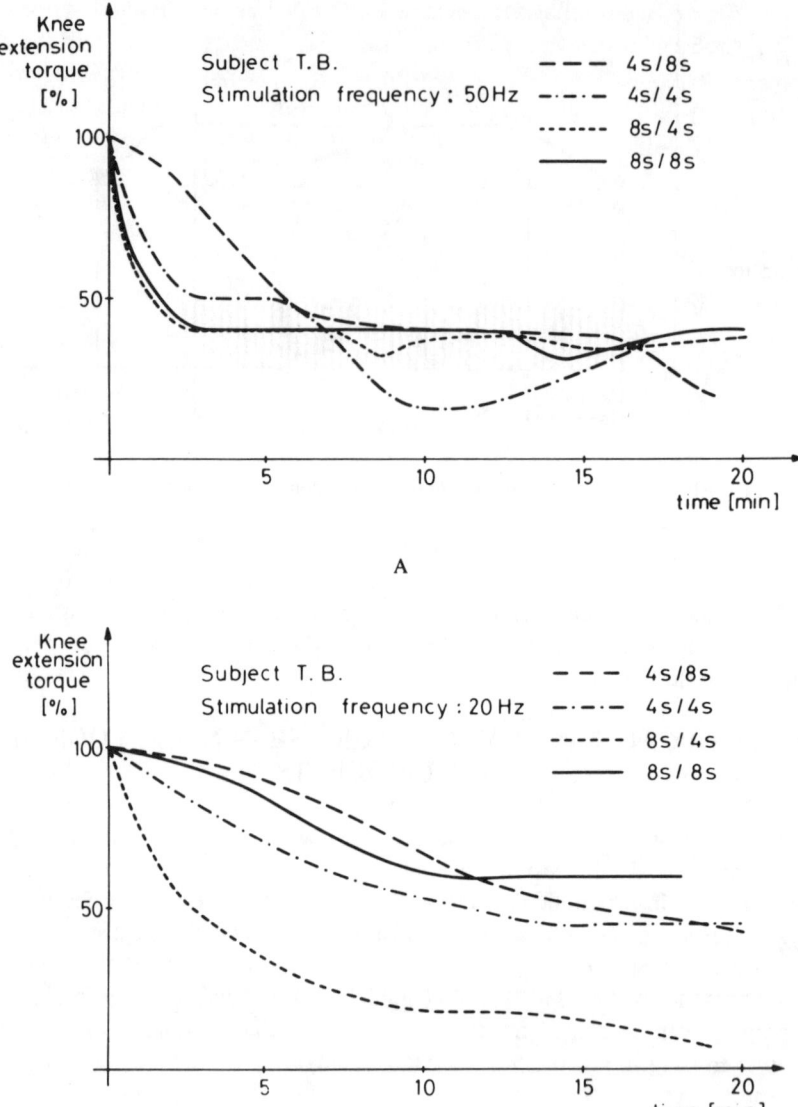

FIGURE 9. Effects of duty cycle at 50 Hz (A) and 20 Hz (B) stimulation frequency on muscle fatigue.

ing.[12] A somewhat higher frequency (200 Hz) was used in electrical stimulation training after knee ligament surgery.[20] A duty cycle of 5 s on and 5 s off was applied for 1 h daily through a period of 4 weeks. Here again, electrical stimulation was compared with isometric training. The results suggested that electrical stimulation was more effective in preventing muscle atrophy occurring after major knee ligament surgery.

A method, used to a large extent in sports training, is the so-called Russian technique of electrical stimulation. It consists of sinusoidal stimuli of 2500 Hz frequency. This waveform is chopped by a rectangular signal. In this way, the pulse cycle is composed of a period of usually 10 to 25 ms of sinusoidal output, followed by a silent period of an equal duration. Subjects with chondromalacia patellae, being a gradual wearing down of the articular cartilage on the undersurface of the patella, were successfully treated by the method described.[21] The mild chondromalacia group showed a 25% increase in quadriceps strength, while the patients having severe damage displayed a minimum of 200% increased strength. Similarly, in a group of healthy subjects, high-frequency electrical stimulation resulted in a statistically significant increase in quadriceps femoris muscle torque, when compared with the nonexercised controls.[22]

No significant difference was noted between this type of electrical stimulation and isometric training. The Russian technique of electrical stimulation also was applied simultaneously with isometric training in a group of healthy subjects.[23] Electrical stimulation combined with maximal isometric contractions had no greater effect on enhancing strength than conventional isometric exercise. Finally, the Russian technique was compared to low-frequency (25 Hz) stimulation, consisting of rectangular pulses.[24] The maximal voluntary isometric torque increased to 25% in a group of patients stimulated with a 25-Hz stimulation frequency and 13% in healthy subjects treated with sinusoidal high-frequency stimuli. It appeared that the presence of fatigue during the high-frequency sinusoidal stimulation diminished the strengthening effects.

IV. ANIMAL MODELS

A considerable body of information is given by low-frequency stimulation studies performed in animals. Here, mostly the influences on muscle contractile properties were studied. Chronic electrical stimulation results in a significant increase of fatigue resistance, while there is little or no improvement in muscle strength. Chronic low-frequency stimulation is, therefore, compatible, to some extent, with endurance training, such as treadmill running.

When a phasic motoneuron is forced to innervate a slow muscle, the muscle is transformed to a fast muscle, even in an adult animal.[25] The decrease of muscle speed is demonstrated, not only by the time course of the rising and falling phases of the twitch contraction, but can also be observed during tetanic contraction. Similarly, the slow or tonic motoneuron converts fast muscle into slow. The slow or fast muscle with alien innervation has no influence in the reverse direction, i.e., on the motoneuron.

The same effects as those obtained by cross-innervation of slow motoneuron to fast muscle can be obtained by simply stimulating a fast muscle with a low electrical stimulation frequency (5 to 10 Hz), corresponding to the frequency naturally occurring in the nerves to slow muscles. When this low-frequency stimulation is applied continuously for 24 h daily, a fast muscle undergoes a sequence of changes that ultimately result in a complete transformation to a slow-twitch muscle.[13] In the first week of the chronic stimulation program, an increased resistance to fatigue is already observable. It appears in parallel to increase in capillary density and changes in capillary blood flow. Changes in isometric contractile properties become important after approximately 2 weeks of the electrical stimulation program. They result in a decrease in the rate of development of both twitch and tetanic tension. After 8 weeks, the maximal velocity of contraction recorded under isotonic conditions is also significantly reduced. Together with the described changes that can be assessed with the help of biomechanical measuring techniques, significant metabolic changes occur, along with morphologic changes at the ultrastructural level. The response of fast muscle to continuous low-frequency stimulation appears to be a reversible phenomenon when the stimulation program is discontinued.

In experiments with continuous low-frequency stimulation, the amplitude of twitch tension does not alter significantly, and the tetanic tension of the stimulated muscles is usually reduced.[26] While there is no significant change in the number of fibers, continuous stimulation results in significant reduction in the weight and cross-sectional area of the muscle fibers.[27] It is also hypothesized that reduction in fiber diameters facilitates the diffusion of oxygen from the capillaries to the centers of the fibers.[28]

When a low frequency of stimulation is applied for 8 h daily, instead of 24 h some differences in the effects of both stimulation regimens occur. Again, slowing of contraction is observed, but it is accompanied by an increase of tetanic tension as well. Thus, it appears that intermittent stimulation affects the ability of a muscle to develop tension in a more marked way than continuous activity.[26]

In another experiment, a 10-Hz stimulation frequency was applied in trains of 4 s every 100 s for 8 h/d.[29] Here, the changes took longer to develop, when compared to continuously delivered stimulation of the same frequency.

No changes in capillary density and fatigue resistance were observed after 4 d of high-frequency stimulation (40 Hz).[29] Both fast and slow muscles were stimulated for 8 h daily with the duty cycle 5 s on and 20 s off. An increase in capillary density appears to occur only when the muscle can take the advantage of an increased blood supply while it is working. It seems that the blood flow is not occluded at low-frequency activity, while it is prevented by the muscle contractions produced at higher stimulation frequencies. It is possible that an increased supply of blood to the muscle cells is important in changing muscle metabolism.

Nerve-mediated influences are not the sole means of changing the muscle fiber properties. Muscular work, whether produced voluntarily or with the help of electrical stimulation, is not absolutely necessary to achieve muscle hypertrophy. Muscle stretch itself is a major factor in determining the properties of skeletal muscle. Denervation hypertrophy is a phenomenon helping to separate the effects of the motor innervation from the effects of stretch. Although most skeletal muscles begin to atrophy shortly after losing the innervation, the denervated hemidiaphragm of the rat undergoes a gross hypertrophy.[30] This transient hypertrophy (enlargement of muscle fibers) has been attributed to the repetitive stretching of the denervated hemidiaphragm, resulting from the rhythmic contractions of the intact contralateral hemidiaphragm. Similarly, tenotomy of the chicken anterior latissimus dorsi leads to hypertrophy (increase in muscle weight) of the same muscle because the wing is stretched with the help of antagonist muscle.[31] In general, muscles hypertrophy by an increase in fiber size rather than in total number of fibers. Nevertheless, it was observed in denervation hypertrophy that new fibers are also obtained by longitudinal splitting. Most of these fibers degenerate.

Considerable efforts will be necessary to bring all the relevant observations and conclusions regarding the influence of electrical currents on the state of a skeletal muscle from the animal laboratory into clinical practice. It appears that FES can be further improved with the help of this knowledge.

V. THE RESTRENGTHENING METHODOLOGY, TRAINING, AND MONITORING

A. Training Modalities

SCI patients with upper motor neuron lesion are candidates for a restrengthening program of their disuse-atrophied paralyzed muscles. This criterion results in the selection of patients with thoracic and cervical spinal cord lesion. Quite often, knee extensor muscles cannot be excited by the described type of stimulation in low-thoracic patients. Here, these muscles suffered lower motor neuron lesion. Nevertheless, the muscle groups governing motion around the ankle joint are usually spastic and can be trained with the use of electrical stimuli. The criteria for patient selection also include the following: adequately preserved skin, good psychosocial condition, motivation, and cooperation.

Our strengthening program consists of applying cyclic electrical stimulation to the knee extensor muscles, resulting in isotonic contractions.[32] Usually several months have passed after the injury, when the patients arrive from the clinic to the Ljubljana Rehabilitation

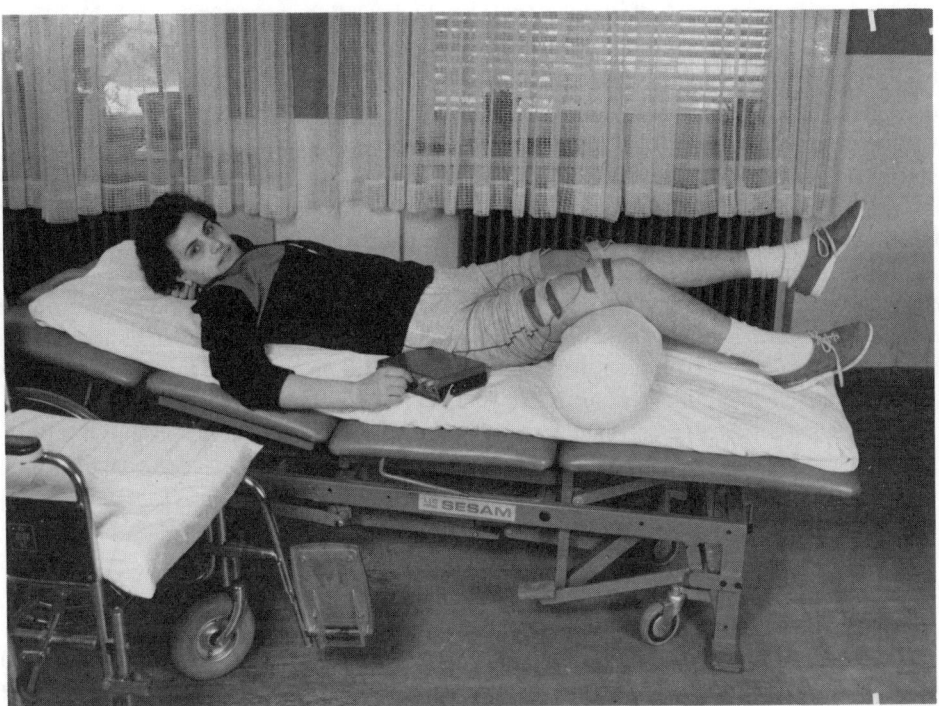

FIGURE 10. Paraplegic patient during muscle-strengthening program.

Engineering Center (REC). The electrical stimulation training program also is equally effective with subjects in cases where several years have passed after the accident.[33] Electrical stimulation of the knee extensors is delivered through large (e.g., 6 × 4 cm) surface electrodes. The stimulation periods of 4 s are followed by a pause of 4 or 8 s. The electrical pulses used are rectangular and monophasic. A stimulation frequency of 20 pulses per second (Hz), a pulse duration of 0.3 ms, and a stimulation amplitude of sufficient intensity to bring the legs into full extension are used. Polarity of the electrodes has some effect on knee joint torque when applying monophasic wave-forms, but has no effect with biphasic electrical stimuli.[34]

During the training, the patients are positioned supine, with both lower extremities semiflexed to approximately 30° by a pillow under the knees (Figure 10). During the first week of the program, the FES sessions last 30 min/d, 5 d/week. As a result of this FES training program, the muscle force is increased and the muscle fatigability is lessened.[11] Because of this, 30 min of FES is added each week thereafter. The FES muscle strengthening is usually divided into two or three sessions each day, which together do not exceed 3 h. Paraplegic subjects easily learn how to use the stimulator, so that the training program is performed by themselves. Quite often, electrical stimulation restrengthening takes place at the patients' homes.

The training modality described is called isotonic. Isometric training, where the extremity being trained is fixed, is used to a lesser extent. If the position of the extremity trained is predetermined with the help of a closed-loop control system, we deal with the so-called isokinetic type of muscle training. Such an example is the isokinetic leg trainer.[35] Here, a position sensor is placed at the knee joint to provide angle information utilized by a computer. A computer controls the shape of electrical stimulation trains delivered to the knee extensors.

The patient can read or be occupied by some manual work while exercising. Nevertheless, paraplegic patients often find electrical stimulation training rather boring. An interesting solution to this problem is presented by the exercise bicycle ergometer.[36] An exercise bicycle was modified by the addition of a pedal sensor to indicate the position of the pedals. The four stimulation channels were computer controlled.

Another approach, which is only applicable to incomplete SCI patients, is presented by biofeedback in conjunction with electrical stimulation. By applying biofeedback, these patients develop a high degree of motivation. The instrumentation includes an electronic unit producing visual and acoustical signals (light and loudspeaker), while an analog or digital instrument displays the value of the joint angle measured by means of a potentiometer. When the patient begins moving the leg in the direction of extension, the pointer of the instrument declines and the sound of the loudspeaker increases. After the angle has reached the threshold value preset by the therapist, the light goes on, which means "reward". At that moment, an intermittent acoustical signal sets in and electrical stimulation of, e.g., knee extensors is switched on, completing the movement to maximal extension. The therapeutic method as described provides not only acoustic and visual information on the position of the joint, but also exteroceptive and proprioceptive information when electrical stimulation excites the skin under the electrodes causing muscle contraction and joint movement.[37]

B. Measuring Methods

There are two biomechanical approaches to the assessment of the effects of skeletal muscle exercising: isometric and isokinetic modality. One of the basic parameters measured when applying electrical stimulation to the extremities is isometric torque. With respect to the measuring equipment available, the isometric torques in lower extremities are usually measured in the knee and ankle joint, but rarely in the hip. Manufacturers of rehabilitation aids sometimes also produce measuring instruments for forces and torques in joints. Such an instrument consists of a brace for fixing an extremity and a dynamometer, whereby a display of static forces is made possible. If we wish to analyze also dynamic properties of the stimulated paralyzed extremity (increase and decrease of isometric torque), we make use of braces where isometric torque is measured as electric voltage with the help of a strain-gauge transducer and led either to analog and digital instruments, or to plotters, or smaller computers recording the time courses of the torque measured. Quite often, such measuring devices are built in research laboratories and used for the purposes of a particular investigation.[38,39] Figure 11 shows a measuring device for the knee torque assessment. To ensure standardization of position and fixation of limb during assessment, a special chair was designed. A subject is seated on a chair in such a way that the long horizontal bar passes below both knee joints. In this way, approximate joint rotation comes into the vicinity of rotation of a special triangular structure. One leg of this triangle is fixed to the chair through a strain-guage transducer. The lower limb is fixed at the ankle joint to the other leg of the triangle. The angle of the triangular metal structure can be adjusted, thus allowing assessment of the knee joint isometric torque at different joint angles. The device described provides a constant lever of the torque measured (distance between joint rotation and transducer position), which makes the measuring procedure simpler. Attachment of the lower extremity to the device is also fast and uncomplicated.

Joint torque can also be assessed with the help of an isokinetic dynamometer.[40] The aim of this device is to keep the speed of movement at a preset level. It consists of a motor that rotates at a controlled constant speed. The motor axis is connected through a clutch coupling to a lever arm. The subject is asked to perform movement against this lever arm. The clutch coupling inhibits the lever arm from rotating faster than the motor axis. When the velocity of the limb movement reaches the speed of the motor axis, the lever arm starts to resist the movement. The rotation of the lever arm can never be faster than that of the motor axis. It was found that the strength of isokinetic contractions is significantly less than that of isometric

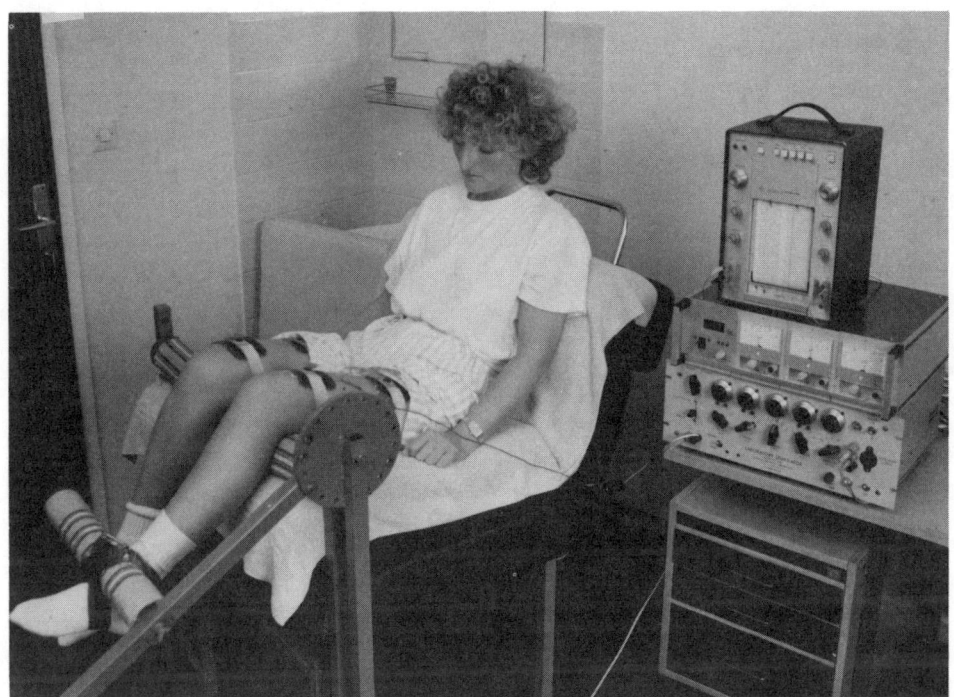

FIGURE 11. Isometric measuring device for the knee joint.

contractions.[41] Isokinetic measurement is, therefore, preferable in patients where, because of osteoporosis, damage to joints or bones can occur because of the high forces obtained under isometric conditions.[42]

Among other modalities of assessment of the effects of muscle exercising, the simplest approach is, by far, measurement of limb circumference. It was observed that quadriceps hypertrophy was underestimated by measurements of thigh circumference, and could, therefore, not be predicted from them.[43]

A much better estimation of muscle mass increase resulting from a restrengthening program can be obtained by studying the whole muscle cross-sectional area. Ultrasound[43] and magnetic resonance imaging (MRI) appear to be especially appropriate.[44] Here, the cross-sectional area of each individual muscle can be measured with the aid of planimeter techniques.

Even closer insight into the phenomena of muscle restrengthening can be achieved by examination of muscle tissue specimens. Such specimens can be obtained by surgical intervention or by needle biopsy. A needle biopsy is safe and rapid. As there is no permanent scar, repeat biopsies allowing follow-up studies can be performed.[45] Muscle biopsy specimen can be histologically and histochemically analyzed. With the help of light and electron microscopy, type I and II fibers are identified and a cross-sectional area of a particular muscle fiber can be determined. Apart from structure, muscle metabolism is studied as well. Specific histochemical methods give insight into distribution of particular molecules within muscle tissue: electrolytes, enzymes, amino acids, and pH.

C. Effects of Exercise on Strength Increase and Fatigue Resistance

When starting a strengthening program for disuse-atrophied thigh muscles, usually at least several months have passed after the injury. This is the time period that patients have spent in a traumatology clinical environment before coming to the rehabilitation unit. Electrical stimulation exercising is sometimes started several years after the injury. A training program

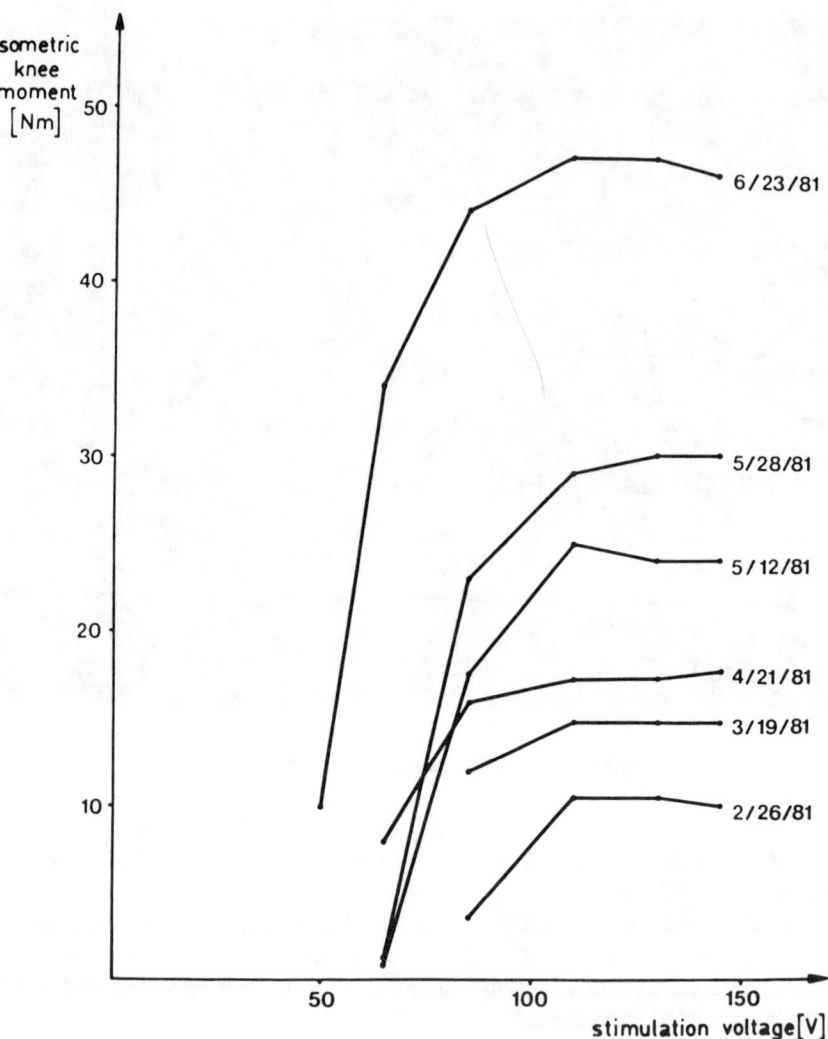

FIGURE 12. Improvement in muscle torque due to the electrical stimulation training program.

also is effective in such cases. Apparently, these are the spasms that are helpful in maintaining the muscle in a viable state for electrical stimulation.[11] In Figure 12, the results of the strengthening program are shown for T-10,11 completely paralyzed paraplegic patient. They are presented by knee joint torques plotted vs. amplitude of stimulation voltage. The curves correspond to control measurements performed at different dates during the muscle-strengthening program. Quite often, at the start of the training program, not more than 10 Nm can be obtained by surface electrical stimulation exceeding 100 V. According to our experiences, knee joint torques around 50 Nm are sufficient to begin standing and walking maneuvers in completely paraplegic patients. In the case presented in Figure 12, 4 months were necessary to increase the knee joint torque five times and reach a functional level. It is interesting to note that maximal knee joint torques that are voluntarily produced by healthy subjects, range around 250 Nm. When stimulating knee extensors of healthy subjects with the help of surface electrodes, no more than 150 Nm are produced. Values exceeding 100 Nm are also often encountered in paraplegic patients after a successful electrical stimulation training program.[46]

The knee joint torques obtained in five randomly chosen completely paraplegic patients before and after electrical stimulation training are shown in Figure 13. The strengthening

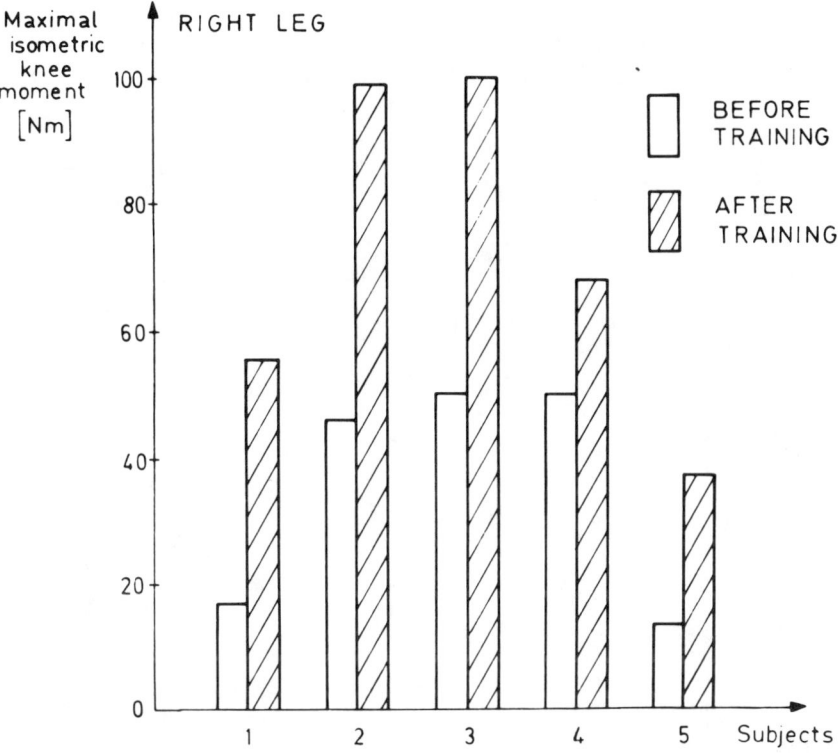

FIGURE 13. Maximal isometric knee joint torques assessed before and after the electrical stimulation training program.

program consisted of 30 min daily sessions of cyclic electrical stimulation. The duty cycle was 4 s of stimulation followed by 4 s of pause. The stimulation frequency was 20 Hz and pulse duration 0.3 ms. The type of training was isotonic. An increase of joint torque can be observed in all five subjects. The general data on five completely paraplegic patients are collected in Table 1, which also includes the duration of the overall training period.

Similar strengthening results of disuse-atrophied muscles in SCI patients also are found with other authors. An increase in muscle force of almost five times was observed by Kralj and Grobelnik.[47] Here, the following electrical stimulation parameters were chosen: 50 Hz stimulation frequency, 0.3 ms pulse duration, 5 s on/5 s off duty cycle. The stimulation sessions, lasting 10 min, were performed three times daily, and after 2 months, three times for 30 min/d. The training program lasted for 6 months. Substantial increase in muscle force was also observed by Phillips et al.[36] and Fournier et al.[48] Isokinetic training and bicycle exercising were used. The stimulation frequency of 50 Hz was chosen. FES training sessions were held 3 d/week for a period of 12 weeks. The exercise period was 15 min. A tenfold increase in knee torque was noted in one patient by Marsolais and Kobetič.[42] In this investigation, implanted percutaneous electrodes were used. The electrical stimulation frequency was 50 Hz and pulse width 0.1 ms. An exercise program of 3 h/d, lasting almost 10 months was carried out by the patient at his home. Implantation of the stimulation electrodes to the femoral and gluteal nerve was performed by Holle et al.[49] Here, electrical stimulation of 30 Hz and 0.6 ms pulse duration was delivered to the atrophied muscle. Two patients were stimulated daily for 30 min. The duty cycle used was 5 s on and 10 s off. After 1 month of training, the muscle force was increased by up to 200%. In the investigation described by Robinson et al.[50,51], out of eight paraplegic patients with complete injury, six had bilateral

Table 1
GENERAL DATA ON THE COMPLETE PARAPLEGIC PATIENTS PARTICIPATING IN THE ELECTRICAL STIMULATION TRAINING PROGRAM

No.	Initials	Sex	Age	Lesion	Time postinjury (months)	Training period (months)
1	D. O.	F	16	T-12	12	3
2	D .D.	M	18	T-5,6	20	7
3	W. H.	M	24	T-4,5	18	1
4	Z. K.	M	26	T-8	23	2
5	G. T.	M	18	T-10	3	6

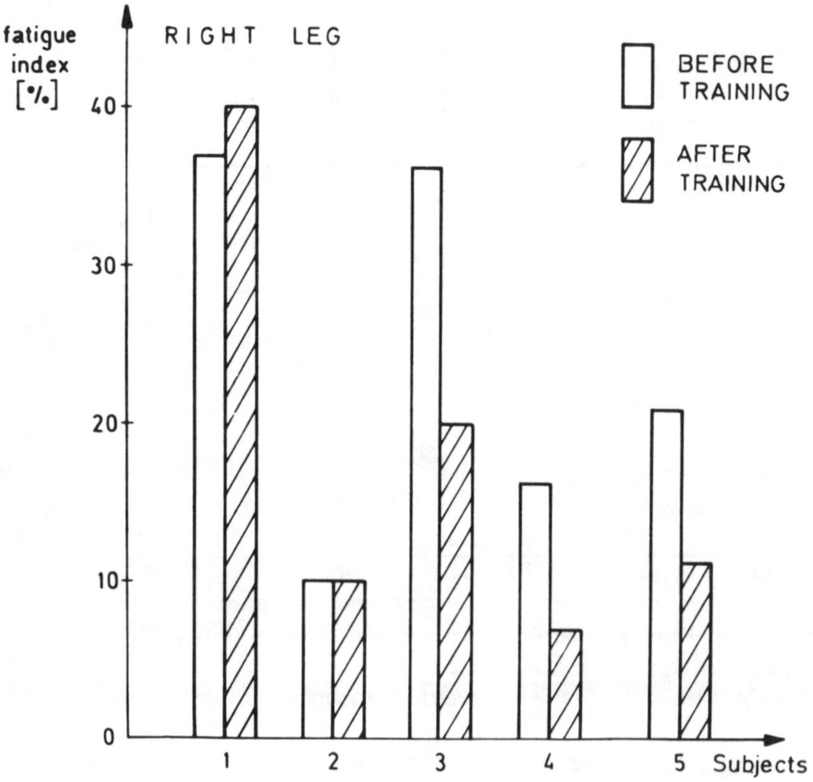

FIGURE 14. Fatigue index assessed in knee extensors before and after the electrical stimulation training program.

increases in peak torque, while two had bilateral decreases. The electrical exercise of the quadriceps was induced twice daily for 20 min through 3 to 8 weeks. The other electrical stimulation parameters were 20 Hz frequency, 0.4 ms pulse duration, and 2.25 s on and 2.25 s off duty cycle.

In Figure 14, fatigue indices, such as previously defined in this chapter, are presented for the same group of patients (Table 1). It can be observed that the type of training described[32,52] is not as effective in increasing muscle endurance as it is in improving muscle strength. Electrically stimulated muscle fatiguing measured over 30 s was improved in only three out of five subjects. In one patient (subject no. 2), low muscle fatiguing was observed already at the beginning of the training program.

Increased maximal force and fatigue resistance were both observed by Peckham et al. while exercising forearm-finger flexor muscles.[11] The main difference between their FES training program and those described previously is lower stimulation frequency, being 10 Hz. Pulse duration used was 0.1 ms and duty cycle 2.5 s on/2.5 s off. The usage of FES generally exceeded 2 h/d and commonly was 4 to 6 h/d. The training program lasted from 2 weeks to 15 months. It is also interesting to note that the fatigue was measured as percent of initial force following 10 min of continuous 10-Hz stimulation. A significant increase in fatigue resistance was obtained by Scott et al.[39] while training tibialis anterior muscles of normal adult subjects. Here again, a 10-Hz stimulation frequency was used. Electrical stimulation was applied continuously for 1 h three times daily through 6 weeks. With this type of stimulation, only a small increase in tetanic tension was found.

Neuromuscular fatigue is defined as the inability of a muscle or group of muscles to sustain the required or expected force.[16,53] With respect to origin, fatigue may be central fatigue (brain and spinal cord), fatigue concerned with neural transmission from the CNS to the muscle, and fatigue within the individual muscle fiber. An important factor related to muscle fatigue is blood flow limitation. Procedures promoting greater blood flow to the stimulated skeletal muscles could possibly increase fatigue resistance for FES-induced exercise.[54] From animal experiments and also from the two last-mentioned investigations performed in tetraplegic[11] and normal subjects,[39] it is evident that low-frequency chronic electrical stimulation is effective in increasing fatigue resistance. This further proves that muscle fatigue associated with low-frequency electrical stimulation is of peripheral origin and that the loss of force is probably due to fatigue of fast-contracting glycolytic fatiguable type II motor fibers and is not caused by failure of neuromuscular transmission or conduction of the peripheral nerve.

Apart from influencing muscle strength and endurance, cyclic therapeutic eletrical stimulation also brings other benefits to SCI patients. It was observed, e.g., that blood pressure during FES exercising was reduced.[36] Improved blood flow may improve skin condition and prevent development of pressure sores. Electrical stimulation can be also an effective treatment against ossifications and contractures. Reversal of disuse osteoporosis was also observed as a side effect of FES exercising.[36] Decreased spasticity, more regular defecations, and even improved sexual abilities were reported by some patients.

The scientific fundamentals of muscle restrengthening and the corresponding physiological mechanisms are not yet elaborated in detail. Similarly, optimal training procedures, together with appropriate screening and prediction of results, are not yet determined.

REFERENCES

1. **Edwards, R. H. T.**, Weakness and fatigue of skeletal muscles, *Advanced Medicine*, Sarmer, M., Ed., Royal College of Physicians, Pitman McOill, London, 1982, 100.
2. **Vodovnik, L., Bajd, T., Kralj, A., Gračanin, F., and Strojnik, P.**, Functional electrical stimulation for control of locomotor systems, CRC *Crit. Rev. Bioeng.*, 6, 63, 1981.
3. **Salmons, S.**, The adaptive capacity of skeletal muscle and its relevance to some therapeutic uses of electrical stimulation, Proc. Int. Symp. Cell Biology and Clinical Management, in *Functional Electro Stimulation of Neurones and Muscles*, Abano Terme, Italy, August 28 to 30, 1985, 71.
4. **Mortimer, J. T.**, Motor prostheses, in *Handbook of Physiology — The Nervous System II*, Brooks, V. B., Ed., American Physiology Society, Williams & Wilkins, Baltimore, MD, 1985, 155.
5. **Reggie, E. V., Smith, J. L., and Simpson, D. R.**, Muscle fibre type populations of human leg muscles, *Histochem. J.*, 7, 259, 1975.
6. **Salmons, S. and Vrbova, G.**, The influence of activity in some contractile characteristics of mammalian fast and slow muscles, *J. Physiol. (London)*, 206, 535, 1969.

7. Eccles, J. C., Eccles, R. M., and Lundberg, A., The action potentials of the alpha motoneurones supplying fast and slow muscles, *J. Physiol. (London)*, 142, 275, 1958.
8. McMiken, D. F., Todd-Smith, M., and Thompson, C., Strengthening of human quadriceps muscles by cutaneous electrical stimulation, *Scand. J. Rehabil. Med.*, 15, 25, 1983.
9. Kovanen, V., Suominen, H., and Heikkinen, E., Mechanical properties of fast and slow skeletal muscles with special reference to collagen and endurance training, *J. Biomech.*, 17, 725, 1984.
10. Fischbach, G. D. and Robbins, N., Changes in contractile properties of disused soleus muscles, *J. Physiol. (London)*, 201, 305, 1984.
11. Peckham, P. H., Mortimer, J. T., and Marsolais, E. B., Alteration in the force and fatigability of skeletal muscle in quadriplegic humans following exercise induced by chronic electrical stimulation, *Clin. Orthop. Relat. Res.*, 114, 326, 1976.
12. Halkjaer-Kristensen, J. and Ingemann-Hansen, T., Wasting and training of the human quadriceps muscle during the treatment of knee ligaments injury, *Scand. J. Rehabil. Med. (Suppl.)*, 13, 1985.
13. Salmons, S. and Henriksson, J., The adaptive response of skeletal muscle to increased use, *Muscle Nerve*, 4, 94, 1981.
14. Stilwill, E. W. and Sahgal, V., Histochemical and morphological changes in skeletal muscle following cervical cord injury, a study of upper and lower motor neuron lesion, *Arch. Phys. Med. Rehabil.*, 58, 201, 1977.
15. Grimby, G., Bromberg, C., Krotkiewska, I., and Krotkiewski, M., Muscle fiber composition in patients with spinal cord lesion, *Scand. J. Rehabil. Med.*, 8, 37, 1976.
16. Bigland-Ritchie, B., Jones, D. A., and Woods, J. J., Excitation frequency and muscle fatigue: electrical responses during human voluntary and stimulated contractions, *Exp. Neurol.*, 64, 414, 1979.
17. Kralj, A., Bajd, T., and Turk, R., Electrical stimulation providing functional use of paraplegic patient muscle, *Med. Prog. Technol.*, 7, 3, 1980.
18. Halbach, J. W. and Don Strauss, A. T., Comparison of electromyostimulation to isokinetic training in increasing power of the knee extensor mechanism, *J. Orthop. Sports Phys. Ther.*, 2, 20, 1980.
19. Godfrey, C. M., Jayawardena, H., Quance, T. A., and Welsh, P., Comparison of electrostimulation and isometric exercise in strengthening the quadriceps muscle, *Physiother. Can.*, 31, 265, 1979.
20. Eriksson, E. and Häggmark, T., Comparison of isometric muscle training and electrical stimulation supplementing isometric muscle training in the recovery after major knee ligament surgery, *Am. J. Sports Med.*, 7, 169, 1979.
21. Johnson, D. H., Thurston, P., and Ashcroft, P. J., The Russian technique of faradism in the treatment of chondromalacia patellae, *Physiother. Can.*, 29, 2, 1977.
22. Laughman, R. K., Youdas, J. W., Garrett, T. R., and Chao, E. Y. S., Strength changes in the normal quadriceps femoris muscle as a result of electrical stimulation, *Phys. Ther.*, 63, 494, 1983.
23. Currier, D. P., Lehman, J., and Lightfoot, P., Electrical stimulation in exercise of the quadriceps femoris muscle, *Phys. Ther.*, 59, 1508, 1979.
24. Stefanovska, A. and Vodovnik, L., Change in muscle force following electrical stimulation, *Scand. J. Rehabil. Med.*, 17, 141, 1985.
25. Buller, A. J., Eccles, J. C., and Eccles, R. M., Interactions between motoneurones and muscles in respect of the characteristic speeds of their responses, *J. Physiol. (London)*, 150, 417, 1960.
26. Pette, D., Smith, M. E., Staudte, H. W., and Vrbova, G., Effects of long-term electrical stimulation on some contractile and metabolic characteristics of fast rabbit muscles, *Pfluegers Arch.*, 338, 257, 1973.
27. Pette, D., Ramirez, B. U., Müller, W., Simon, R., Exner, G. U., and Hildebrand, R., Influence of intermittent long-term stimulation in contractile, histochemical, and metabolic properties in fibre populations in fast and slow rabbit muscles, *Pfluegers Arch.*, 361, 1, 1975.
28. Hudlicka, O., Brown, M., Cotter, M., Smith, M., and Vrbova, G., The effect of long-term stimulation of fast muscles on their blood flow metabolism and ability to withstand fatigue, *Pfluegers Arch.*, 369, 141, 1977.
29. Brown, M. D., Cotter, M. A., Hudlicka, O., and Vrbova, G., The effects of different patterns of muscle activity on capillary density, mechanical properties and structures of slow and fast rabbit muscles, *Pfluegers Arch.*, 361, 241, 1976.
30. Yellin, H., Changes in fiber types of the hypertrophying denervated hemidiaphragm, *Exp. Neurol.*, 42, 412, 1974.
31. Sola, O. M., Christensen, D. L., and Martin, A. W., Hypertrophy and hyperplasia of adult chicken anterior latissimus dorsi muscles following stretch with and without denervation, *Exp. Neurol.*, 41, 76, 1973.
32. Bajd, T., Kralj, A., Turk, R., Benko, H., and Šega, J., The use of a four-channel electrical stimulator as an ambulatory aid for paraplegic patients, *Phys. Ther.*, 63, 1116, 1983.
33. Bajd, T., Kralj, A., and Turk, R., Standing-up of a healthy subject and a paraplegic patient, *J. Biomech.*, 15, 1, 1982.

34. **McNeal, D. R. and Baker, L. L.**, Stimulating the quadriceps and hamstrings with surface electrodes, in *Proc. 8th Ann. RESNA Conf.*, RESNA Association for the Advancement of Rehabilitation Technology, Washington, D.C., 1985, 237.
35. **Petrofsky, J. S., Heaton, H. H., III, and Phillips, C. A.**, Leg exerciser for training of paralysed muscle by closed-loop control, *Med. Biol. Eng. Comput.*, 22, 298, 1984.
36. **Phillips, C. A., Petrofsky, J. S., Hendershot, D. M., and Stafford, D.**, Functional electrical exercise — a comprehensive approach for physical conditioning of the spinal cord injured patient, *Orthopedics*, 7, 1112, 1984.
37. **Winchester, P., Montgomery, J., Bowman, B., and Hislop, H.**, Effects of feedback stimulation training on knee extension in hemiparetic patients, *Phys. Ther.*, 63, 1096, 1983.
38. **Bajd, T., Kralj, A., Šega, J., Turk, R., and Benko, H.**, Muscle strengthening in paraplegic patients by cyclic electrical stimulation, in Proc. 3rd Mediterranean Conf. Biomedical Engineering, Portorož, Yugoslavia, September 5 to 9, 1983, 3.6.
39. **Scott, O. M., Vrbova, G., Hyde, S. A., and Dubowitz, V.**, Effects of chronic low frequency electrical stimulation on normal human tibialis anterior muscle, *J. Neurol. Neurosurg. Psychiatry*, 48, 774, 1985.
40. **Knutsson, E.**, Assessment of motor function in spastic paresis and its dependence on paresis and different types of restraint, in *Recent Achievements in Restorative Neurology, Upper Motor Neuron Functions and Dysfunctions*, Eccles, Sir J. and Dimitrijević, M. R., Eds., S. Karger, Basel, 1985, 199.
41. **Murray, M. P., Gardner, G. M., Mollinger, L. A., and Sepic, S. B.**, Strength of isometric and isokinetic contractions, *Phys. Ther.*, 60, 412, 1980.
42. **Marsolais, E. B. and Kobetič, R.**, Functional walking in paralyzed patients by means of electrical stimulation, *Clin. Orthop. Relat. Res.*, 175, 30, 1983.
43. **Young, A., Stokes, M., Round, J. M., and Edwards, R. H. T.**, The effect of high-resistance training on the strength and cross-sectional area of the human quadriceps, *Eur. J. Clin. Invest.*, 13, 411, 1983.
44. **Fisher, M., Kralj, A., and Jaeger, R.**, MRI studies of the lower extremities in spinal cord injury: effects of long-term electrical stimulation, in Proc. 5th Annu. Meet. Soc. Magnetic Resonance Medicine, Montreal, August 18 to 22, 1986.
45. **Edwards, R. H. T., Round, J. M., and Jones, D. A.**, Needle biopsy of skeletal muscle: a review of 10 years experience, *Muscle Nerve*, 6, 676, 1983.
46. **Bajd, T., Kralj, A., Krajnik, J., Turk, R., Benko, H., and Šega, J.**, Standing by FES in paraplegic patients, in Proc. 8th Int. Symp. External Control Human Extremities, Dubrovnik, Yugoslavia, September 3 to 7, 1984, 51.
47. **Kralj, A. and Grobelnik, S.**, Functional electrical stimulation — a new hope for paraplegic patients, *Bull. Prosthet. Res.*, BPR 10-20, 75, 1973.
48. **Fournier, A., Goldberg, M., Green, B., Brucker, B., Petrofsky, J., Eismont, F., Quencer, R., Sosenko, J., Pina, I., Shebert, R., Kessler, K., MacDonald, A., Fiore, P., and Burnett, B.**, A medical evaluation of the effect of computer assisted muscle stimulation in paraplegic patients, *Orthopedics*, 7, 1129, 1984.
49. **Holle, J., Frey, M., Gruber, H., Kern, H., Stöhr, H., and Thoma, H.**, Functional electrostimulation of paraplegics — experimental investigations and first clinical experience with an implantable stimulation device, *Orthopedics*, 7, 1145, 1984.
50. **Robinson, C. J., Wurster, R., Bolam, J., Engelmeier, P., Nemechausky, B., Fruin, M., Gratzer, M., and Jaeger, R.**, Initial assessment of responses to surface electrical stimulation of the quadriceps in individuals with spinal cord injury, in Functional Electro Stimulation of Neurons and Muscles, Abano Terme, Italy, August 28 to 30, 1985, 159.
51. **Robinson, C. J., Bolam, J., Chinoy, M., Engelmeier, P., Fruin, R., Johnson, N., Ketl, N., Nemachusky, B., and Wurster, R.**, Response to surface electrical stimulation of the quadriceps in individuals with spinal cord injury, in *Proc. 9th Annu. RESNA Conf.*, RESNA Association for the Advancement of Rehabilitation Technology, Washington, D.C., 1986, 282.
52. **Kralj, A., Bajd, T., Turk, R., Krajnik, J., and Benko, H.**, Gait restoration in paraplegic patients: a feasibility demonstration using multichannel surface electrode FES, *J. Rehabil.*, 20, 3, 1983.
53. **Bigland-Ritchie, B. and Woods, J. J.**, Changes in muscle contractile properties and neural control during human muscular fatigue, *Muscle Nerve*, 7, 691, 1984.
54. **Glaser, R.M., Strayer, J. R., and May, K. P.**, Combined FES leg and voluntary arm exercise of SCI patients, in *Proc. Institute of Electrical and Electronic Engineers 7th Ann. Conf. Engineering Medicine Biology*, IEEE Service Center, Piscataway, NJ, 1985, 308.

Chapter 3

INFLUENCE OF ELECTRICAL STIMULATION ON SPASTICITY IN SPINAL CORD INJURED PATIENTS

I. CHARACTERISTICS OF SPINAL SPASTICITY

The word spasticity is often used simply as a single term to describe the complex results occurring after spinal cord lesion or other neurological disorders.[1] It represents a multitude of dysfunctions of the motor system, such as exaggeration of normal phasic proprioceptive reflexes, tonic proprioceptive reflexes, and polysynaptic flexion reflexes. Clinical experience has shown that electrical stimulation can affect spasticity. In some cases, decreased spasticity was observed, while in other cases patients have reported subjective descriptions of increased muscle spasticity. It is the aim of this chapter to present some evidence with regard to the influence of electrical stimulation on spinal spasticity.

Immediately after transection of the spinal cord, there is a phase of depression of reflexes in spinal cord injured (SCI) patients. This phase is called spinal shock and may last for several weeks.[2] The stretch reflex and cutaneous reflexes cannot be obtained and the muscles innervated from the segments below the level of the lesion are hypotonic. This initial phase is followed by a period when reflexes gradually return in the cases of upper motoneuron lesion. First, the flexion response returns. At the very beginning, it is demonstrated as the Babinski response, occurring after stimulation of the sole of the foot. By the third or fourth week, it increases into the so-called flexion synergy, where all flexor muscles of the lower extremity are strongly contracted during the withdrawal response, usually obtained by innocuous stimulation. In addition, the zone where the reflex can be triggered is significantly enlarged, extending up to the thigh region. A mass reflex often is obtained with strong stimuli, resulting in brisk bilateral withdrawal, as well as emptying of the bladder.

In the case of correct nursing, extensor reflex activity also returns. Correct posture, with the paralyzed limbs abducted and extended at the hips and knees, is of utmost importance. Reflex activity returns first to the distal muscles of the lower extremity. Ankle jerks are usually the first of the stretch reflexes to recover. The extensor thrust reflex can be produced by firm pressure on the sole of the foot. Extensor hypertonus usually develops only several months after spinal transection.

At a certain stage, both flexion and extension types of spasticity are present. In the spinal patient, there is a tendency for flexion spasticity, developing troublesome flexion contractures and making rehabilitation difficult. Adequate nursing, including correct posture in bed, early passive movements of the limbs, and early restoration of upright posture, results predominantly in the extension type of spasticity.

Spasticity can be more strictly defined as a motor disorder characterized by a velocity-dependent increase in tonic stretch reflexes with exaggerated tendon jerks, the latter resulting from a hyperexcitability of the stretch reflex, as one component of the upper motor neuron syndrome.[3] The term "spasticity" should, therefore, be used exclusively in those conditions of increased muscle tone in which velocity sensitivity is present. This velocity dependence results from the dynamic sensitivity of the muscle spindle.[4] Nevertheless, spindle input is not sufficient by itself to produce spasticity. Direct recordings from muscle spindle afferents in humans show that muscle spindle sensitivity is not a principal factor in determining the strength of stretch reflexes in normal subjects and spastic patients. Exaggeration of stretch reflexes in spasticity is believed to reflect central overactivity to an essentially normal spindle input.[5]

The pyramidal tract exerts a tonic excitatory effect on fusimotor neurons, while the extrapyramidal fibers have an inhibitory effect. Interruption of this inhibitory pathway would be expected to cause extensor hypertonus in the lower limbs of man.[6] Flexor reflex afferents are subject to tonic inhibition from the brainstem. Damage to this pathway can release flexor reflexes. It appears, therefore, that destruction of interneurons in the spinal cord removes an inhibitory influence from the higher central nervous system (CNS) centers and results in the state of hyperactivity. Here, it is interesting to note also that in clinically complete spinal cord lesion, some supraspinal descending pathways may be preserved. Their presence can be proved by the presence of the tonic vibration reflex, sustained clonus, and responsiveness to the Jendrassik maneuver,[5] consisting of strong sustained activation of a selected muscle group.

The lumbosacral spinal cord, separated from the influence of the brain, generates unsustained phasic reflexes. Residual brain influence will contribute to the tonic features of segmental reflexes.[7] Remaining functional pathways of the injured spinal cord can also be determined with the help of sensory-evoked potentials.[8] Somatosensory-evoked potentials are usually elicited by electrical stimuli delivered to a peripheral nerve. They are recorded along the somatosensory spinal pathway. Somatosensory-evoked potentials primarily reflect dorsal column function and provide no direct evidence of intact motor function. It is possible that motor tracts may be damaged, leaving sensory pathways and sensory-evoked potentials unharmed.[9] Usually, in acute spinal trauma, sensory and motor changes usually correspond closely. Spinal cord monitoring of evoked potentials can therefore provide information on completeness of the spinal cord lesion.

The skeletal muscle spasticity may be divided into phasic and tonic spasticity. The difference is evident from the electromyogram (EMG) activity assessed during imposed passive movements. Phasic spasticity is demonstrated by single bursts of EMG activity, where an integrated EMG signal is linearly related to the rate of stretch. In tonic spasticity, there is sustained evoked EMG activity present throughout the passively induced movement.

The importance of the increased stretch reflexes can be appreciated by the observation that in normal people, the tension generated by a phasically evoked stretch reflex is only 5% of the maximal voluntary effort, whereas the stretch reflex in spastic patients can generate up to 40% of maximal voluntary activity.[10] The degree of spasticity is also largely dependent on external influences. Upright posture, for example, doubles the tone of the extensor muscles over that found with the supine patient. Environmental temperature, pain sources, and emotion can also affect the degree of spasticity to a significant extent.

With regard to functional electrical stimulation (FES)-approached standing and ambulation, flexion spasticity certainly represents a disadvantage. Moderate extension spasticity can be helpful during prolonged standing. Severe spasticity of both types may seriously hinder completely paralyzed paraplegic patients while performing different daily activities, such as transfers from the wheelchair, dressing, or physical therapy exercises. Satisfactory upright standing posture is often difficult to maintain with patients who experience strong abdominal spasticity. Some patients have useful spasticity during the daytime, but are kept awake by flexor spasms at night. A spasm is an uncontrolled activity of muscle in response to a stimulus. Such stimuli may come from a number of different sources: pressure sores, contractures, urinary tract infection, extreme temperatures, or discomfort from tight clothing. Treatment of spasms involves treatment of the cause, while spasticity itself can be approached through pharmacological, surgical, and physical treatment modalities.

II. CLINICAL ASSESSMENT OF SPASTICITY

The existing methods for quantitative measurement of spasticity can be divided into neurophysiological and biomechanical procedures. Neurophysiological measurements are rather complicated. Standardization of testing is difficult to perform and long training is required to enable the examiner to obtain reproducible results. To have a satisfactory picture of the spasticity of a given patient, it is recommended to rely on a battery of complementary tests.[11] These tests are based on reflexology as a tool for exploring the motor system. Main reflexes elicited in clinical neurophysiology can be divided into monosynaptic and polysynaptic reflexes. Monosynaptic reflexes, such as is the phasic stretch reflex, can be clinically assessed in an efficient way by testing the tendon reflex, the Hoffmann reflex, and the tonic vibration reflex. The tendon reflex can be elicited in a standardized way by using an electromechanical hammer. To record the reflex response, an electromyographic recording is usually applied. The Hoffmann reflex is electrically evoked by stimulation of the tibial nerve. The response is assessed in soleus muscle after a latency of about 35 ms. Vibration of a tendon results in low-amplitude continuous electromyographic activity in the vibrated muscle. This activity is known as the tonic vibration reflex. In the lower extremity, several polysynaptic reflexes can be obtained following stimulation of the plantar surface of the foot, medial sole of the foot, or mixed nerves, such as the sural nerve and the tibial nerve at the ankle. The study of polysynaptic reflexes further reveals how the CNS processes and directs the afferent impulses after damage to the spinal cord.

Spasticity of muscles of the upper and lower extremities is usually assessed by physical therapists as increased resistance of a particular muscle group to manually induced passive movement. All the biomechanical procedures are based on measurement of resistance of the spastic limb to passive joint movement. Passive movements are induced manually or by means of electrical or hydraulic motors. The parameters measured are, in most cases, joint forces or torques, joint angles, and EMG potentials. An extensive study of spasticity was performed by Burke et al.[4] Passive flexion of the knee was manually induced by the examiner. Tension, goniogram, and velocity were recorded, together with EMG. In the study performed by Nashold,[12] movement of the forearm was provided by a constant speed motor. The angle of movement was measured by a potentiometer and the amount of resistance to passive motion by a torque meter. Similar instrumentation was used in the experiment performed by Webster.[13] Linear passive motions of the forearm or lower leg were obtained by a special active turntable. Strain gauges attached to the turntable detected the patient's muscular reaction to induced movement. The author reports disadvantages of the measuring machine, such as complexity, unphysiologic testing position, and speed limitations.

Joint compliance, defined as the ratio of joint rotation to applied torque, has been measured at sinusoidal torques with frequencies between 3 and 12 Hz.[14] The torques were provided by a computer-controlled direct current (DC) torque motor. The EMG of the antagonistic muscles was also measured in the experiment. In the study conducted by Reberšek et al.,[15] the joint movements were performed by an electrohydraulic position-controlled servosystem. The position of the ankle was measured by means of a potentiometer, while the resistive torque was assessed by a strain-gauge bridge. EMG activity in ankle joint muscles was also detected. In the study, sinusoidal test movements were used. Testing movements were performed at different velocities. Five different frequencies of sinusoidal movements (0.2, 0.5, 1, 1.5, and 2 Hz) were chosen to detect the velocity dependence of the stretch reflex hyperactivity. According to these parameters, the lowest velocity of the joint movement was $9.4° \text{ s}^{-1}$ and the highest velocity $188° \text{ s}^{-1}$.

A simple and convenient approach to the measurement and evaluation of spasticity is represented by eliciting the abnormal stretch reflexes during passive swing manuevers of a limb. Such an approach is called a pendulum test.[16,17] Spasticity of the knee extensor muscles was tested by placing the patient on a tilt-table in a supine position with both legs bent over the edge hanging free at the knee. The incomplete SCI patients were asked to relax as much as possible. The examiner grasped the foot and brought one leg to a horizontal position. The limb was allowed to fall freely, while recording knee angle with an electrogoniometer (Figure 1) and quadriceps EMG.

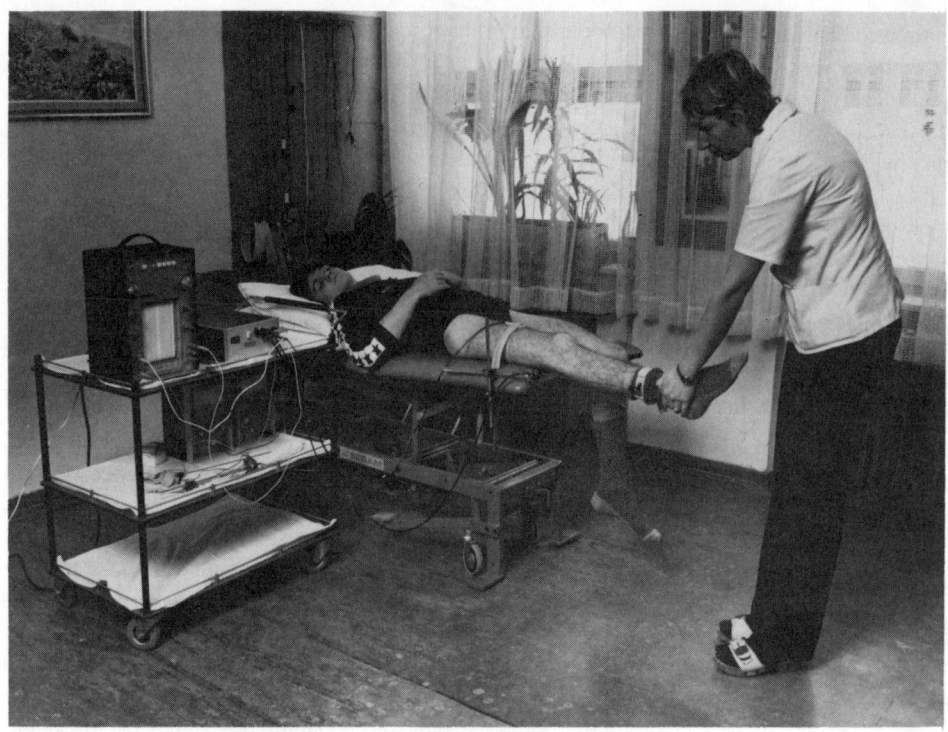

FIGURE 1. Patient's position during testing of knee extensors spasticity.

Figure 2 shows how different degrees of spasticity are manifested in the knee goniogram and quadriceps EMG potentials.[18] Figure 2A belongs to a healthy subject. The leg swings around the resting position and no EMG is present when the subject is fully relaxed. The maximal velocity of the freely swinging leg is $210°$ s^{-1}. Figure 2B shows a patient with only slight spasticity. There is an irregularity in only the first minimum of the knee goniogram, and it is preceded by a small amount of EMG activity. Figure 2C shows the knee goniogram never reaching $0°$ and the EMG occurs at each negative slope of the knee joint angle. Figure 2D is an example of severe spasticity. Even less oscillation occurs and high EMG activity is apparent throughout the trace. In a patient with extreme spasticity, the lower leg does not move at all from the fully extended initial position.

The level of spasticity was evaluated from the first minimum of the knee goniogram. This corresponds to the angle at which the spasticity stops the natural backward swing. To eliminate the influence of different resting angles belonging to different subjects or to the same subject on different testing days, the amplitude of the first backward swing ϕ_1 was normalized by the difference in angles between the resting and starting position ϕ_0 (Figure 3). In normal subjects, this ratio displayed a value around 1.6. A relaxation index was therefore defined as follows: $R = \phi_1/(1.6 \phi_0)$. Thus, $R > 1$ would signify a nonspastic limb, whereas $R < 1$ would quantify various degrees of spasticity. A relaxation index of zero signifies no motion of the knee from an extended position, and therefore, extreme spasticity. A relaxation index of one signifies a normal limb swing, and therefore, no spasticity. Special importance was assigned to this parameter because it belongs to the first "burst" of spastic activity that is the most cumbersome to paraplegic patients while performing daily activities such as dressing, transfers from the wheelchair, etc.

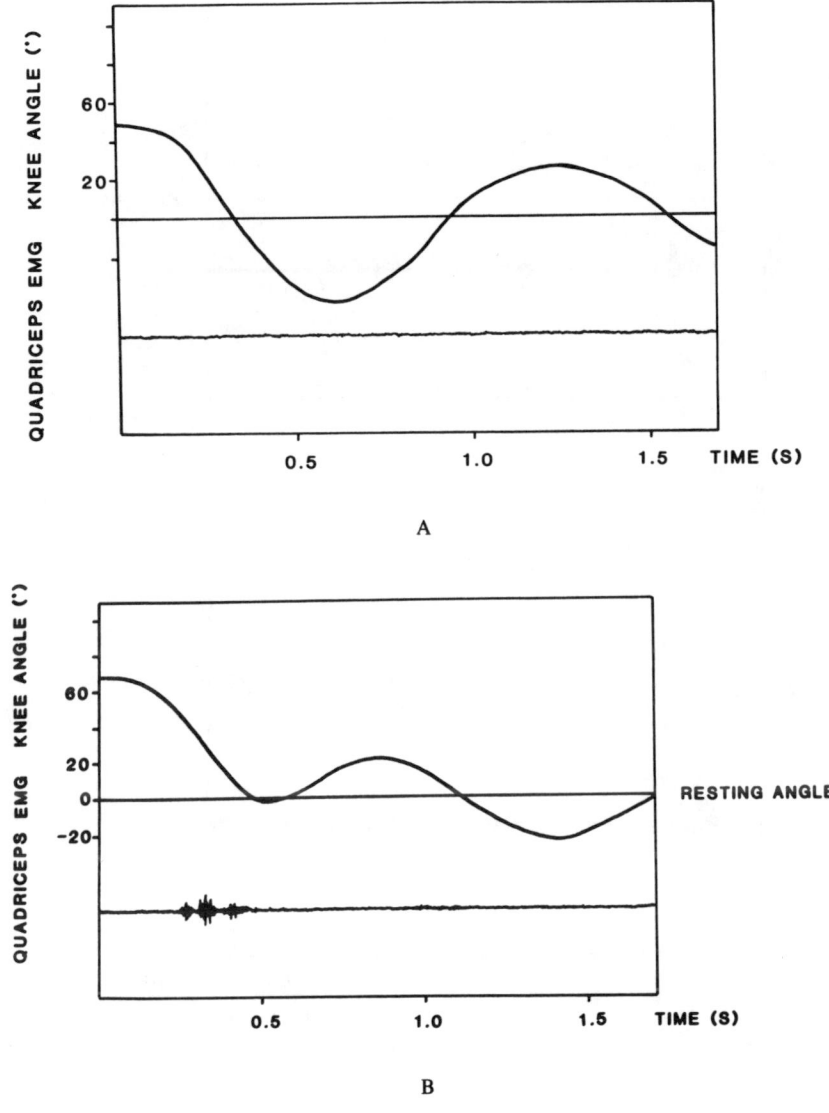

FIGURE 2. Examples of different degrees of spasticity: (A) absent, (B) slight, (C) moderate, and (D) severe.

III. TREATMENT OF SPASTICITY AND INFLUENCE OF ELECTRICAL STIMULATION ON AGONIST AND ANTAGONIST MUSCLE SPASTICITY

There are three major approaches currently used as treatment procedures for spasticity: pharmacological, surgical, and physical.[19] The pharmacological procedures can be divided into those acting centrally and others that are influencing peripheral nerve pathways. The spasmolytic action of the first type of drugs is thought to be due either to an increase in presynaptic inhibition or to depression of interneuron activity in polysynaptic pathways in the spinal cord. Peripherally acting drugs are aiming to block small nerve fibers, or neuromuscular junctions, or interfere with the contractile response of the spastic muscle itself.

The older surgical methods (rhizotomy, cordectomy) involved an operation on the spinal cord. Surgery is nowadays limited to peripheral procedures such as tenotomies, myotomies, neurectomies, neurotomies, tendon transfers, and tendon and muscle lengthening.

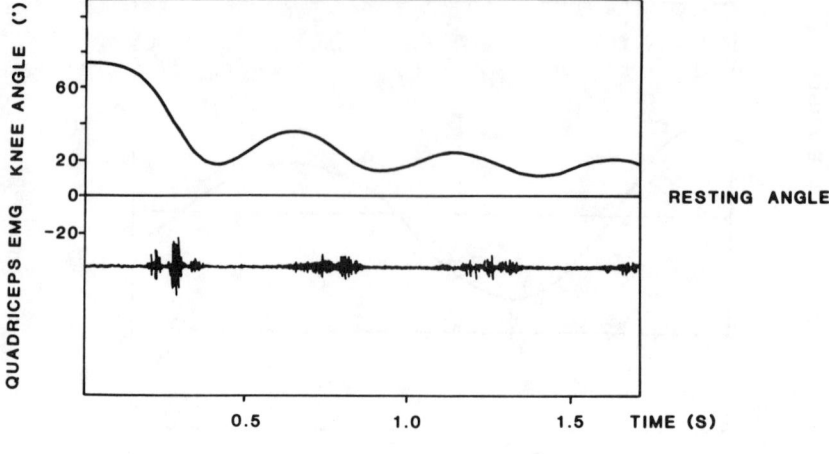

FIGURE 2C.

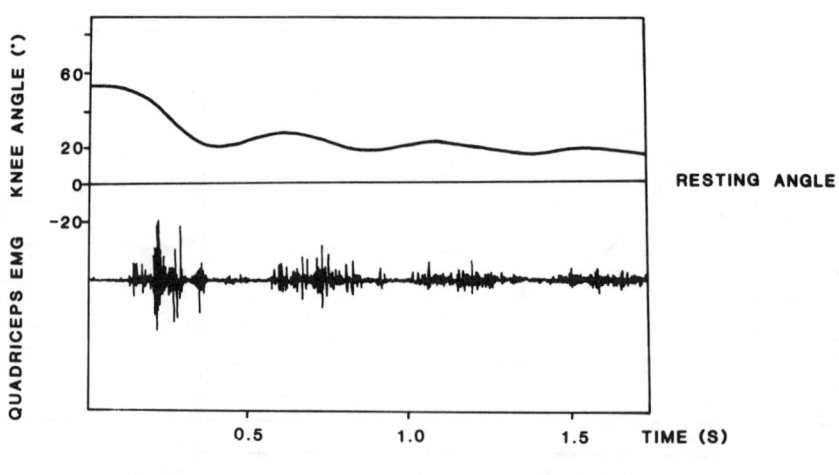

FIGURE 2D.

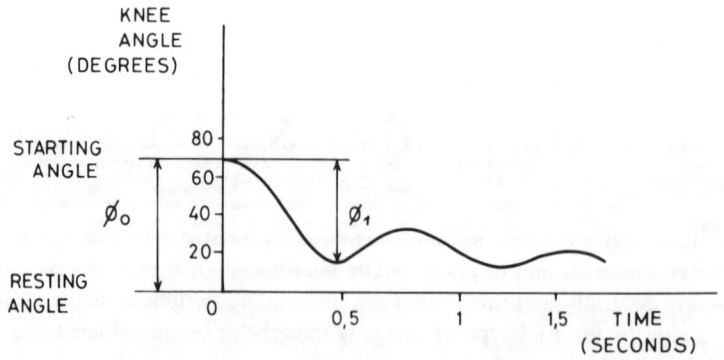

FIGURE 3. Knee joint goniogram displaying moderate spasticity of knee extensors. Starting angle (horizontal position of the lower leg), resting angle (vertical position of the lower leg), and amplitude of first swing are denoted.

Table 1
GENERAL DATA ON THE PATIENTS IN WHOM THE INFLUENCE OF ELECTRICAL STIMULATION ON AGONIST SPASTICITY WAS EXAMINED

No.	Initials	Sex	Age	Lesion	Time postinjury (months)
1	C. P.	F	33	C-2,3 incomplete	4
2	A. O.	M	31	C-5 incomplete	4
3	E. R.	M	22	T-5 incomplete	1
4	R. S.	M	27	C-7,8 complete	4
5	L. D.	M	11	T-5 incomplete	3
6	M. H.	M	25	T-7 incomplete	1
7	T. T.	M	51	C-5,6 incomplete	21
8	R. S.	M	19	C-5 incomplete	2
9	D. D.	M	27	T-6 incomplete	3
10	G. L.	M	42	T-3 incomplete	42

A very important mode for managing spasticity is physical therapy. Among therapists' approaches are passive joint ranging, spastic muscle cooling, and reeducation therapeutic exercising, including use of biofeedback.

It was observed as early as 1871 that electricity has an effect on spasticity.[20] Clinical reports of electrically stimulated SCI patients have claimed reduction in spasticity,[21,22] with only a few reports of heightened spasticity.[23] More recently, the authors report mostly about beneficial effects, but the specific techniques and stimulation sites do not seem to be of primary importance.[24,25,26] Spinal cord stimulation[27] and cerebellar stimulation[10] are also used for relieving spasticity.

In our studies, the influence of cyclic electrical stimulation on agonist and antagonist muscle spasticity was examined.[28] The effect of electrical stimulation of the knee extensors on the spasticity of the same muscle group was tested in ten SCI patients (Table 1). The measurements were performed in the morning, before other physical therapy exercises. No stimulation was applied to the patients during the first 3 d, when only one pendulum testing was performed. Two measurements were performed on the 4th d, the first before and the second after 30 min of stimulation therapy. Cyclic surface electrical stimulation of knee extensors with 6 s of stimulation followed by 12 s of rest was applied. The stimulation frequency was 33 Hz, and the duration of rectangular pulses was 0.3 ms. The electrical stimulation exercise was isotonic.

In Figure 4, the results are shown from ten patients where knee extensors were stimulated and the spasticity tested in the same muscle group. The white columns represent the average of four spasticity measurements performed on four different days. The standard deviations show the fluctuations of spasticity from day-to-day. The black columns belong to the level of relaxation after the application of electrical stimulation on the 4th d. In three patients (A. O., E. R., and R. S. — patient No. 8 in Table 1), spasticity was significantly decreased. In four other patients (R. S. — patient No. 4 in Table 1, L. D., M. H., and T. T.), the spastic activity demonstrated by the pendulum test was only slightly lessened. In the rest of the patients, the differences after the stimulation were smaller than the natural fluctuations of spasticity, showing in one patient (D. D.), a tendency to increase spasticity after stimulation therapy.

Five SCI patients (Table 2) participated in the investigation of the effects of cyclical neuromuscular stimulation of knee extensors on the spasticity of knee flexors. The same method and instrumentation were also successfully used for measurement of knee flexor spasticity. Patients were seated on a high chair, their lower leg was flexed maximally, and

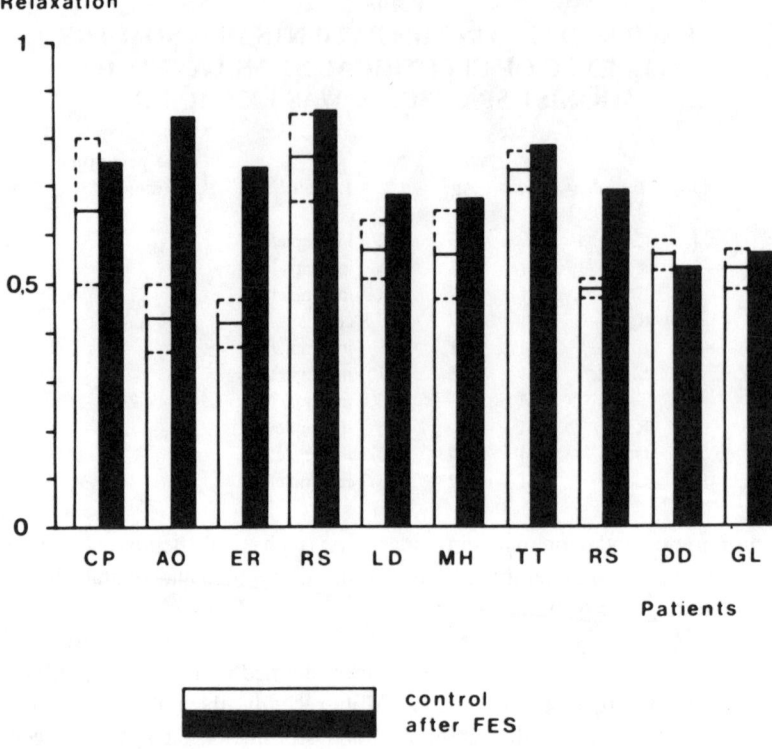

FIGURE 4. Influence of electrical stimulation on the spasticity of stimulated muscle.

Table 2
GENERAL DATA ON THE PATIENTS IN WHOM THE INFLUENCE OF ELECTRICAL STIMULATION ON ANTAGONIST SPASTICITY WAS EXAMINED

No.	Initials	Sex	Age	Lesion	Time postinjury (months)
1	V. S.	F	35	C-5 complete	4
2	M. G.	F	15	C-5 complete	3
3	F. C.	M	17	C-6 incomplete	9
4	T. M.	M	23	C-5 incomplete	5
5	G. D.	F	21	C-4 complete	4

then dropped. The same electrical stimulation treatment protocol described earlier was also applied in this study. Here, in three patients (V. S., M. G., and T. M.), spasticity was decreased, while no significant changes were recorded in two other patients (Figure 5).

Although the population studied was limited in numbers, it was shown that electrical stimulation is not increasing spasticity, so that it can be safely used for therapeutic exercises or functional activities. The trend, however, was toward a reduction in spasticity following electrical stimulation.

IV. TRANSCUTANEOUS ELECTRICAL STIMULATION OF DERMATOMES

Since spinal cord stimulation[27] and cerebellar stimulation[10] have already been used to reduce spasticity, it seemed worthwhile to apply cutaneous stimulation for reduction of

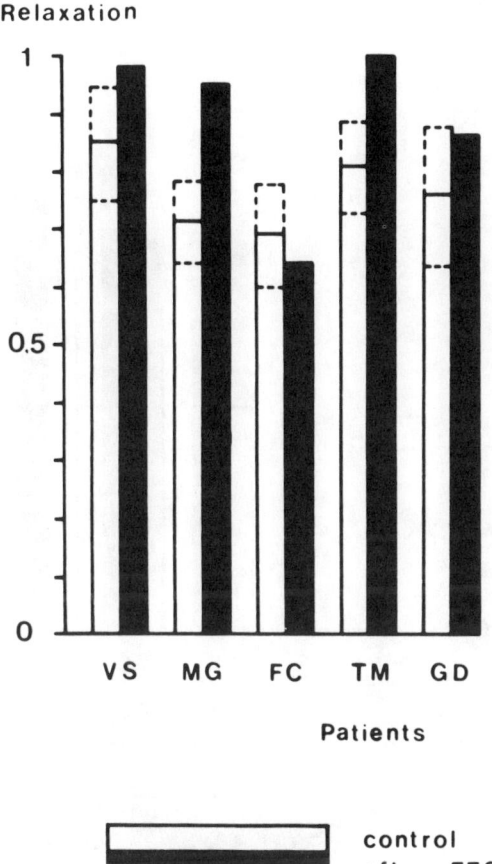

FIGURE 5. Influence of electrical stimulation on the spasticity of antagonistic muscle.

spasticity. With transcutaneous electrical stimulation, no motor response was obtained, so that sensory information was predominantly delivered through the large-diameter afferent fibers, conveying information from the mechanoreceptors and pressoreceptors to the spinal neuronal pool, mediating there the imbalance between excitation and inhibition which presumably causes the state of spasticity.[29]

The pendulum test was generating an extensor pattern of spasticity in the quadriceps muscle group, whose motoneurons lie in the L-3,4 segments of the spinal cord. Therefore, it was hypothesized that transcutaneous electrical stimulation applied to the L-3,4 dermatomes, corresponding to the same spinal segmental level as the spastic muscle group under consideration, will produce the greatest reduction of spasticity.

Dermatomes L-3,4 were excited by electrodes placed on the lateral aspect of the leg just above the knee and on the medial aspect just below the knee. Cutaneous electrical stimulation was delivered through large (6 × 4 cm) electrodes covered with water-soaked layers of gauze. A monophasic rectangular stimulus wave-form was used with a pulse repetition frequency of 50 Hz, pulse duration of 0.3 ms, and current pulse amplitudes up to 50 mA. Stimulation did not produce muscle contraction, as the electrodes were not positioned over a single muscle. Such a stimulation wave-form was applied continuously for 20 min. During the electrical stimulation treatment, the patients were in a supine position, with both lower extremities extended. The stimulation of dermatomes was performed bilaterally.

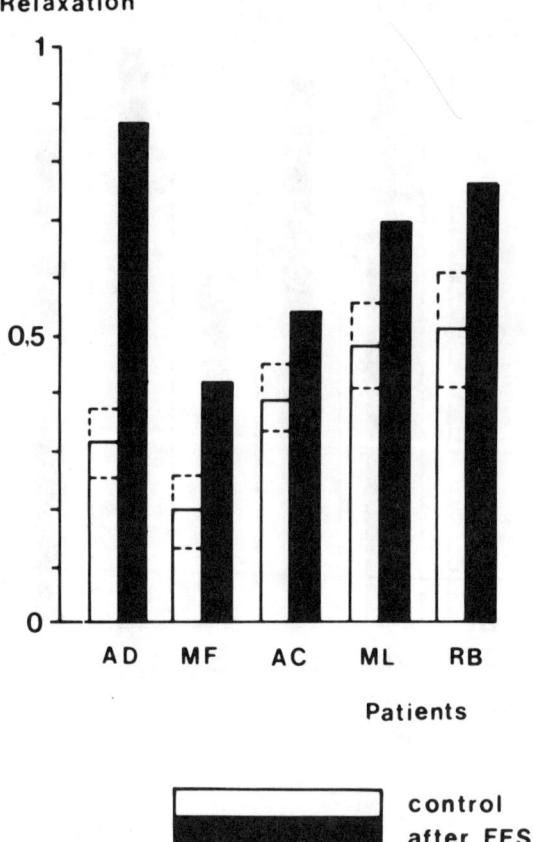

FIGURE 6. Influence of transcutaneous electrical stimulation of the dermatomes on spasticity in the muscle innervated from the same spinal level as the corresponding dermatome.

The intensity of spasticity was assessed immediately before and after the treatment. In addition, single-control pendulum tests were performed on seven different days. The results obtained from the group of five SCI patients having severe extension spasticity are presented in Figure 6. The white columns represent the average of eight spasticity measurements performed on eight different days. All the subjects were in good general health without decubiti or bladder infections (Table 3). It can be observed that the degree of spasticity was reduced to a noticeable extent in all subjects tested. In addition, the subjects were asked to describe their state of spasticity. All five subjects reported a decrease of spasticity after stimulation of L-3,4 dermatomes.

The quantitative data and the subjects' descriptions mainly differ on the short-term carryover effects of electrical stimulation. The patients reported a relief from spasticity lasting for 1 to 3 h following the application of L-3,4 dermatomes stimulation. However, the results of the pendulum tests showed only a very limited decrease in spasticity already after 30 min. According to the patients' descriptions, electrical stimulation provoked not only a relief of spasticity resulting in more easily manageable lower limbs, but also in less frequent spasms. Typically, this was described by the subjects as less "jumping" of the legs. Less flexor spasms at night was also reported by one of the subjects.

A remarkable decrease in spasticity was evident in patient M. F. Upon arrival at the rehabilitation center, her legs were fully extended while she was sitting in the wheelchair.

Table 3
GENERAL DATA ON THE PATIENTS IN WHOM EFFICACY OF THE STIMULATION OF DERMATOMES WAS TESTED

No.	Initials	Sex	Age	Lesion	Time postinjury (months)
1	A. D.	M	25	T-9 complete	38
2	M. F.	F	23	T-11 complete	13
3	A. C.	M	31	T-12 incomplete	5
4	M. L.	M	30	C-5,6 incomplete	53
5	R. B.	M	28	C-6,7 complete	11

After the stimulation of L-3,4 dermatomes, her legs could be easily manipulated into any desired position and could be placed on the footrests of the wheelchair.

The patients were supplied with inexpensive two-channel stimulators. It is hoped that after using electrical stimulation regularly, the patients will be less dependent on the antispastic drugs which also result in some unwanted effects, such as drowsiness, sedation, and hypotonia, which definitely hinder the rehabilitation of spastic patients. It was suggested to the patients that they apply the stimulator three times daily for 20 min. A stronger decrease of spasticity can be achieved by a more permanent use of cutaneous electrical stimulation.

In conclusion, it can be stated that FES is not worsening the state of spinal spasticity. The electrical stimulation rehabilitative approach results in restrengthening of disuse-atrophied paralyzed muscles. As the force of electrically stimulated muscle is considerably increased during the training program, patients may, in the beginning, have a subjective feeling of heightened spasticity. Regular pendulum testing performed in paraplegic patients who are already using electrical stimulation daily for standing and walking for several years, revealed a rather low level of spasticity (See also Figure 40B in Chapter 4). These data are in accordance with the reports of patients. The patients also report that the degree of spasticity is immediately higher when they, for various reasons, discontinue the stimulation program for several days. Severe spasticity is, in general, a contraindication for FES-assisted standing and ambulation. In these patients, the only purpose of applying electrical stimulation, is to decrease the degree of spasticity.

REFERENCES

1. **Young, R. R. and Shahani, B. T.**, A clinical neurophysiological analysis of single motor unit discharge patterns in spasticity, in *Spasticity. Disordered Motor Control,* Feldman, R. G., Young, R. R., and Koella, W. P., Eds., Year Book Medical Publishing, Chicago, 1981, 219.
2. **Bedbrook, G. M., Ed.,** *Care & Management of Spinal Cord Injuries,* Springer-Verlag, Berlin, 1981.
3. **Lance, J. W.,** Symposium synopsis, in *Spasticity. Disordered Motor Control,* Feldman, R. G., Young, R. R., and Koella, W. P., Eds., Year Book Medical Publishing, Chicago, 1981, 485.
4. **Burke, D., Gilliels, J. D., and Lance, J. W.,** The quadriceps stretch reflex in human spasticity, *J. Neurol. Neurosurg. Psychiatry,* 33, 216, 1970.
5. **Dimitrijević, M. R. and Lenman, J. A. R.,** Neural control of gait in patients with upper motor neuron lesions, in *Spasticity. Disordered Motor Control,* Feldman, R. G., Young, R. R., and Koella, W. P., Eds., Year Book Medical Publishing, Chicago, 1981, 101.
6. **Lance, J. W.,** Pathophysiology of spasticity and clinical experience with baclofen, in *Spasticity. Disordered Motor Control,* Feldman, R. G., Young, R. R., and Koella, W. P., Eds., Year Book Medical Publishing, Chicago, 1981, 185.

7. **Dimitrijević, M. R. and Faganel, J.**, Motor control in the spinal cord, in *Recent Achievements in Restorative Neurology, Upper Motor Neuron Functions and Dysfunctions*, Eccles, Sir J. and Dimitrijević, M. R., Eds., S. Karger, Basel, 1985, 150.
8. **Grundy, B. L.**, Monitoring of sensory evoked potentials during neurosurgical operations: methods and applications, *Neurosurgery*, 11, 556, 1982.
9. **Hacke, W.**, Neuromonitoring, *J. Neurol.*, 232, 125, 1985.
10. **Bloedel, J. R. and Ebner, T. J.**, Cerebellar stimulation for spasticity, *IEEE Eng. Med. Biol.*, 2, 36, 1983.
11. **Delwaide, P. J., Martinelli, P., and Crenna, P.**, Clinical neurophysiological measurement of spinal reflex activity, in *Spasticity. Disordered Motor Control*, Feldman, R. G., Young, R. R., and Koella, W. P., Eds., Year Book Medical Publishing, Chicago, 1981, 345.
12. **Nashold, B. S.**, An electronic method of measuring and recording resistance to passive muscle stretch, *J. Neurol. Neurosurg. Psychiatry*, 26, 310, 1966.
13. **Webster, D. D.**, The dynamic quantitation of spasticity with automated integrals of passive motion resistance, *Clin. Pharmacol. Ther.*, 5, 900, 1964.
14. **Gottlieb, G. L, Agarwal, G. C., and Penn, R.**, Sinusoidal oscillation of the ankle as a means of evaluating the spastic patient, *J. Neurol. Neurosurg. Psychiatry*, 61, 32, 1978.
15. **Reberšek, S., Stefanovska, A., Vodovnik, L., and Gros, N.**, Some properties of spastic ankle joint muscles in hemiplegia, *Med. Biol. Eng. Comput.*, 24, 19, 1986.
16. **Wartenberg, R.**, Pendulousness of the legs as a diagnostic test, *Neurology*, 1, 18, 1951.
17. **Bajd, T. and Vodovnik, L.**, Pendulum testing of spasticity, *Biomed. Eng.*, 6, 9, 1984.
18. **Bajd, T. and Bowman, B.**, Testing and modelling of spasticity, *J. Biomed. Eng.*, 4, 90, 1982.
19. **Bishop, B.**, Spasticity: its physiology and management. IV. Current and projected treatment procedures for spasticity, *Phys. Ther.*, 57, 396, 1977.
20. **Duchenne de Boulogne, G. B. A.**, *Electrophysiology*, R. Hardwicke, London, 1871.
21. **Levine, M. G., Knott, M., and Kobat, H.**, Relaxation of spasticity by electrical stimulation of antagonist muscles, *Arch. Phys. Med.*, 33, 668, 1952.
22. **Vogel, M., Weinstein, L., and Abramion, A.**, Use of tetanizing current for spasticity, *Phys. Ther. Rev.*, 35, 435, 1955.
23. **Lee, W. J., McGovern, J. P., and Duvall, E. N.**, Continuous tetanizing (low voltage) currents for relief of spasms, *Arch. Phys. Med.*, 31, 766, 1950.
24. **Hufschmidt, H. J.**, Die Spastik — Theoretische Überlegungen zu einer neuen Therapie, *Ther. Nervenartz*, 39, 2, 1968.
25. **Alfieri, V.**, Electrical treatment of spasticity, *Scand. J. Rehabil. Med.*, 14, 177, 1982.
26. **Vodovnik, L., Bowman, B. R., and Hufford, P.**, Effects of electrical stimulation on spinal spasticity, *Scand. J. Rehabil. Med.*, 16, 29, 1984.
27. **Cook, A. W., Taylor, K., and Nidzgorski, F.**, Functional stimulation of the spinal cord in multiple sclerosis, *J. Med. Eng. Technol.*, 3, 18, 1979.
28. **Bowman, B. and Bajd, T.**, Influence of electrical stimulation on skeletal muscle spasticity, in Proc. 7th Int. Symp. External Control Human Extremities, Dubrovnik, Yugoslavia, September 7 to 12, 1981, 567.
29. **Bajd, T., Gregorič, M., Vodovnik, L., and Benko, H.**, Electrical stimulation in treating spasticity due to spinal cord injury, *Arch. Phys. Med.*, 66, 515, 1985.

Chapter 4

RESTORATION OF STANDING

I. INTRODUCTION

The material of this chapter is arranged in logical order according to the FES utilization phases as they occur during the practical implementation of FES-enabled standing. For better understanding and to make the text simpler and also for the readers not familiar with the mechanics, at the beginning of the chapter, brief recapitulation of selected topics of mechanics is presented. Following the biomechanical principles and rules of FES standing-up and standing, the fundamental biomechanical principles for solid and segmented structures standing together with the requirements and limitations of standing are explained. The terms of posture, as related to standing, and postural space are defined. Postural movements are discussed in regard to constraints given by joint contractures and osteoporosis. The biomechanical principles of bone stressing, resulting from body segments weight and muscular function, are explained, representing the base for understanding synthesis and composition of stimulation patterns. Terms, like amuscular standing, intrinsic, and extrinsic stability, are explained together with the presentation of biomechanics of transitions from the sitting to standing position. Descriptions of standing-up and sitting-down maneuvers and definitions of particular phases and events with related terms are given. The transition maneuvers are displayed by the stand/sit trajectories. The diagnostic value of these trajectories is also demonstrated. The strategy of stand/sit movements is related to optimal stand/sit trajectories representing minimal energy expenditure. The stand/sit strategy with appropriate trajectory selection is discussed with regard to the principles and problems of FES sequences synthesis. Next, the patients' selection is presented according to lesion, neurological, physical, and physiological status. In further text, practical FES standing is explained, including training of standing together with the possibilities of how to prolong the duration of standing by utilizing the posture switching principle. Here, also the experiences and assessment results obtained in training of FES standing and its daily use are presented. The benefits of daily FES standing are also described. Paraplegic subjects, while standing and maintaining balance by holding with one hand the handles of the wheelchair attached folding frame, are able to perform with the other hand simple functional tasks. At the end of the chapter, hybrid concepts of FES standing, balance, and safety of standing, in general, are briefly discussed.

II. MECHANICS OF STANDING

A. Forces and Movements

On Earth, gravitational acceleration ($g = 9.89$ ms^{-2}) encompassed in Newton's second law[1,2] (Equation 1) is forcing the objects to reassume a position where the potential energy (Equation 2) will exhibit minimal value.

$$F = m \cdot a \quad (1)$$

$$E_p = m \cdot g \cdot h \quad (2)$$

In Equation 1, F represents force in Newtons N, m is mass in kg, and a is acceleration in ms^{-2}, while in Equation 2, E_p belongs to potential energy and h to the height of position of an object. It is known from mechanics that an object will start to move when the sum of all forces in any direction (usually we are using the Cartesian rectangular coordinate

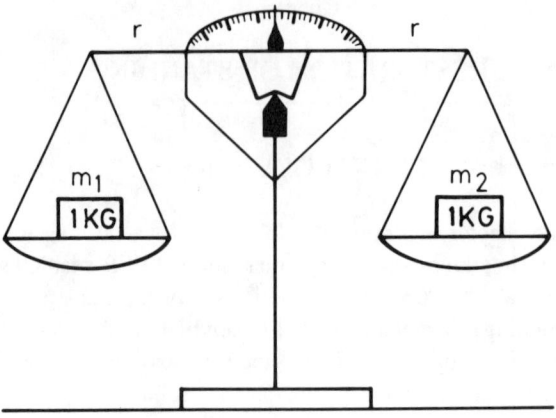

FIGURE 1. Example of steady balance.

system [x, y, z]) will differ from zero (Equation 3). The object will then move in the direction in which the sum of forces started to be larger than zero.

$$F_{x_1} + F_{x_2} + \ldots F_{x_i} + \ldots F_{x_n} = \sum_{i=1}^{n} F_{x_i} = 0$$

$$F_{y_1} + F_{y_2} + \ldots F_{y_j} + \ldots F_{y_n} = \sum_{j=1}^{n} F_{y_j} = 0$$

$$F_{z_1} + F_{z_2} + \ldots + F_{z_k} + \ldots F_{z_n} = \sum_{k=1}^{n} F_{z_k} = 0$$

or

$$\sum_{i=1}^{n} \vec{F}_i = 0$$

$$\vec{F}_i = [F_x, F_y, F_z]^T \tag{3}$$

Because of gravity, an object can also turn around an axis of rotation. This will occur when the sum of torques around any selected axis will be different from zero (Equation 4).

$$\vec{M}_1 + \vec{M}_2 + \ldots \vec{M}_i + \ldots \vec{M}_n = \sum_{i=1}^{n} \vec{M}_i = 0 \tag{4}$$

If we take an example of a balance (Figure 1) where we have on both sides equal weights, the balance will be steady and will not move. After removing one weight, it will start to dip around the axis. As we know, the torque M [Nm] is proportional to the moment lever, r, and to the force, F (Equation 5):

$$M = r \cdot F \tag{5}$$

For the steady balance with both weights in place and using Equation 4, we can write the following equations:

$$M_1 + M_2 = 0 \tag{6}$$

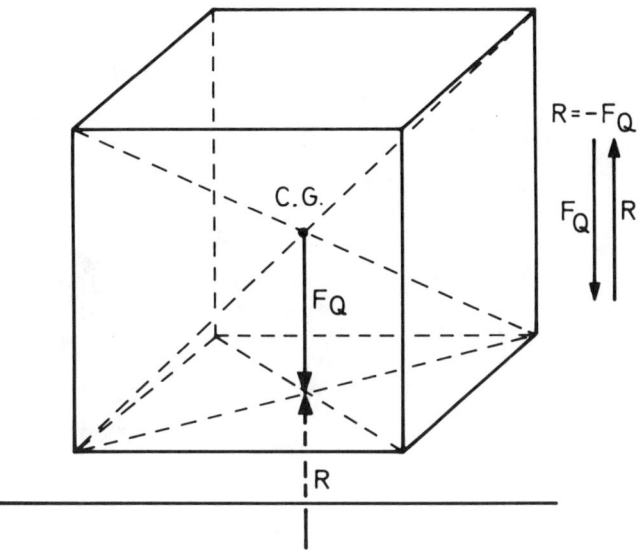

FIGURE 2. Example of steady cube.

$$m_1 \, g \, r + m_2 \, g \, r = 0$$

$$m_1 \, g \, r = -m_2 \, g \, r$$

$$M_1 = -M_2 \tag{6 con't}$$

Equation 6 describes the equilibrium state. Any motion of the balance is impossible and is stopped when Equation 6 is satisfied. An object in space is in steady state and will not move or turn when force equations and torque equations around all main axes (Equation 7) are satisfied.

$$\sum_{i=1}^{n} F_{xi} = 0$$

$$\sum_{j=1}^{n} F_{yj} = 0$$

$$\sum_{k=1}^{n} F_{zk} = 0$$

$$\sum_{i=1}^{n} M_{xi} = 0$$

$$\sum_{i=1}^{n} M_{yj} = 0$$

$$\sum_{k=1}^{n} M_{zk} = 0 \tag{7}$$

It is evident that an object, e.g., a cube placed on a table, is steady and does not fall due to the gravitational forces. The gravitational pull is resisted by an equal push force exerted by the table and floor (Figure 2), and Equation 3 is again satisfied. This is the content of

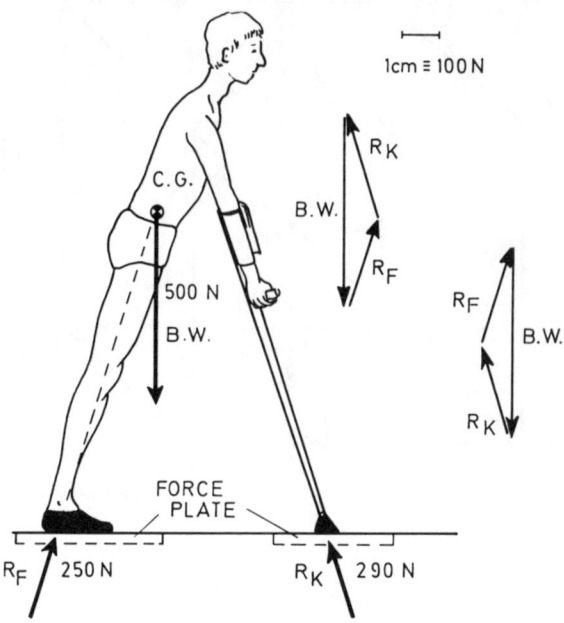

FIGURE 3. Sagittal view of a subject standing with the help of crutches on the force plate.

Newton's third law that each action has its reaction. The weight of the cube is acting downwards to the table (action F_Q), while the table is resisting with an opposite equal force called the reaction (R). The reaction acts in opposite direction with regard to F_Q, therefore, R is equal to F_Q. When a force is acting along a line, it has its direction, magnitude, and origin.[2,3,4,6] Therefore, the force may be graphically represented by an arrow — where the length represents, through a scaling factor, its magnitude. The origin of the gravitational force of an object is, according to the mechanical laws represented and placed into the center of the mass of the object, also called the center of gravity (C.G.).

For muscle activity, the force application point is evident from the anatomical landmarks and is acting along the tendon at the insertion point. For static equilibrium the action and reaction must be equal (Equation 3 satisfied), but this requirement does not specify the exact point in space where this equality has to take place. In regard to Figure 2, it must be valid for any table height.

From this observation, a useful rule may be deducted. Each force may be moved along its line of action for mechanical presentation without affecting its mechanical action. This is quite useful in cases where many forces are acting and one would like to use a simple method for depicturing the static situation. For this reason, a force vector diagram can be drawn. The arrow representation of forces, as used in Figure 2, is called vector diagram, because in mathematical language, an arrow with its direction, magnitude, and point of origin is called a vector. For a static, stationary setup where no movement takes place (such as in Figure 2), the vector diagram is a very useful tool. According to (Equation 3), the sum of all acting forces in a statically stable situation is zero, therefore, the sum of all forces in the vector diagram must be zero. This can be verified in Figure 2. In Figure 3, the utilization of the explained vector diagram is illustrated. By means of a force plate, the foot reaction force is measured, while it is our intention to find the crutch reaction force. The directions and magnitudes for all forces are given in Figure 3. Two of the forces are known, body weight (B.W.) and foot reaction force (R_F) measured by the force plate. For static stability, the sum of the vectors must be zero which results in finding the crutch reaction

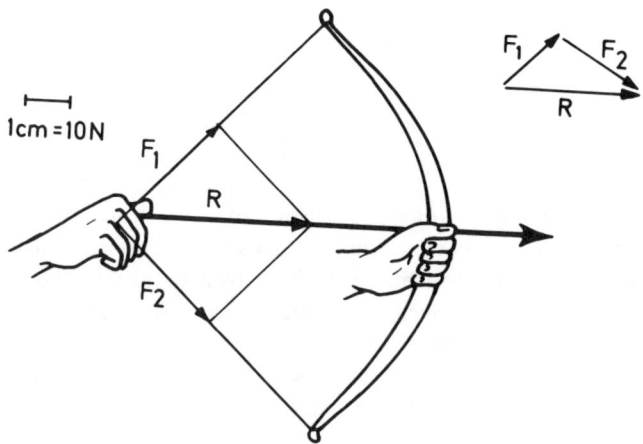

FIGURE 4. Force diagram of a stretched bow.

force, R_K (e.g., starting with B.W., continuing by R_K, brings us to the starting point of R_F, which must end in starting point of B.W.). This graphic summation of forces is useful also in cases where we are interested in substituting two acting forces with one force which will exert the same action (resultant force) as shown in Figure 4. Here, the action of both forces, F_1 and F_2, was simply added, therefore, the resultant force is drawn from the starting point of the first force to the end of the second force in the vector diagram.

In Figure 3, the friction components of the forces R_F and R_K prevented sliding of crutch tips and moving the feet apart. Suppose that we are horizontal to the table surface pushing an iron cube. In the first trial, the table surface is highly polished (low pushing force required), and in the next case, the table is rubber surfaced (very high pushing force required). The iron cube-rubber surface contact property is responsible for the higher force required. One can explain the increase in the pushing force by an opposing horizontal force created by the contact surface. The force which is resistant to the sliding is called the shear force, F_S. It can be easily understood that the contact property and the weight of the iron cube, pressing both surfaces together, are determining the magnitude of the shear force. This resistant force against sliding will be larger in static circumstances, while it is abruptly decreased once sliding starts. The ratio of F_S and the maximal pushing force, F_N, before sliding starts, defines static coefficient of friction, τ_s. For the static friction coefficient Equation 8 is valid. The coefficient τ_s may have values between zero and one and the value for a given material

$$\tau_s \leq \frac{F_S}{F_N} \tag{8}$$

interface depends on the force F_N. The dynamic behaviour of the shear force and friction coefficient is not important for the explanation of static standing and therefore, will not be reviewed here further.

B. Work, Energy, and Power

The gravitational forces are constantly working and trying to flatten the surface of the Earth. Therefore, all objects, like stones, soil, and sand, are constantly being pulled toward lower places of the landscape. For overcoming the gravitational forces, forces acting in the opposite direction are required. For a given rectangular coordinate system, to prevent sliding along a line and tipping around an axis, the set of equations in Equation 7 must be satisfied. This fulfillment is here written in a shorter form (Equation 9):

$$\sum_{i=1}^{n} \vec{F}_i (x, y, z) = 0$$

$$\sum_{i=1}^{n} \vec{M}_i (x, y, z) = 0 \qquad (9)$$

and is representing also the criteria for examination of static steadiness or stability. In case all the sums of Equation 9 are not zero, translational and/or rotational movements are taking place. We are dealing with an unstable, changing, dynamic event. The part of mechanics which studies how forces (movements) accelerate and move masses or bodies is called dynamics and requires rather complex mathematical background. Because of that, and owing to the sufficiently accurate presentation and description of the biomechanics as needed for most rehabilitation purposes, here, only the static mechanical tools will be used throughout the presentations.

Before the fundamentals of human standing can be explained, the terms of work and energy must be defined. In physics, work, A, is measured in Joules [J] or [kg m² s⁻²] and is defined according to the Equation 10:

$$A = F \cdot s \qquad (10)$$

Regarding Equation 10, a horizontal force F has pushed along its action line an object for a distance of s. In this case, positive work was performed, such as pushing the cube in Figure 2 on the table for a distance of s. Our muscles, by pushing, produced the force F which overcame the resisting friction force. For doing so, the muscles used the stored metabolic energy. Therefore, the work performed is also a measure of how much energy was used from the energy storage. Energy and work have the same measure [kg m² s⁻²]. According to Equation 10, for lifting a cube in Figure 2 from the table of the height, h_1, to a higher position h_2, the muscles have to perform work by overcoming the gravitational force. Accordingly, the potential energy E_P is rising and Equation 11 is obtained from Equation 10.

$$A = F (h_2 - h_1) = m \cdot g \cdot (h_2 - h_1) = E_P \qquad (11)$$

When rewriting Equation 11 into the form of Equation 12, it can be noticed that the cube already had certain energy at the table level.

$$A = (mg\ h_2 - mg\ h_1) = mg\Delta h = E_P$$
$$\Delta h = h_2 - h_1 = E_P \qquad (12)$$
$$\Delta E_P = E_{P2} - E_{P1}$$

The muscular work, exerted by lifting the cube, increased the initial energy level of $mg\ h_1$ to a higher energy level $mg\ h_2$ by adding $mg\ \Delta h$ of energy. It seems like the cube has accumulated the energy and, because of that, has a potential of returning this stored energy which also is called gravitational potential energy. In the case of pushing the cube across the table, the invested energy was dissipated, while by lifting the cube against the gravitational pull, the invested work is conserved and hence, it can be returned. The latter will happen when the cube is dropped from h_2 back to h_1 for a distance $\Delta h = h_2 - h_1$.

At each level, the body has a given potential energy. When gravity (gravitational force) is pushing an object downwards, the force and displacement vector have the same direction, and the work performed is positive. When the object is moved against the gravitational force (displacement and force vector of the gravitational force have different directions), the work exerted by gravity is negative and the potential energy is increasing. When the lifted object is released and starts to fall, the gravitational force is acting on the body, and it is accelerating the object according to the Newton's second law (Equation 1). The velocity of the object will start, because of the constant acceleration, to increase and the distance Δh can be calculated by the Equation 13.

$$s = \Delta h = \tfrac{1}{2} g t^2 \tag{13}$$

Utilizing Equation 10 and substituting s by expression in Equation 13, we obtain Equation 14:

$$A = \tfrac{1}{2} m g^2 t^2 \tag{14}$$

From elementary physics, we know that velocity is proportional to the acceleration and time (Equation 15):

$$v = g \cdot t \tag{15}$$

By substituting Equation 15 into Equation 14, a new expression is obtained for energy (Equation 16).

$$A_K = \tfrac{1}{2} m v^2 = E_K \tag{16}$$

This energy is called kinetic energy E_K. Comparing Equations 11, 12, and 16, we can write Equation 17:

$$E_P = mg\Delta h = \tfrac{1}{2} m v^2 = E_K \tag{17}$$

Equation 17 shows that potential energy, E_P, can be transformed in the form of kinetic energy and vice versa. When a highly placed object is falling, its velocity is increasing and hence, its kinetic energy. At the instance of the impact on the table, this energy will be released as collision work (falling object may break). Particularly important is the conservational property, as the invested work in the gravitational field (conservative force) can be completely regained. Energy cannot be destroyed; it can only be transformed (principle of conservation of energy).

Most functions like standing-up, standing, walking, manipulation movements, and sitting-down are performed in the gravitational field. The body and muscles are working against the gravitational forces. Therefore, it is important to understand the fundamental laws and properties of work performed by a conservative force, and how the body recuperates the invested work. The basic laws governing an event in the gravitational field are the following:

1. The work performed against the conservative force (e.g., gravity) is completely recoverable. For performing this work, we may use kinetic energy of the object under consideration, or we may act on the object with an active lifting force (muscle force).
2. The work performed in the gravitational field is proportional to the difference of the initial and final vertical distance covered.
3. Because of no. 2, no gravitational work is performed for moving an object horizontally (equipotential movement).

Related to work is power P [J s^{-1}] which describes the rate in performing work and is defined by Equation 18:

$$P = \frac{A}{t} \qquad (18)$$

In Equation 18, t stands for time. Also note that 1 J s^{-1} is the power of 1 Watt [W]. To accomplish the same amount of work A, one may use different power P, but the corresponding time of working must satisfy Equation 18 so that the product of P · t equals A. In reality, this means that one may reach a given height by walking over different slopes requiring different muscle power, but the walking time will be longer for lower slopes of the same height. Patients with weak muscles may accomplish given work, but because of weaker muscles, they will need more time.

C. Fundamentals of Standing

The word standing is used to describe an upright position of a human body, or the state of maintaining an upright extended position of trunk and lower extremities. The opposite meaning is the word laying, expressing that a subject is in a recumbent position. We talk about standing and laying not only with subjects, but also with objects. The dimension of an object exceeding the other two dimensions is called length, and to put an object to the standing or upright position means that the long axis is perpendicular to the horizontal surface. When the object remains in this upright position, we call its state to be stable, expressing the resistance to overthrow or the ability not to fall. The opposite term to stable is unstable, expressing a tendency to change or alteration of position or state. Similar meaning has the term labile, describing an object which is very likely to change its position or liable to displacement. For understanding human standing and the requirements for its stability, in addition to the understanding of physical or more specifically mechanical laws, it is useful to be acquainted with the process of human evolution and adaptation. In most living species and also in humans, the locomotion and standing functions are of vital importance. From here on, we are focusing our discussion on fundamentals of human locomotion functions. Because of being in a gravitational field, the evolution encountered in its optimization process of the locomotor system and also the gravitational laws. For humans, the upright standing position and walking are important for finding food and shelter and for having improved surveillance of the surroundings because of safety reasons. There are many reasons why a longish upright body construction is useful, but there are also many reasons and conditions in which the longish body shape is inadequate and a ball type shape becomes optimal (like sneaking into a narrow shelter, resisting cold, etc.). It is not difficult to realize that the only solution which allows taking of different shapes is given by a segmented structure interconnected by joints between segments. It is interesting to question what would be an optimal number of joints, and how to determine the segments lengths of such an upright body structure to optimize mobility, dexterity, and working space. To be higher from the ground means improved surveillance and to be further away from possible dangerous attacking of some other species. Therefore, the evolution process has placed most of the body parts vital for living on higher levels (brain, eyes, ears). Furthermore, close to these higher levels, food is more likely to be found. Placing so many vital body organs highly up from the ground resulted in a structure where the body weight center was moved also higher above the ground. It seems that some compromises were made during the evolution, but the main goals were multifunctionality, simplicity, high effectiveness, and adaptability, while taking into account physical, mainly mechanical, and other laws with different constraints to the maximal extent. The criteria which nature used throughout the evolution process are not

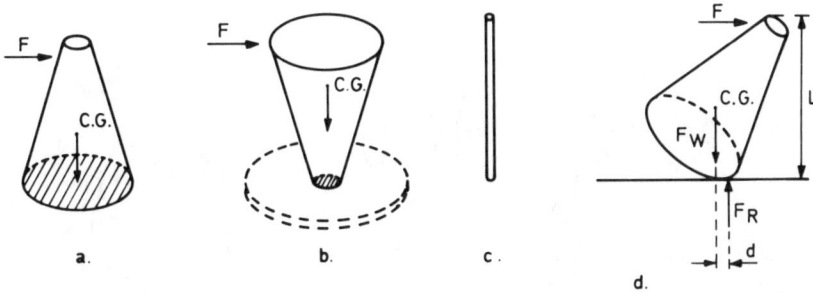

FIGURE 5. Stable and unstable objects.

completely known, but the end product, man, is here and ready for study. Let us, at this instance, post the following hypothesis: the human biomechanical and neuromuscular structure with its function reflects the evolution process together with the criteria and constraints utilized in the neuromuscular and musculoskeletal system control and functioning. Combining the mechanical laws from previous sections and the explained here thinking, the fundamentals associated with standing and later also with walking will be explained.

D. Stability and Energy Criteria Related to Standing
1. Solid Objects

From daily life experience, we know that a cone placed on its base is stable, but placed upside down (Figure 5a, b), it becomes unstable or labile. In a similar way, a stick (Figure 5c) can be placed into an upright standing position, characterized by unstable state or labile equilibrium. The upright standing in Figure 5b, c substantially differs from the stable standing in Figure 5a. Note, that the cone presented in Figure 5a is stable, while the previously mentioned standing structures are very likely to fall over. For good stability and stable standing, the center of gravity (weight force vector) shall be passing well within the boundary of the support area (shaded area in Figure 5a). In unstable standing, the support area is small (Figure 5b) and any slight induced lateral movement will cause the weight force vector to leave the support area. The object will already dip over at small pushing forces. On the contrary, the setup in Figure 5a will tolerate rather large pushing forces. It displays high resistance also to forces being sufficient to lift the base, which after cessation of the lateral force returns into stable standing (Figure 5d). The structure in Figure 5a has good stability, while the cone in Figure 5b is rather unstable and has poor resistance to perturbations. For the stick in Figure 5c, the supporting area is reduced to a point and therefore, only in one given well-balanced position, stable standing is possible. According to Figure 5d, the force F is producing a tipping moment by acting upon the lever L (distance to the point of action of the reaction force F_R), while the weight force F_w originating at the C.G. is acting across the lever d, is producing an opposite stabilizing torque. In the case when both torques are equal, the object will remain standing as shown in Figure 5d. Equation 19 is giving, according to the cone structure and induced lateral force, the range of magnitude of the force F for which the structure will remain in an upright position:

$$F \leq \frac{F_w \cdot d}{L} \qquad (19)$$

The balance of the tipping and resisting moments results in "freezing" of the cone in a resulting position (quiet upright position). Here, let us write the following lemma: in stable upright standing, the body weight line must pass within the support area. If outside, the body will fall and standing will not be possible. Observing Figures 5 a to d and taking into

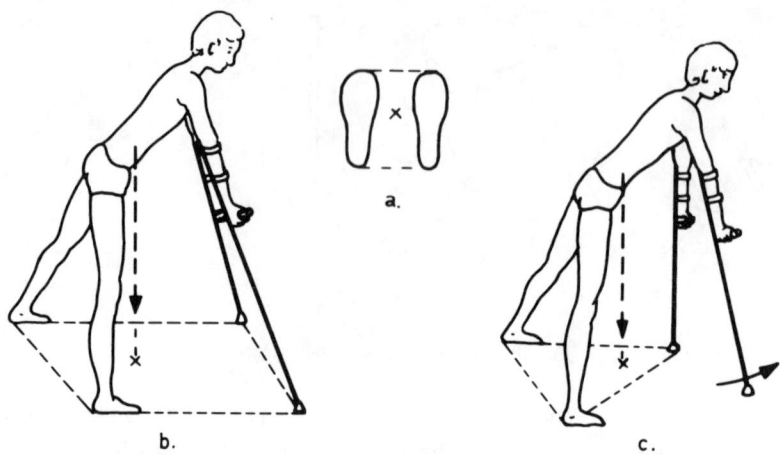

FIGURE 6. Support area during free standing (a), during standing by the help of crutches (b), and reduced support area because of one crutch support only (c).

account Equation 19, the following additional lemma is given: increasing of support area for a given object results in increasing the stability — resistance against outside tipping force. Consider the effect of a firm attachement of a round base plate drawn by the dashed line in Figure 5b to the cone base. Applying the principles mentioned, Figure 6 is explaining the static area of support and changed stability for different modes of a standing man. Note how the support area is changing.[5]

2. Segmented Structures

Up to now, we have been dealing mostly with solid nonsegmented objects. The human body is utilizing the segmented structure. Any segmented structure can be "converted" into a solid body by fixing or locking the joints. If the joints are stabilized — locked — the structure is intrinsically stable.[5] Intrinsic joint stability and stabilization of the human body can be obtained by using active muscle force (for maintaining the locking torques). Locking torques can be produced also by the body weight force, creating opposing torques because of a limited range of joint motion. Locking of joints can be obtained also because of ligaments function (hyperextension of the hip or knee) or by external fixation (passive orthotic devices like: AFO — Ankle-Foot Orthosis or KAFO — Knee-Ankle-Foot Orthosis). In analogy to the term intrinsic (related to the joints) stability, one may define the stability preventing falling of a structure as extrinsic stability. The intrinsic stability prevents the segmented structure from collapsing at joints, and it is a measure of the rigidity of structure. It also represents resistance to collapsing under the weight or load carried by the segmented structure.

Figure 7 is presenting such a structure which represents human standing in the sagittal plane. Because of simplicity, the trunk, arms, and head are represented as a single segment. For intrinsic stability, joint collapsing must be prevented. The body weight produced torques have the tendency to bend the joints, while by the muscle activity produced torques must resist the body weight passive torques during standing. At this instance, we must be aware that the definition of biological work differs from that in physics. Muscle is performing work (biological work) when it is contracting and resisting an external force regardless whether shortening or lengthening of the muscle is taking place or not. For resisting an external force — isometric contraction (e.g., holding a weight in quietly extended hand) — the muscle must produce contraction force and hence, use metabolic energy. Mechanically, muscle is able to perform work in several modes, depending how the direction of muscle filaments sliding relates to the direction of muscle force. Muscle is producing external work

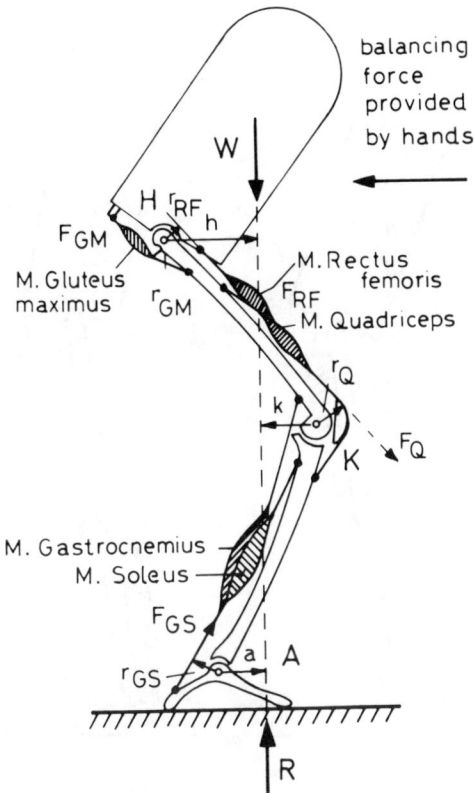

FIGURE 7. Segmented structure representing human standing in sagittal plane.

in active shortening and in active lengthening when it is stretched by external force acting in the opposite direction. Such a situation frequently occurs in gait. For static standing, Equation 20 can be written according to Figure 7, and the following observations can be made. The body weight (B.W.) is producing a torque at each joint (the shank and thigh weight is neglected because of simplicity), according to the lever given as the perpendicular distance from the joint center of rotation to the weight vector line. At the hip, for instance, the weight torque is B.W. · h and must be balanced in the state of equilibrium by m. gluteus maximus torque produced by F_{GM} acting over the r_{GM} lever. Note that the m. rectus femoris torque is also adding to the total hip weight torque. In principle, at each joint, to ensure stability, the torques produced in the joint by the weight and by all acting muscles must be balanced (Equation 20).[20-22]

$$\begin{aligned} \text{Hip:} \quad & \text{B.W.} \cdot h + F_{GM} \cdot r_{GM} + F_{RF} \cdot r_{RF} = 0 \\ \text{Knee:} \quad & \text{B.W.} \cdot k + F_Q \cdot r_Q + F_{GS} \cdot r_{GS} = 0 \\ \text{Ankle:} \quad & \text{B.W.} \cdot a + F_{GS} \cdot r_{GS} = 0 \end{aligned} \quad (20)$$

For different joint angles at the hip, knee, and ankle, the torque values in Equation 20 will vary accordingly. As it is well known, different joint angles of a standing subject are related to the term posture. Man is able to assume different standing postures. The standing postures requiring the least muscle energy and effort are the most interesting because these

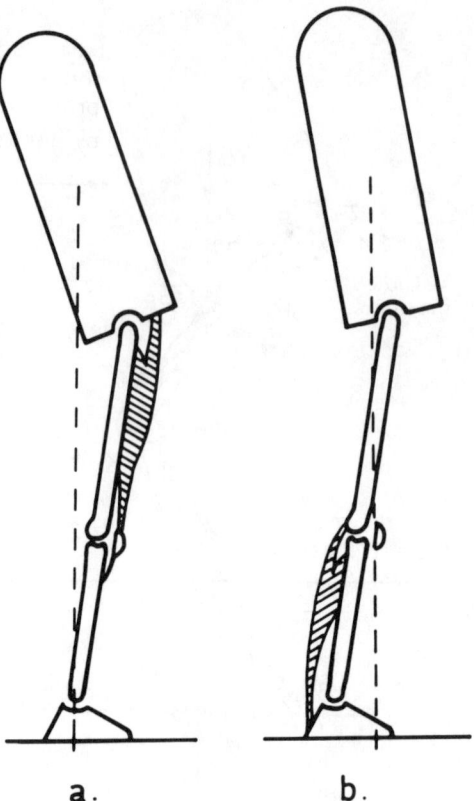

FIGURE 8. One muscle standing postures.

postures will require the least energy for standing. Equation 20 indicates that in the case when the moment levers of the weight force are all zero, then all the muscle forces should be zero. In other words, if one assumes standing posture in such a manner that the body weight line is passing through all the joint rotation centers, no muscle effort is necessary for standing. Let us denote this special example of posture as amuscular standing, being analogous to a structure of sticks placed one upon another. (see also Figure 39 in Chapter 6). Any slight lateral external force can disturb this posture. The neuromuscular control of posture is resisting during relaxed standing to all the perturbations in a manner to maintain standing as close as possible to amuscular standing posture. The evolution process adapted in man a refined musculoskeletal segmental structure with an unique body weight distribution all tuned for optimizing locomotion functions (standing-up, standing, gait, sitting-down). Each standing posture is, according to the actual joint angles, external weight, or forces applied, characterized by weight line which is vertical and is passing through the C.G. In standing, it is within the supporting area. The extrinsic stability (resistance to falling of the standing structure) is proportional to the distance between the ground reaction vector application point and the boundary of the support area. The stability margin is, according to Figure 7, low in the anterior direction, but in the posterior direction, it is substantially greater. Human subjects assume their posture according to the required work performance, expected distrubing forces, extrinsic stability desired, and many other criteria like effort, terrain, etc.

Similar to amuscular standing, the postures displayed in Figure 8 are characterized by the minimal muscular effort requiring only one muscle group of each extremity to be active.[7]

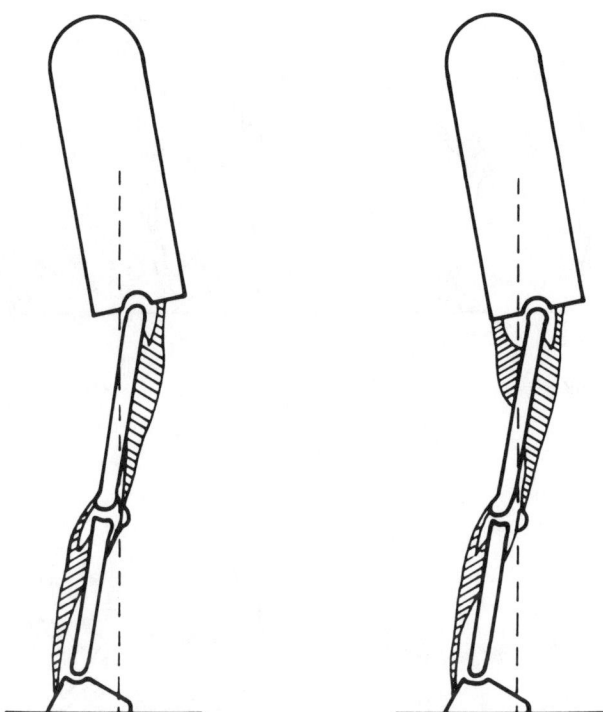

FIGURE 9. Two and three muscle groups standing postures.

In Figure 8a, this is m. quadriceps. The hip joint is locked by the weight torque, and tipping back is prevented by the hip joint ligaments, while the ankle joint is stabilized in the amuscular mode. By the hand exerted balancing forces, the upright stability is maintained. In a similar, way Figure 8b posture requires activity of the calf muscles, while the hip and knee joints are locked by gravity torque against the joint ligaments. The postures presented in Figure 9 are stabilized by the action of two and three muscle groups. Up to now, only the sagittal plane postures have been considered, but it is easy to understand that the same principles apply also for the frontal plane, for double and single limb standing, also thus allowing, mixed left/right activation of selected muscles for ensuring intrinsic stability. The arsenal of postures is unlimited and what is found very useful in cases of injury to selected muscles. In the latter case, standing is still feasible, only that some postures are not possible (allowed).[95] It can be concluded that each inactive muscle imposes prescribed and known constraints to the selection of possible postures. Even more severe constraints apply in cases when several muscles are not usable because of injury. Similar are the constraints which apply because of joint damage or limited range of motion (ROM). The latter deficiency is very common in elderly people and in patients having developed contractures. The consequences of limited range of motion provoke constraints regarding the possibilities of obtaining intrinsic stability as well as to the extrinsic stabilization. As seen from Figure 10, ankle (A), knee (B), and hip (C) contractures can lead to such severe limitations where standing is not possible.[8] Consequently, if contracture effects are compensated by excessive muscular efforts, pathologies may develop in other joints like hyperextended knee (Figure 10A, ankle, b) and lordosis (Figure 10C, hip, d). Generally, all cases of constraints imposed by limited ROM consequently, increase muscular effort as a logical necessity for achieving intrinsic stabilization. In summary, the effect of limited ROM is devastating and considerably limits the available postures:

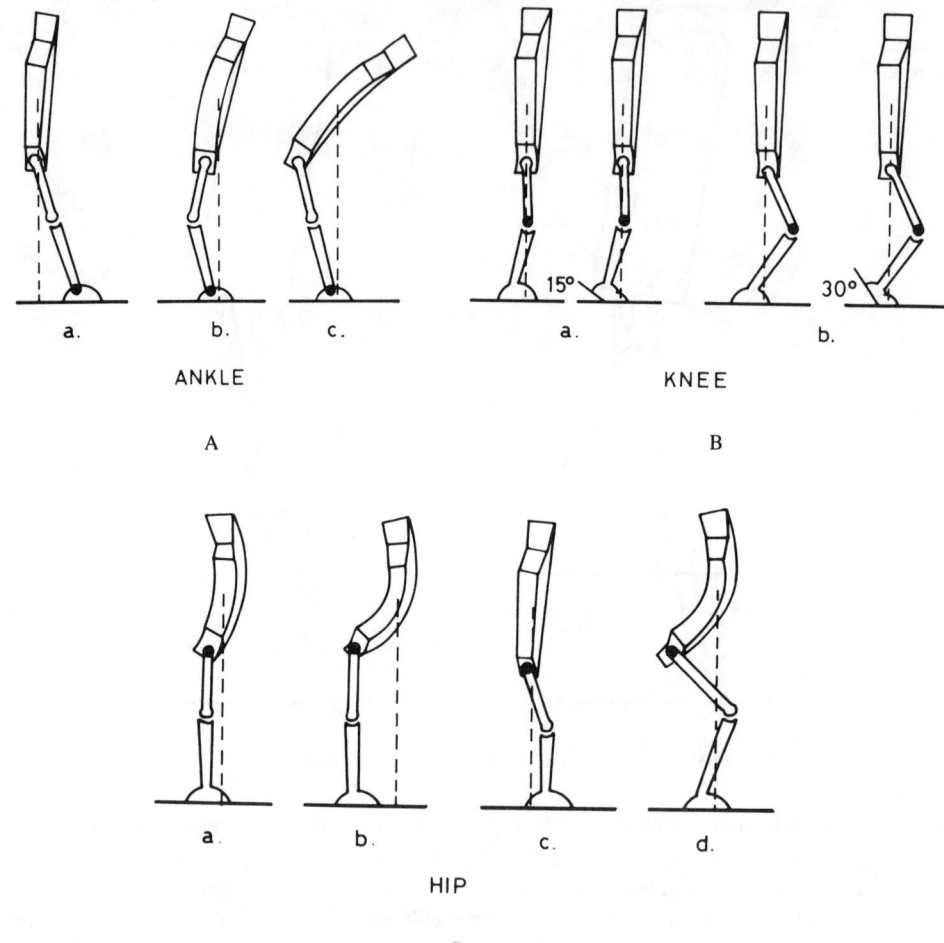

FIGURE 10. (A) Ankle, (B) knee, and (C) hip contractures imposing limitations to standing.

1. Because of required high muscle forces which are often not available in patients
2. Because of secondary pathological deviations development
3. Because of not allowing to adjust the weight vector line into the support area

There are some external means given for compensating limited ROM, like the possibility for compensating the limited ROM of plantar flexion by heel inserts (consider a heel insert in Figure 10A, Ankle, a). With hip flexion contractures (Figure 10C), standing is often not feasible, but can be accomplished by using arm supporting aids like walkers or crutches (Figure 10C, Hip, b). Disadvantage of such standing or walking is, consequently, high body weight force supported by arms.

Interesting to note is toe standing. Observing Figure 8b posture, let us suppose a sufficient forward lean for bringing the weight line under the great toe. It is easy to realize that in the case when the body weight line is at the top of the toes, the line is passing the border of the support area. At this standing, with the body weight line being in front at the tip of the great toes, the calf muscles have to resist the tipping moment of the body weight (Figure 11 and Figure 8b). In Figure 11, a simpler model of the posture shown in Figure 8b is used for presenting the mathematical expression for defining and calculating the extrinsic stability, S [%]. Equation 21 applies for cases where no external supporting devices are used. For a

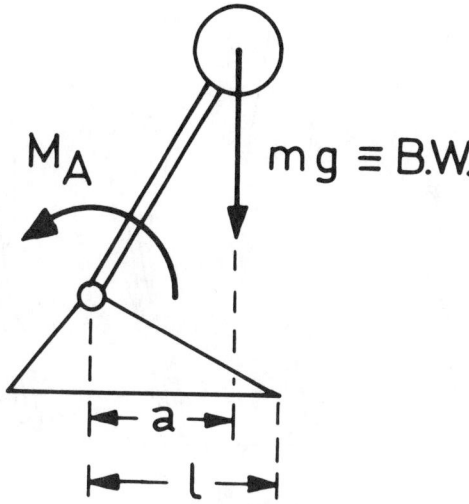

FIGURE 11. Definition of extrinsic stability.

given strength of calf muscles, corresponding torque M_A can be obtained, allowing certain forward lean resulting in displacement of the body weight line. The maximal possible forward displacement ℓ is describing 100% of forward lean extrinsic stability. The following equation for joint locking can be written:

$$a = \frac{M_A}{B.W.}$$

$$\text{for } M_A < M_A\text{max} \qquad (21)$$

The definition of the extrinsic stability therefore, would be,

$$S = \frac{a}{\ell} = \frac{M_A/B.W.}{\ell}; \quad 0 \leq S \leq 1$$

and the estimate of extrinsic stability expressed in percents:

$$S\,[\%] = \frac{M_A/B.W.}{\ell} \cdot 100 \qquad (22)$$

Increased strength of calf muscles and reduced body weight contribute to improved extrinsic stabilizing capabilities, while obesity is reducing the extrinsic stabilizing abilities. Here the term sway will be introduced,[9,11,13,15] describing the range of postures which can be periodically adopted by chance in an oscillating manner during standing of an individual. We distinguish between maximal voluntary sway and unpredictable subconscious swaying[10,12] while a subject is asked to stand quietly. The latter is a consequence of neuromuscular regulation in man. Maintaining selected posture is a dynamic process carried, supervised, and controlled by the neural control in man.

E. Posture Selection and Standing

The human structure with its segments and joints was perfected during the evolution process by numerous compromised requirements and criteria and resulted in a universal adaptability and functionality. The locomotion functionality of man is evident also from the

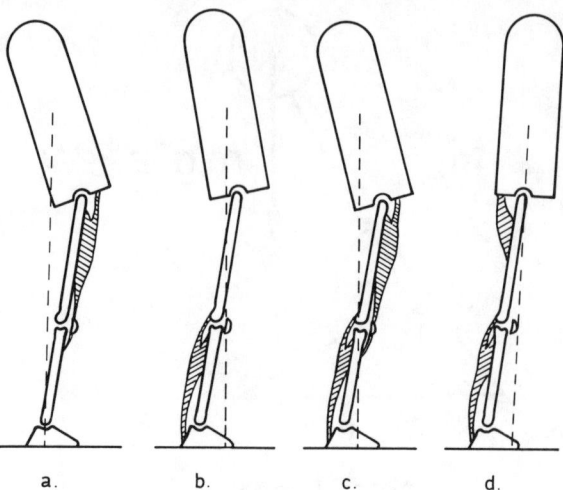

FIGURE 12. Activity of different muscle groups for bilateral standing in different postures.

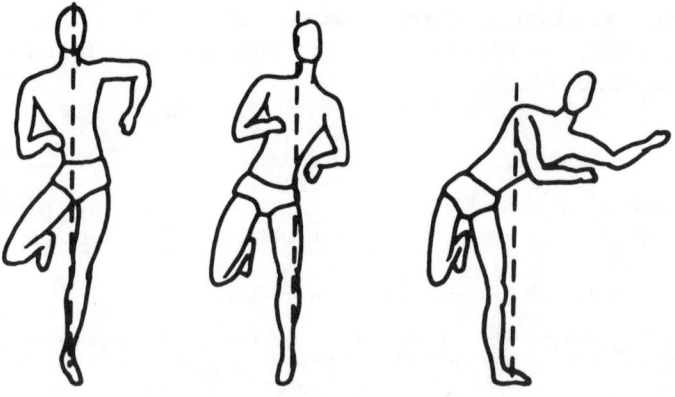

FIGURE 13. Postures of single limb standing.

reach aresnal of possible postures.[40] For any posture of static standing, two rules can be applied:

1. The segmented structure must be locked in joints (frozen) ensuring intrinsic stability
2. The body center weight line must pass within the support area (requirement for extrinsic stability)

Obviously, there are many postures possible for standing. They may be divided in two larger groups bilateral and single limb standing postures. In 1982, it was proposed[7] that the advantage of variety of postures may also be aimed at reducing fatigue by giving intermittent rest to selected muscles during prolonged standing. As seen in Figure 12, different muscles are activated for different postures. Also, it is possible to activate different muscles at each body segment for different single limb postures shown in Figure 13. Here, we recognize that there does exist a relationship between the positions of the body weight line and the joints, indicating required activation of different muscles. Also note that in joints which are passed by the body weight line, no stabilizing torque is necessary, resulting in zero muscle

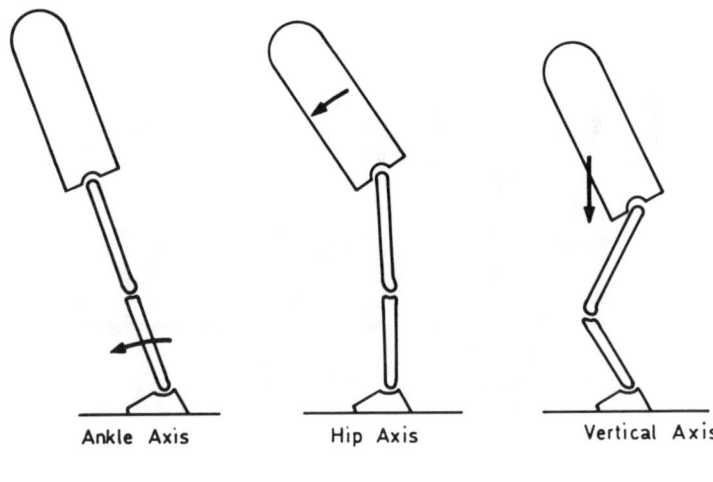

FIGURE 14. Influences of ankle, hip, and knee movement on location of center of gravity (a). Vertical displacement of center of gravity with respect to ankle and hip locus (b).

activity. One may wonder whether there are ways how muscles are able to collaborate, help each other, or substitute a weak muscle by sharing work and power. It also appears that at different postures the stress and load on the joints and bones is quite different. It is important to understand when and how to activate different muscles by FES for maintaining standing and switching among different postures. For coping with the explained problems nature has arranged several muscles across most of the joints and foreseen a complex activation strategy utilized by human neural control.

F. Postural Space

All postural adjustments deal with required changing of joint angles and positions in respect to the body weight line. An adequate control strategy would tend not to displace, if it is not required, the center of body mass in the vertical direction. The latter means losing and wasting of energy. To minimize or avoid vertical displacements, nature has selected the three joint arrangement with the knee, which separates the two long leg segments, with the aim to enable a large set of posture adjustments with minimal or no vertical displacement of the C.G.[14] Observing Figure 13, this is evident as considerably different postures are possible without any knee joint involvement, while the C.G. is extensively horizontally, but minimally vertically displaced. The ankle and hip joint work together when adjusting postures in a large space domain (frontal and sagittal plane), while the knee is fully extended. Bending of the knee is predominantly adjusting the height and hence, moving the C.G. vertically in space. The vertical body movements against gravity can be called suspensory movements.[15] From Figure 14a, the influences of each joint movement can be nicely recognized, while from Figure 14b, it is evident that large hip or ankle joint movement is only slightly changing the location of the C.G. in the vertical direction. After Fick,[16] in a 169-cm tall man, the C.G. is located 104 cm above the ground. For ankle angle change of $\pm 10°$, the vertical displacement of C.G. is 16 mm and for a hip angle range of $\pm 20°$, 10 mm (hip joint to C.G. distance is 16 cm). If comparison is made between the three joints of the lower limb structure used for postural adjustments and a rectangular coordinate system, one may associate the knee joint to the vertical (Z) axis, while the hip and ankle joints belong to the two (x,y) horizontal plane axes. This interesting analogy to represent the body position space

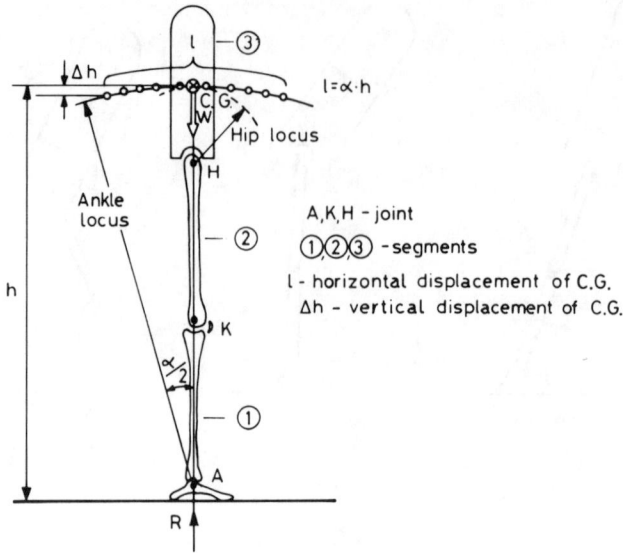

FIGURE 14b.

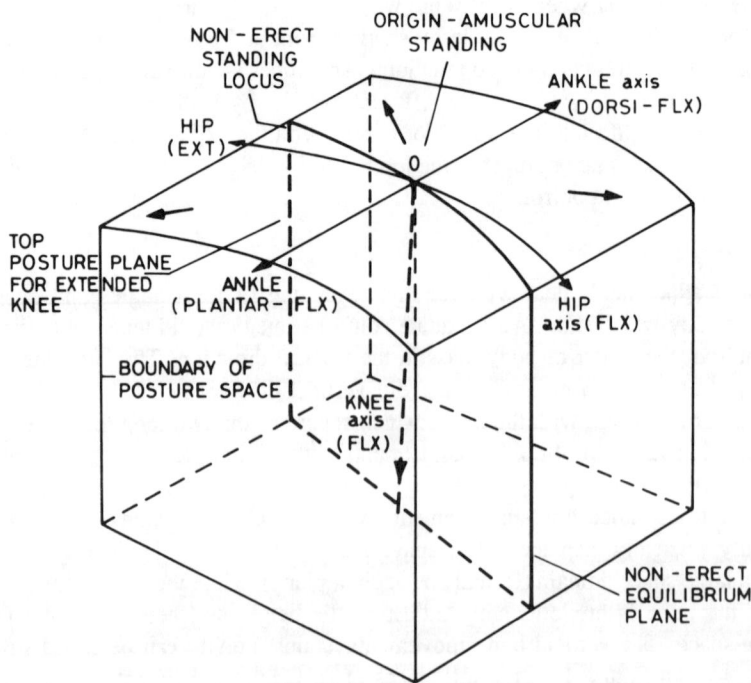

FIGURE 15. Postural space.

was proposed by Nashner and McCollum.[15] We adopted it here to illustrate further the biomechanics and neuromuscular control of standing.

To envisage the whole postural space, the representation of Figure 15 is very helpful. The space is divided by the three axes representing joint movements in four quadrant sections. The origin, O, of the space is given by the amuscular fully erect balanced standing characterized by the body weight line intersecting all the joint axes and passing the foot support area in a point defined as support center of balanced standing. There are numerous possible postures characterized by given hip and ankle angle (for a given knee angle — height), requiring that the C.G. line is passing through the support center of equilibrium. All these postures form the nonerect standing locus in the hip-ankle angle plane. The nonerect standing locus is a plane in the posture space which is displaced for a slight angle in the clockwise direction out of the hip axis and drawn in Figure 15 with a heavier line. The plane also bends slightly in the direction of the hip axis because hip movements are lowering the height of the C.G. The ankle movements also result in lowering of the plane, but can be for practical considerations neglected. The described hip-ankle plane is lowered along the vertical axis according to the knee angle movements to form the postural space.

Of course, the thoracic and lumbar spine extension and flexion add to the complexity, because their flexion/extension range is $\pm 20°$ to $\pm 30°$. The thoracic and lumbar spine flexion/extension range creates an area of possible postures around each point in the posture space. This space is used for compensation of slight limitation of ROM in the main joints. The posture space is limited along the axes by the constraints of ROM. For the hip joint, these constraints are flexion 120°, extension 30°, for the knee 135° flexion and for the ankle joint 20° dorsiflexion and 50° plantar flexion. Note that for standing-up and erect standing, only a very narrow section of the posture space is utilized. All the remaining space is used only in gait, running, and some not very frequently used postures, such as kneeling.

It is interesting to observe how the body is going to fall if for any posture in the postural space the muscle forces, constantly ensuring intrinsic stability, are released. For postures along the nonerect equilibrium standing line, gravity will pull the body downwards into stooping. For all postures being out of the locus of equilibrium, after releasing the active muscular forces required for standing, the body will start to fall because of the gravity in a given direction associated with its posture in postural space.[15] Some of these vectors of falling are drawn as arrows in the posture plane in Figure 15. The possible hip-ankle postures can also be studied and distinguished, according to the required muscle actions for maintaining intrinsic stability. The arrangement of muscles in humans and its control ensure that, while the muscles are adjusting a new posture by selecting new hip and ankle joint angles, the locking (equilibrium of torques) at the knee joint is maintained. This orchestrated muscle actions are called muscle synergies. Any postural movement along a trajectory in postural space reflects in an analogous "muscular activation space" where constraints and rules are imposed with criteria for the selection of muscular synergies, timing, and amplitude of contraction for each muscle required to excute the given standing posture. It is not the scope of this work to study in details the strategies and muscular synergies with their neural control. The reader is referred to the references for additional reading.[13,15,17-19,40] At this point, however, a remark must be made regarding the control of FES. The biomechanical knowledge and functions described must be to the maximal extent incorporated into the FES control system for standing-up and standing, assuming different postures selected. Patterns for FES-enabled standing and posture exchange (posture switching) are rather simple and make use of preset and constant amplitudes, while the timing is under the patient's control. The FES control required for transition among postures is an active research area.[19] The choice and adjustment of stimulation sequences (patterns) for a particular patient and posture is a demanding task. Advanced solutions in this respect are a matter of future research and will require collaboration of workers specialized in different disciplines.

G. Postural Movements and Bone Functions

Until now we have considered the bones (segments) and joints in a simplified manner. Mechanically, the joints were simply presented as hinges, while in reality, the joints are complicated structures, sustaining high pressure forces in addition to the ability of moving in several degrees of freedom under the influences of torques produced by body weight and muscular forces. In locomotor rehabilitation (also when applying FES), it has to be ensured that only patients with intact bones and joints are admitted to the rehabilitation program. This can be verified by different methods (X-rays, magnetic resonance imaging, bone density study). The pathological developments in different patients like SCI, stroke, and CP patients, leading towards pathological destruction of joints, are prevented by various, in most cases external, means restricting the joint motion to a safe range. FES has added new possibility for preventing joints damages by utilization of active muscle force controlled by FES. This natural way of preventing damages to joints cannot be presently utilized in all examples of FES application and also not in synthesis of human locomotion. The main reason is lack of knowledge. Therefore, careful studies and very subtle use of FES is recommended in all occasions where damage to joints could occur by improper use of FES. Experimental data about influence of employed FES on the joints during standing and gait are rare and missing.

Contracture represents serious constraint in joint mobility. It is a condition associated with the altered contracting properties of muscles. Contractures can be caused by fibrosis of the tissue supporting the muscles or joints. Contracture is manifested by a rigid or contracted joint, resulting frequently from agonist-antagonist muscles disbalance in muscle strength as the consequence of neural damage. Overstretching of muscular tissue is also a common cause of contracture development. Contractures of all kinds are seriously hindering the use of FES. In the case of severe contractures, FES is not indicated.[23]

Ossification is a common post-traumatic development affecting up to 20% of patients and is severly influencing and damaging to the mobility of joints.[25] Ossification of a joint may start 1 to 4 months postinjury, and it is a consequence of conversion of joint surrounding tissue and cartilage into bone or bony substances. Cartilaginous ossificated tissue replaces cartilage, and ectopic ossification results from formation of bone in tissue normally not belonging to osseous system and in connective tissue normally not manifesting osteogenic properties. Ossification is also a common post-traumatic development in SCI, preventing the application of FES. Ossification is hard to prevent, and exact causes and mechanisms of development are not yet known. However, it was observed that ossification will progress and take place if joints are not mobilized frequently. It can also be speculated that specific damage to the autonomous nervous system caused at the incidence of the SCI may facilitate additionally the ossification of joints. Joint ossification is a contraindication for FES application, and only at onset and very early in not progressing stage, FES may be administered with caution.

Osteoporosis or demineralization of bones is associated with decreased osteoblastic activity in the bone. Less than the normal rate of bone deposition is believed to be caused by: (1) lack of bone stressing; (2) malnutrition caused by different reasons, such as insufficient calcium intake, altered metabolic functions, lack of C-vitamin, lack of estrogen secretion needed for osteoblastic stimulating activity, etc.; (3) age factors related to physiological changes; and (4) post-traumatic and different disease provoked changes.[24] The consequence of osteoporosis is severe weakening of bone and, because of it, frequent fractures. Osteoporosis is a common disorder also in normals, in particular, in aged women. The most desirable treatment is its prevention. Adequate dietary intake of calcium, exercise promoting bone loading and stressing, and avoidance of excessive intake of protein and phosphorous food is advised. The causes of osteoporosis are not well understood, but the onset changes are manifested in an increase in bone resorption on the endosteal surfaces of bone with failure of adequate bone substitutional formation. In SCI patients, insufficient exercising and unfavorable metabolic circumstances very frequently cause severe osteoporosis. Osteoporosis is diagnosed by X-ray examination and bone density studies. Once detected, it demands great caution in FES application, and in many cases, osteoporosis will prevent FES to be chronically utilized.

Bone stressing after onset of osteoporosis must be applied with care because osteoporotic

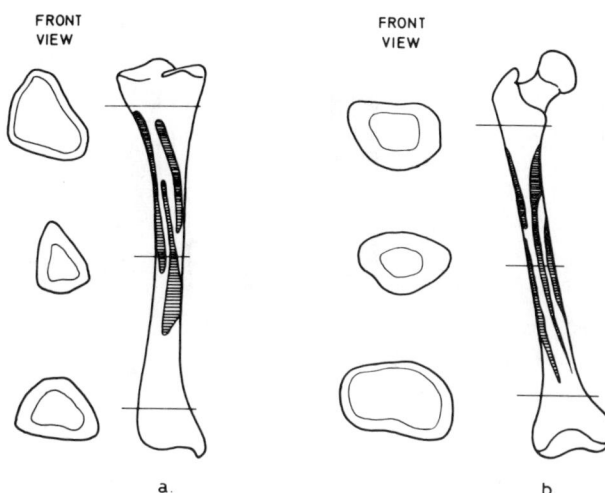

FIGURE 16. Femur and tibia with their cross-sections.

bones are prone to breakages.[26] Bone function in humans was optimized through the evolution process. Loading and stressing of bone is, in most clinical and rehabilitation engineering models, considered in a very simplified manner. The simple and usually adopted model represents bones as stick segments serving as supports to the body weight.[27,28] Establishing a more realistic model and better understanding of bone function is essential for proper FES application. To understand proper determining of FES sequences, the bone mechanics also must be considered. All the following paragraphs are therefore intended to review key issues in bone mechanics, according to the findings published in the literature. For readers wishing more detailed insight, we recommend the following literature.[29-32]

The human skeleton with its shape and attachment of various muscles gives convincing evidence that bones are not just stick shaped segments. Also, it can be noted that neither the body weight vector is passing parallel to the bones, causing therefore, unevenly distributed loading (stressing, bending, compression, torsion, etc.) nor the muscles act parallel to the bones or to the body weight line. Such arrangement was selected by nature in the evolution process; therefore, it is expected that such arrangements provide important advantages. In addition, the so created locomotion apparatus must show evidence of greatest possible use of energy. It is important to know that compressive stressing strength of bone is, by far, greater compared to the bending stressing endurance. For bones, the bending stressing is about 300 to 600 Nm/cm^2 and the compression stressing 10,000 to 30,000 N/cm^2. Therefore, bone can take 30 or up to 50 times more of compressive stressing than bending loading.[29,32,33] If the same amount of material is used to build a tubular and nontubular bone, the tubular bone will provide, by far, better strength with regard to bending stressing. As a rule, long bones in man, which are highly stressed by bending, are utilizing the tubular shape. Consequently, one may conclude that the tubular construction of bones uses less material for the same strength. It is also evident that bending stressing of long bones is dangerous in order to break the bone, while in compressive stressing the same bones may be able to carry very high loads.[29,34] A stick will break at the point of highest bending stress. Therefore, nature has selected, according to the bending stressing occurrence and appropriate distribution of bony material along the long bones, variable and adequate tubular cross-section area. In such a way, high stress regions are built for resisting the high bending torques. In Figure 16a and b, the tibia and femur of man are depictured with cross-sections made at different levels.[35] The femur is most stressed in the frontal plane, while the tibia in the sagittal. The

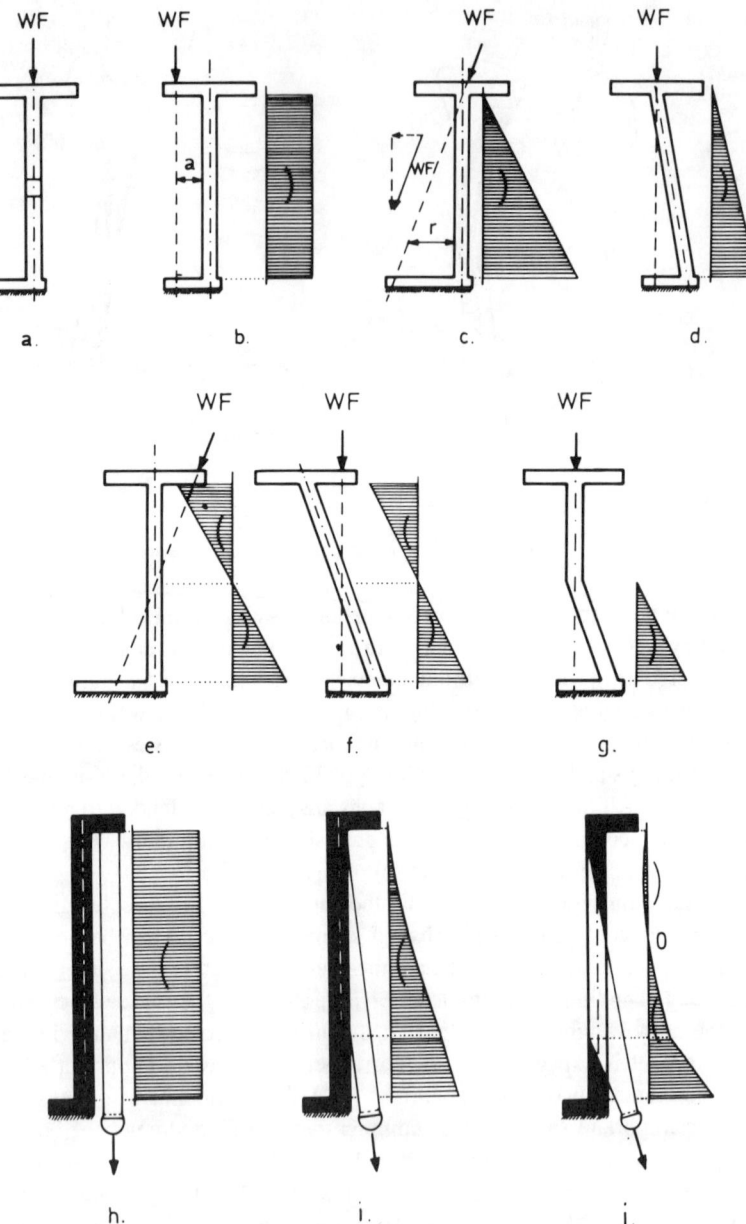

FIGURE 17. Bending stressing diagrams.

cross-sectional shape and area are varied according to the magnitude and direction of bending, torsional, and compressive stressing.

Figure 16 is suggesting that the bones are, regardless to their specific activity in man, nearly always stressed in the same way. The latter is possible only because of indeed ingenious arrangement of the muscles and their control. Pauwels,[29] in his excellent studies, has proved this observation, and he has also analyzed the various underlaying principles employed by nature in the construction of the human locomotor system. In Figure 17, a segment is presented schematically as a stick being stressed in different ways by a weight force WF. If the force is applied centrally to the stick (Figure 17a), compression stressing only is applied to the segment. If the weight force acts out of the center, but in parallel to the segment (Figure 17b), compression and bending torque result. The latter is proportional to the moment arm a. The segment is in addition to the compression stressing also under the influence of bending being constant along the length of the stick. For WF applied at a given angle (Figure 17c), the stick is stressed by compression and bending. The diagram of the bending torque has a triangular shape, according to the varying moment arm r. The WF force in Figure 17c has vertical and horizontal components. The vertical component is stressing the segment in the direction of compression, while the horizontal component represents the shear force. This shear stressing has little influence to bone stressing in general and will be in further text left out of consideration. It is important to note that in a non-perpendicular limb segment, a perpendicular weight force results in a triangular profile of bending (Figure 17d). If the line of action of weight force intersects with the segment, the bending stressing is zero at that point. For this case, the bending stressing diagram has a shape of two triangles, displaying opposite characters of stressing (Figure 17e and f). Let us be aware of the fact that regardless of the bending stressing, the segment is in all cases, also stressed in the direction of compression.

Considering the muscles and their attachments to the bone, Figure 17h, i, and j can be drawn. In each of the cases, the muscle action is stressing the segment (bone) in a specific way as shown by the bending stressing diagrams. In all of these cases, the segment is, because of muscle action, also stressed by compression. The comparison of bending stressing diagram of Figure 17b with the one presented in Figure 17h demonstrates that the diagrams are equal in shape, but represent opposite characters of bending stressing. Let us imagine the situation where a segment is loaded as shown in Figure 17b, while the muscle force acts according to Figure 17h. In this case, the bending torques and hence, the bending stressing are canceled out and zero bending stressing of the segment results (with double compression stressing). In this respect, let us consider also Figure 18 showing the results of stressing[29] of straight and bent bones together with attached muscles m_1, m_2, and m_3. As a result, the bending torques and stressing in joints are zero and the overall bending stressing is considerably reduced. This arrangement demonstrates how appropriate muscle action can substantially reduce the bone bending stressing. The muscle in Figure 17h is presenting a two-joint muscle. For triangular profile of bending stressing represented in Figure 17c and d, the activity of muscle according to Figure 17i is favorable and enables nearly complete compensation of the stressing. The muscle action of Figure 17j is favorable also for compensating bending stressing of bones. These functions are hard to realize at the first sight, because the double triangle shaped bending stressing in Figure 17e and f do not look similar to the profile in Figure 17j. In case the segment is bent, as in Figure 17g, the principle of compensation is again applicable. Human long bones are in general slightly bent (see also Figure 18). The double triangular shape of bending stressing of Figure 17e and f is, when adding the action of a double joint muscle (according to Figure 17h), converted into a triangular shape and then compensated to nearly zero by the action of muscles acting according to the Figure 17i. From this short presentation, we appreciate how evolution has very precisely selected bone shape, curvature, and muscle attachments for ensuring excellent compensation, as long as the muscles are appropriately activated. In this way, very smart utilization of important mechanical principles takes place. These principles have to be understood and also utilized in the FES applications. It is not the intention of this text to prove and explain these principles in detail, but only to make the reader and user of FES aware of them and their influence on the FES applications.

According to Pauwel's findings,[29] these important principles utilized by nature are:

1. Bending stressing of bones is reduced by tension bands. Muscles act as tension bands (e.g., two-joint muscles) as shown in Figure 18a, b, and c.
2. To increase the muscle effect and decrease the weight-provoked bending torque, bones

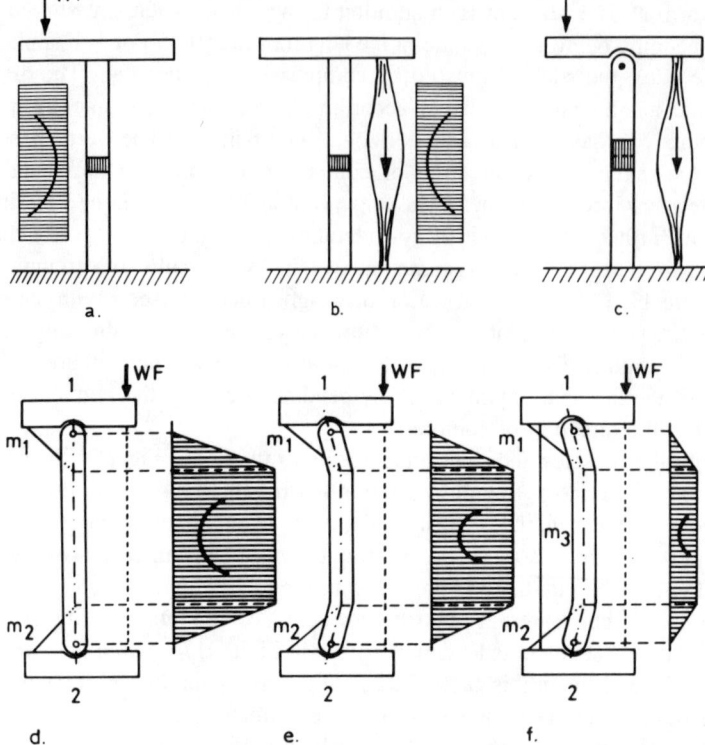

FIGURE 18. The influence of weight force and muscle activity on bone segments (a, b, c). The action of WF is counterbalanced at joints 1 and 2 by monoarticular muscle action, m_1 and m_2, respectively (d). WF is causing substantial bending stress of long bone. The latter is favorably reduced by bending the long bone toward the weight force action line, thus reducing the moment arm for WF (e). In the same time, the moment level of two-joint muscles, m_3, is increased compensating the bending action. The explained arrangements and the applied principles result in considerably reduced bending stress of the long tubular bones in man (f).

are bent toward the weight line, thus reducing the weight force moment lever and increasing at the same time the muscles moment lever. The same muscles (Figure 18d, e, and f) are also locking the joints to provide intrinsic stability.

3. Bending stressing peaks are dangerous. To reduce them, we need monoarticular (one-joint) muscles (Figure 17). The insertions of these monoarticular muscles occur in order to provide the stressing peaks compensation at different locations along the bone, longitudinally and sometimes also along circumferential areas of bones (compensation of torsional bendings). The muscle action in the latter case demonstrates compartmentalization activation according to the needs of stress reduction (consider intermedius insertion area on femur in Figure 16). In Figures 17 and 19 the one-joint muscle action is clearly demonstrated.[36,37]

4. Because the shape of the long bones is fixed, their stressing is also prescribed and determined. The muscles are so wisely attached and controlled according to the weight loading that the bones have almost always the same quantitative distribution of bending stressing over their length and also always the same profile and nature of stressing. This is valid and takes place also during movement of the limbs through the various phases of support. Also to note is the direction of bending which is always the same

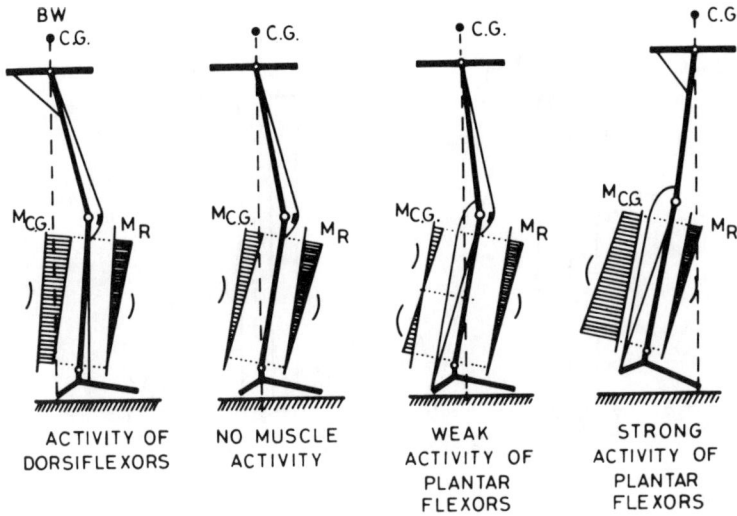

FIGURE 19. Statical presentation of loading in ankle joint which with associated muscle action results in a constant bending profile (M_R) of the tibia, regardless of weight line position.

whatever the position of the limb might be during support, because adequate muscle action prevents excessive bone stressing. The latter is displayed in Figure 19.

5. The requirements for stabilization of joints in order to provide intrinsic stability are demanding equilibrium between the body weight, bending moments, dynamic forces, torques, and the action of muscles. The net moments at joints during static support must be zero in any position. The resultant force and the reaction force must pass through the center of the joint. In this way, the joints are in static standing always loaded only in direction of compression. Figure 20 is clearly illustrating the described arrangement.

6. Owing to the requirements given in no. 6, the moment exerted by the muscles at a joint must have a given value (for balancing the body weight),[38,39] while the forces and moments produced by muscles along the tension tract can have any magnitude sufficient to compensate the bending stressing along the long bone. The latter is accomplished by varying the biarticular and monoarticular muscle forces. (Note that muscles have different moment levers at the joints! See also Chapter 6.)

Figure 19 is a clear and instructive presentation for how the tibial bone is independent of the joint position and direction of the body weight line. The proper muscle action, in respect to long bone loading, ensures that the resultant profile of bone stressing remains the same with respect to its type. This principle applies to all long bones and muscle actions in general.

7. Muscles, together with ligaments, strongly increase the compressive forces which act on tubular bones. In contrast, muscle action reduces high and dangerous bending stressing caused by the body weight. Muscle action and weight forces acting together result in particularly favourable loading of bones and, because of that, in lighter bones and hence, a great economy of material used for bone construction. This results in a very energy efficient construction of the human body carrying minimal mass with very high structural efficiency. Therefore, strong FES muscle activation with missing weight bearing loading is not recommended, since dangerous bending stressing may cause bone breakage.

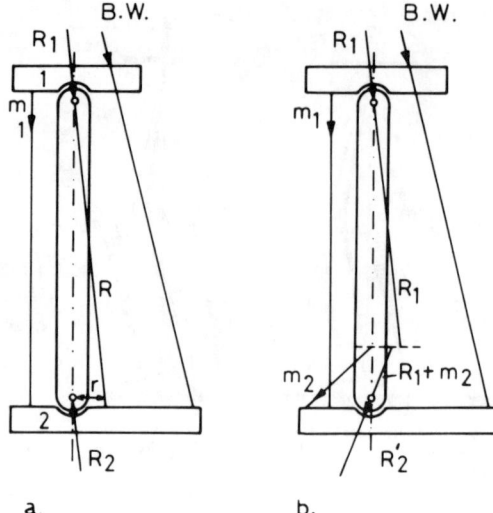

FIGURE 20. Two joints (knee and ankle) structure with one segment displayed during static standing after equilibrium was obtained. In (a), the B.W. action is combined with the m_1 muscle force in a way to ensure equilibrium in joint 1. The joint 1 resultant force is passing through the joint 1 and not through the joint 2. According to the mechanical laws, the reaction force in joint 2 can only pass through joint 2, therefore, the couple R_1-R_2 creates through the lever r a moment in joint 2. To obtain static standing and equilibrium in joint 2, the action of m_2 compensating the moment in joint 2 must be added. The moments in joint 2 are in this way compensated and the joint 2 loading force $R_1 + m_2$ is passing through the joint and is resisted by the R'_2 resultant force. Thus, the joint is stressed in the direction of compression.

8. According to Figure 19, it appears that if the loading profile remains nearly unchanged regardless to the static position (posture), then the same must be true also during the movement (support phase during gait). It can be concluded that in a human subject the static and kinetic effects of muscles are combined for ensuring high efficiency. In contrast, in machines this principle is not yet applied. In other words, the supporting and locomotor system in man are combined to achieve the greatest possible economy of energy. Static action of muscles saves bone mass — weight and hence, indirectly energy.

9. Because of specific mechanical arrangements of muscles to the bones, muscles can safely exert forces — stressing on bones and joints only if a counterbalancing force is present (weight, external force, or contraction of antagonists).

10. In equilibrium of torques, the joint is "locked" and the resultant force is passing through the joint. The same is true also for the reaction force. These forces, according to the joint surface, create joint pressure. In case the resultant force (F) is passing close to the boundary of joint surface (S), then because of reduced surface area, the joint pressure (p) is considerably increased (Equation 23) and can reach levels where joint cartilage may

$$p = \frac{F}{S} \qquad (23)$$

be damaged. At the point of resultant force passing through the joint, the pressure is increased. From the center to the outside area, the pressure is decreasing. Because of mechanical reasons and because the resultant force remains at the same position, the integral of pressure vs. distance multiplied by distance must be equal in all directions. The latter displays that for shorter distances the pressure must build up. Ligaments represent a safety mechanism for preventing the former situation. In joints with loose ligaments, the damage of cartilage is very likely to happen.

Therefore, it is evident that the mechanics of bones and joints in pathological conditions is very important to be considered before and during the application of FES in SCI patients.

H. Biomechanics of Standing-Up and Sitting-Down

The human segmented structure, if no active forces (muscles activity) are applied, is, because of gravity, forced into positions where external reaction forces, provided by the resting surfaces, support the body and ensure a stable steady state. The latter is possible in a seated and recumbent or supine laying position. Any transition of human posture towards standing requires active forces, normally provided by muscles. Knowledge of biomechanics of standing-up, swaying, toe standing, and sitting-down is a prerequisite for understanding and proper FES application in SCI. Standing-up, swaying, posture switching, and toe standing with sitting-down in paraplegic patients using FES is based on the same biomechanical principles as in normals, but in a simplified manner, because by FES usually only the main muscles are activated, while the rest of required active torques and balancing forces is provided by arm support. The problem of controlling stability will not be considered here. The act of standing-up is characterized by the fact that active forces have to overcome the body segments weight and therefore, extensive muscle power and work are required. For sitting-down, similar muscular involvement is required. First, let us consider the kinematics of standing-up and sitting-down.

The biomechanics of standing was, in the past, intensively studied[8,15,17,41] and is rather well elaborated. Also, the clinical issues related to standing pathologies were well correlated with various mechanical results. The biomechanics and control of equilibrium were also considerably studied in the past, while the biomechanics of transitional movements, like standing-up and sitting-down, were only occasionally studied and reported in the literature. As a consequence, the biomechanics of standing-up is poorly elaborated. At present, there are missing even commonly accepted terms for particular phases as related to the transition movements of standing-up and sitting-down. In the following paragraphs, some important knowledge related to standing-up and sitting-down with the help of FES is presented and explained.

The standing-up transition phase is of interest for FES application because FES control and tailoring of adequate FES sequences for individual patients and their pathological state can be utilized. In gait, the terminology and events are very well known and defined, and practically every practitioner describes the gait of the patients treated by the help of terms such as step length, cadence, swing and single limb support time, etc. It is also evident that standing is a prerequisite for gait and hence, standing-up is another important prerequisite before gait restoration can be started. Without standing-up and sitting-down, standing and gait are impossible to accomplished, and yet, the biomechanics of standing-up and sitting-down are not elaborated in-depth or monitored in patients for diagnostic purposes. Learning and training standing-up and sitting-down are performed, to a large extent, in patients on subjective measures and are not based on quantitative study aiming to optimize the required movements. The latter is essential in optimizing the energy expenditure associated with muscular work and power output related to standing-up. For patients, standing-up can be a hard task or a simple and easy one. Rising into standing position is, in principle, related to

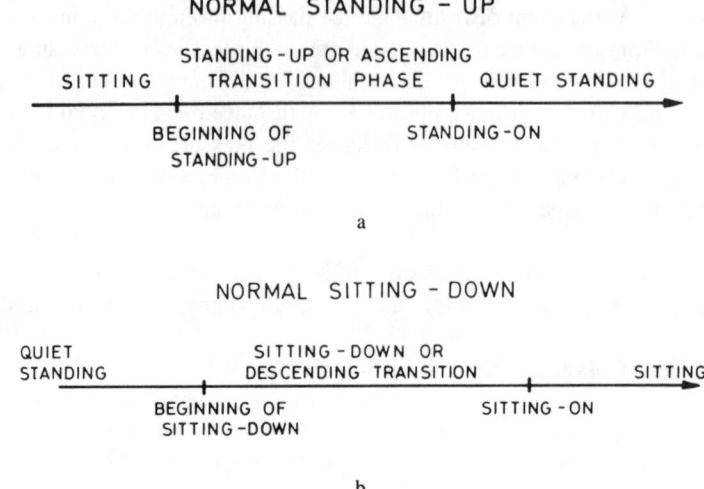

FIGURE 21. Component phases of standing-up (a) and sitting down (b).

how the patient was trained to perform the standing-up maneuver. Particularly, in patients with total loss of proprioception, like in SCI patients using FES for standing-up and standing, appropriate FES administering, control, and synchronization to upper body movements during the ascending and descending phase are important.[42-45] To the maximal extent, the knowledge related to the questions mentioned must be obtained from the biomechanical studies of normals in comparison to patients' performance and results.

1. Standing-Up and Sitting-Down Movements: Definition of Terms

The standing-up phase is a transitional movement which brings a subject from sitting to quiet standing. The standing-up or ascending phase represents our main interest (Figure 21a). Similar are the events only in reversed order for sitting-down (Figure 21b). In standing-up, active muscle forces are lifting the body mass against the gravity, while in sitting the muscles must only resist breaking during descending phase. In principle, the energy used for both transition types should be the same, but in reality, the sitting-down maneuver energy expenditure is, to some extent, smaller because the chair impact also can be used in final breaking phase. During the ascending phase, the muscles perform active work for lifting the body mass against the gravity. If trunk, arms, and head are represented by a single segment, and the main joints contributing to standing-up are presented together with the main extension muscle groups, a model can be obtained such as shown in Figure 7. Here, standing-up and standing employing hands to provide balancing force will be studied. The equality signs in Equation 20 are necessary for quiet standing, as they describe a condition of equality between the gravity torques pushing into stooping and the active muscular torques. When the torques produced by muscles are greater than the gravity torques the segmented structure will start to rise and accelerate in the ascending direction. The opposite happens when gravity torques are surpassing the active joint torques. The structure will start to descend and accelerate in the stooping direction. Therefore, it is not difficult to realize that standing and sitting movements are associated with dynamic accelerating and decelerating balancing events. In a detailed biomechanical kinematic study of stand-sit maneuvers, the setup displayed in Figure 22 was used. Force plate data, including reaction forces and application point of force reaction vector, were recorded together with joint angles data and seat contact force. Stand-sit transition movements were studied for different seat heights and feet placements and with and without hands assistance. The results obtained led to the

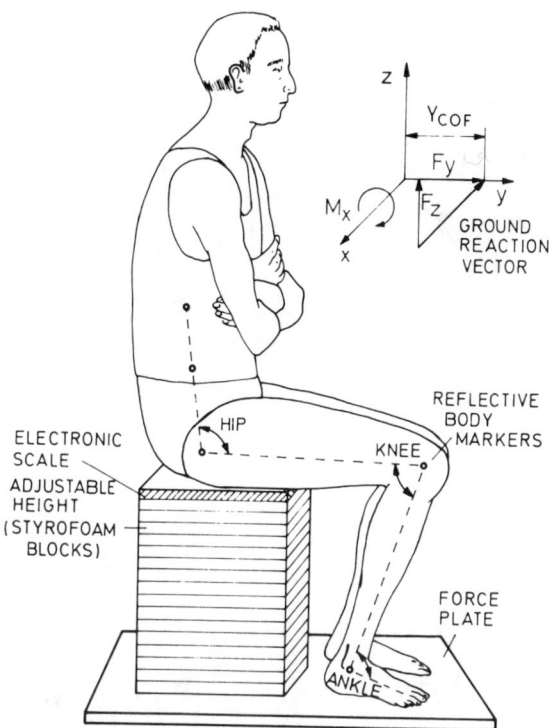

FIGURE 22. Measuring setup required for assessment of standing-up and sitting-down movements.

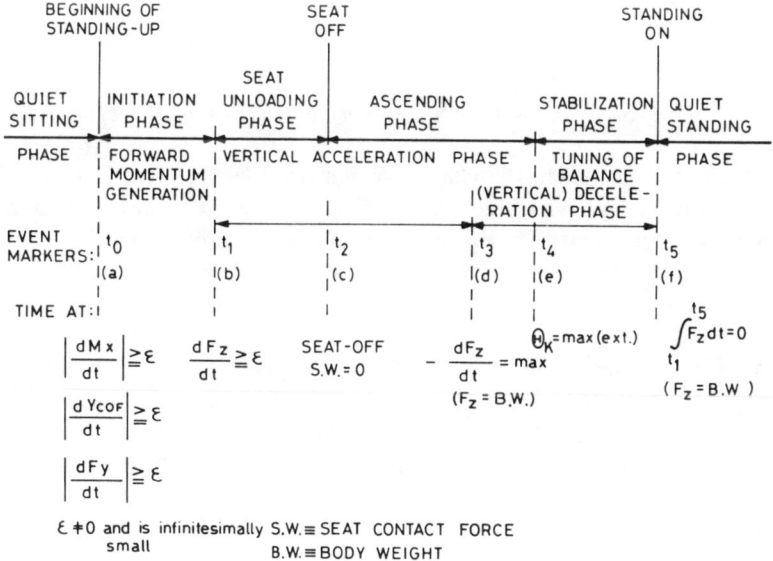

FIGURE 23. Detailed phases of standing-up maneuver together with event markers occurring at characteristic values of relevant biomechanical parameters.

definition of component phases and events for the standing-up in normal man as shown in Figure 23. The standing-up phases are the initiation phase, mainly performed by forward trunk movement, the seat unloading phase, the ascending and stabilization phase which

78 *Functional Electrical Stimulation: Standing and Walking after Spinal Cord Injury*

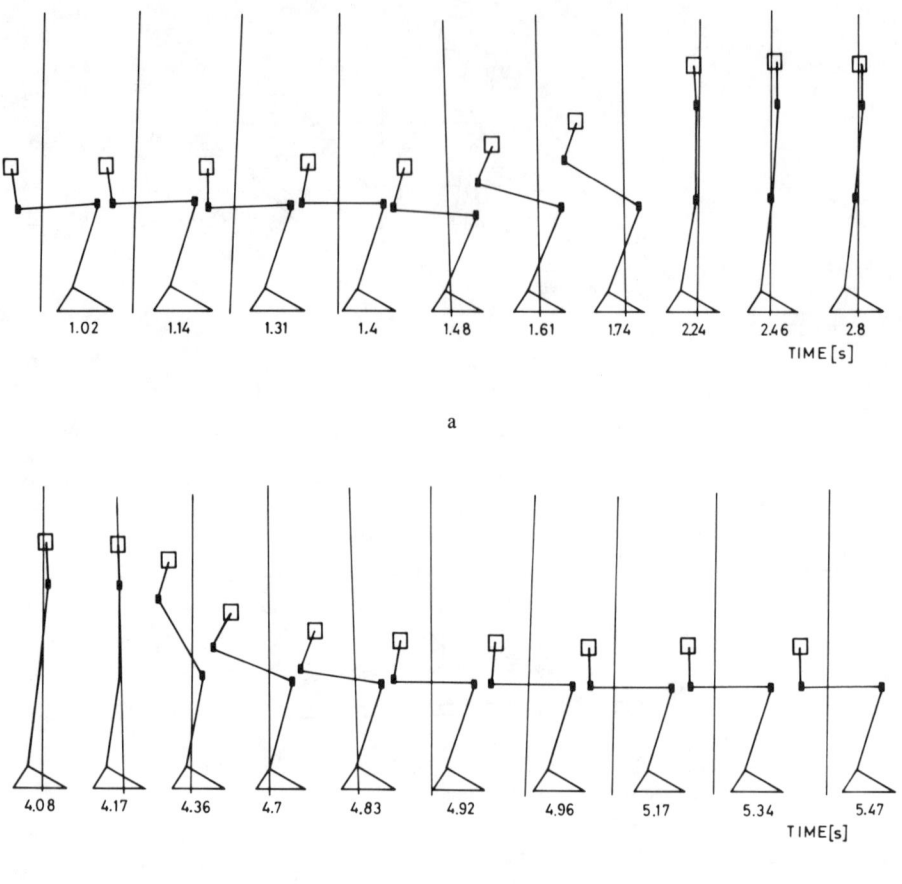

FIGURE 24. Stick diagram visualization of standing-up (a) and sitting-down (b) maneuver.

terminates with quiet standing. The phases are separated by six event markers which are related to characteristic values of biomechanical parameters as defined in Figure 23. For example, the ascending phase is beginning at the event of seat-off and terminates when the knee joints achieve full extension. At this event, the stabilizing phase also starts.[19] During the initiation phase, the trunk moves forward and flexion in hip increases. This movement is necessary for the momentum generation which is, consequently, necessary for accomplishing transfer from the sitting support to the legs supporting area. The sudden increase of body weight (t_1) marks the event when initiation phase terminates and the seat unloading phase starts. This event also represents starting of vertical acceleration.

During hands assisted standing-up the forward momentum generation is not required because with proper leg placement the required displacement of the reaction vector in the forward direction is rather small and can be neglected. Considering the stick figure visualization of the stand-sit maneuver of a normal subject such as given in Figure 24a and b, the trunk movement during the initiation phase can be clearly recognized. The ground reaction vector is represented by the vertical line. Actually, both the trunk and the ground reaction vector are moving rapidly forward, and after 0.46 s, the ascending phase starts. Note that the knee joint hardly moves in the vertical direction. In contrast, the changes in hip and trunk positions are considerable. This finding indicates that the main lifting work and power is provided by the knee extensors together with the hip and trunk extensor muscles. The standing-up movement is completed in normal subjects in 1 to 1.5 seconds. A diagram

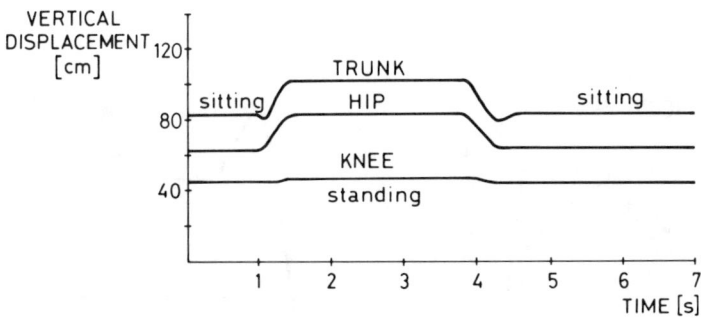

FIGURE 25. Vertical displacements of trunk, hip, and knee during standing-up and sitting-down.

presenting the vertical displacements of knee, hip, and trunk, during the stand-sit maneuver of a normal subject, is instructive for highlighting the biomechanical events described (Figure 25). The force reaction vector is, during the sitting-down maneuver, not displaced behind the ankle joint in the first phase of transition period (Figure 24b; time period from 4.08 to 4.83 s), but the center of gravity is substantially lowered during this time period. After this time (4.83 s), the vector rapidly moves backwards while moderate lowering of the C.G. is still taking place. Strong extension in the trunk and hip sets in thereafter. The complete sitting-down maneuver lasted 1.39 s and took nearly the same time as the standing transition. It is also interesting that each subject has adopted his own time of maneuver which does not vary much in successive stand/sit trials.

2. Biomechanical Parameters of Stand/Sit Maneuvers

According to the Figure 22, an experimental setup provided assessment of joint angles, reaction forces, and displacements of body markers. Observing Figures 24 and 25, we can establish that the ankle joint angle is changing during stand/sit maneuver to a smaller extent, while the hip and knee joint, being the opposite joints at each side of the femur, must provide vertical lifting of the body. Considering also Figure 14b, we can conclude that joint locus or distance from joint to C.G. is largest for the ankle joint. The ankle joint has, therefore, little influence on changing the vertical position of C.G. By similar reasoning, we can conclude that the knee joint has to move a greater extent and the hip joint to the largest extent. Figure 26a to c, display the changes of joint angles vs. time for stand/sit maneuver of a 30-year-old male subject performing the rising and sitting at his freely selected speed. Figure 26d to g and h display records of seat scale data, reaction forces, M_x torque in the sagittal plane, and coordinate Y_{COF} which is calculated from M_x using the equation $M_x = Y_{COF} \cdot F_z$. The seat scale provides seat-off and timing data, while the F_z and F_y reaction forces, as our studies have demonstrated, are very sensitive to changes in speed of standing-up and can be used to calculate the vertical acceleration, momentum, and force impulse provided by the muscles in both vertical and horizontal anterior/posterior direction. With decreasing or increasing the speed of stand-sit maneuver the F_z and F_y forces change substantially. For slow stand-sit transition, they are rather low, and with rapid maneuvers the amplitudes increase considerably. It is also interesting to note that the changes of force vs. time during the stabilizing phase show the influences of the activities performed for achieving stabilization and, as expected, the latter must take place predominantly in the anterior/posterior direction (F_y force). Also during the sit movement, both F_z and F_y forces display stabilizing and regulatory activity influencing the dynamics of maneuver, which can be attributed to the fact that during sitting-down, the only feedback we have regarding the height and location of the seat is visual information, and even this is limited as we do not

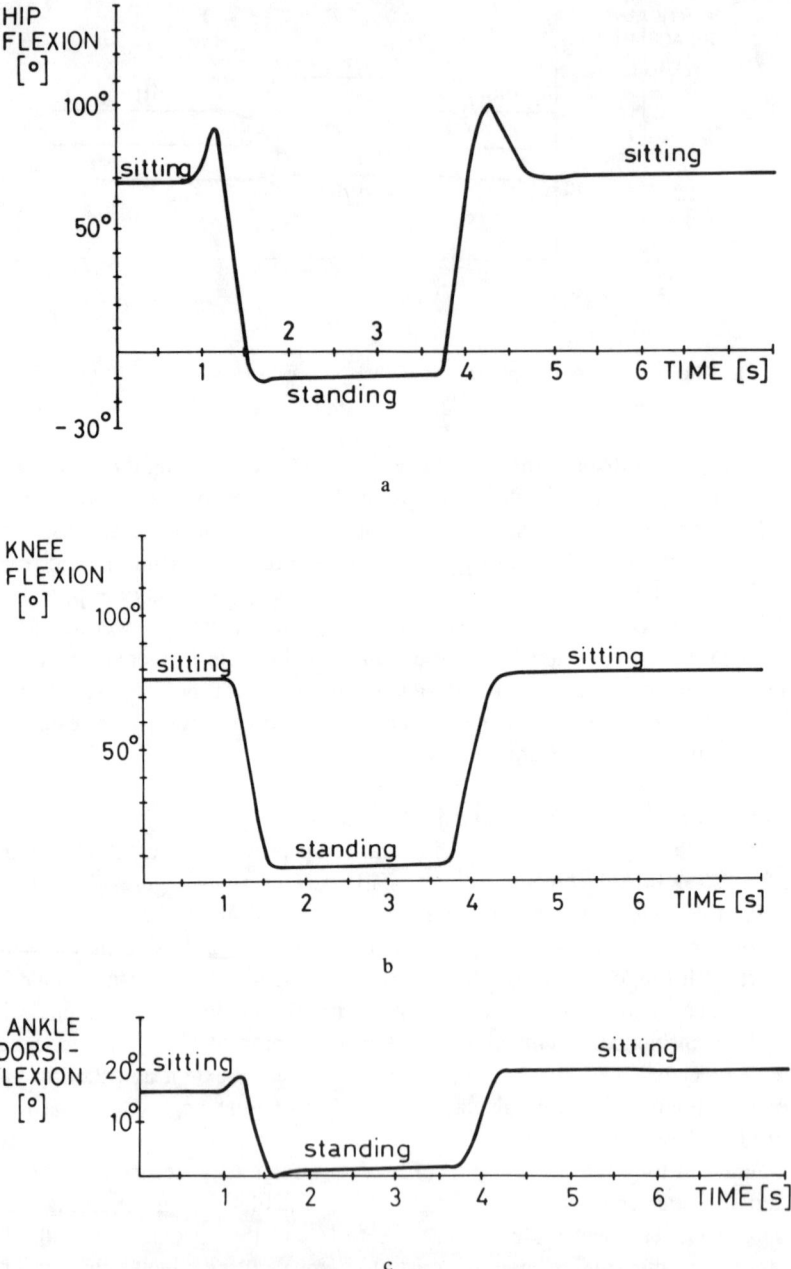

FIGURE 26. Hip (a), knee (b), and ankle (c) joint goniograms during standing-up and sitting-down maneuver together with seat scale data (d), vertical (e) and horizontal (f) reaction force, and torque (g) and reaction force displacement (h) in the sagittal plane.

see adequately behind us. The F_z force is during standing-up first increasing above the body weight, while during sitting-down it first decreases and later increases above the body weight value. The F_y force is changing in respect to the zero line. In the records presented the ankle joint was located within zero line of Y_{COF} displacement.

For a normal subjects standing-up and sitting-down using hand support and the starting posture, such as presented in Figure 33, the measurement records are presented in Figure

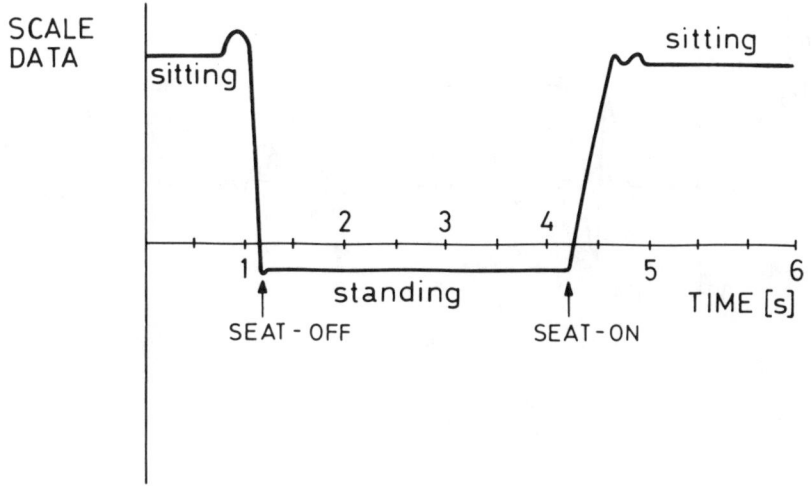

FIGURE 26d.

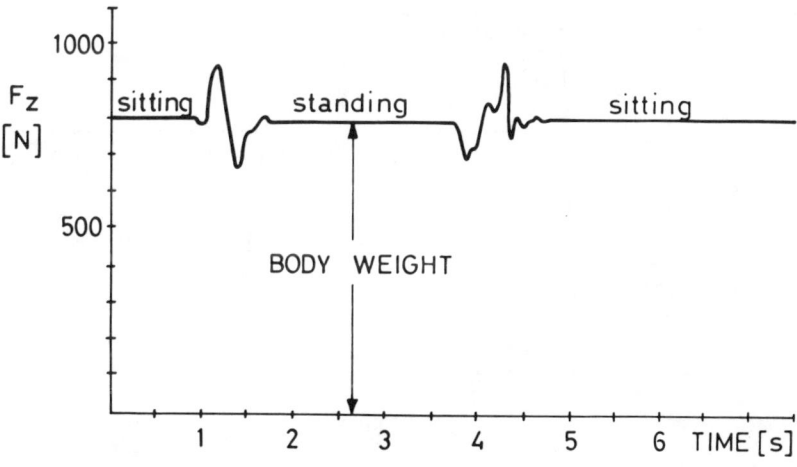

FIGURE 26e.

27. Striking differences are observed in the F_z and F_y plots (Figure 27a and 27b) while the Y_{COF} and joint angle records do not display substantial differences (Figure 27c, 27d, 27e, and 27f). During the hands-assisted stand-sit maneuver the shape of the force records changed and a noticeable drop in F_z force, for instance, clearly indicates that the difference in propulsion required for lifting was delivered by the help of hands. Also interesting to note is that during the normal subject's standing-up, the F_y force occurrence preceded the vertical force changes, while for the hands assisted standing-up this was not the case. The comparision of joint angle records for normal subject's stand/sit maneuver with and without hand support (compare Figure 26a, b, c with Figure 27d, e, and f) does not display any significant differences.

The joint torques in hip, knee, and ankle were measured during the standing-up of a healthy subject. Force plate and stroboscopic photography were used in the experiment.[90] The subject (height 185 cm, weight 82 kg) stood with both legs on the force plate. With the healthy subject it was assumed that, during standing-up, body weight is equally distributed

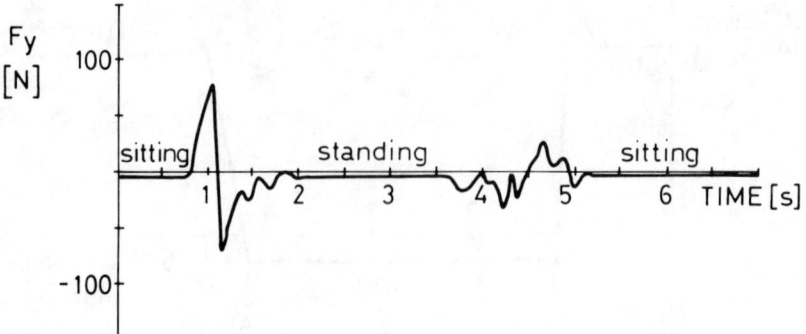

FIGURE 26f.

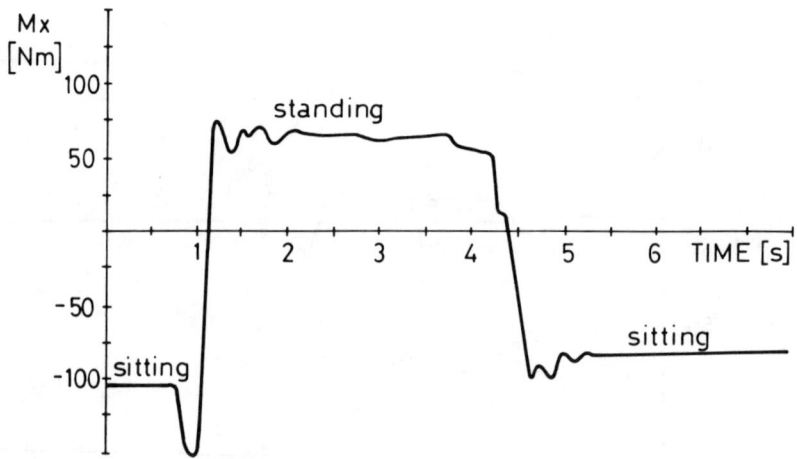

FIGURE 26g.

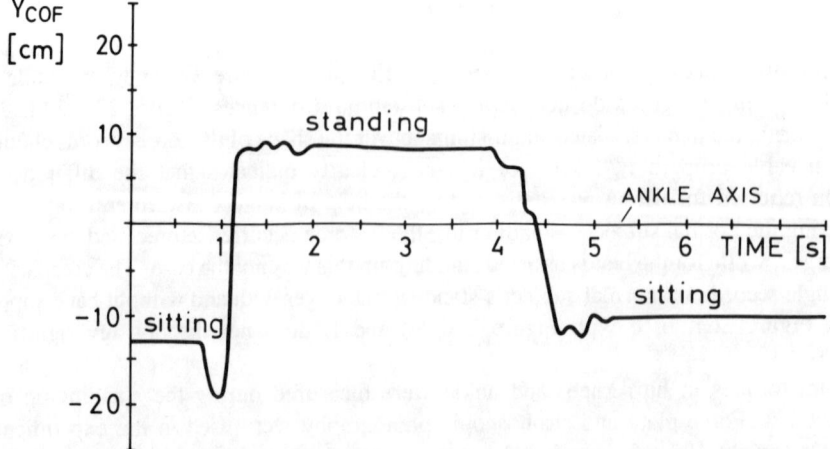

FIGURE 26h.

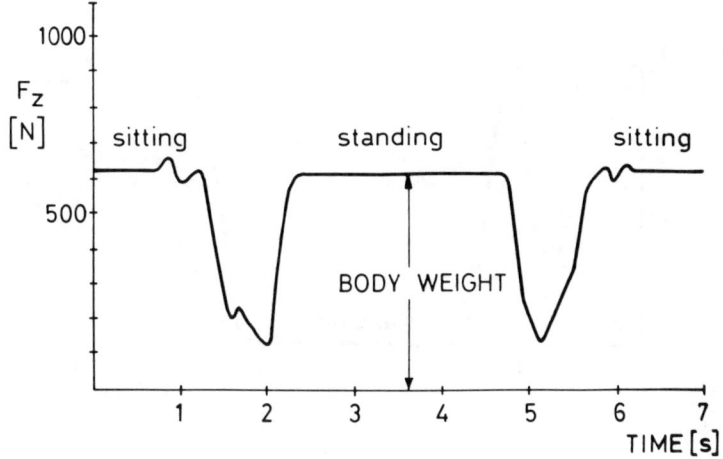
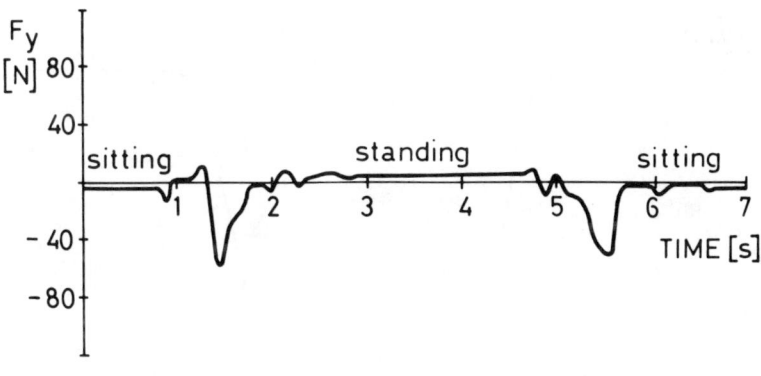
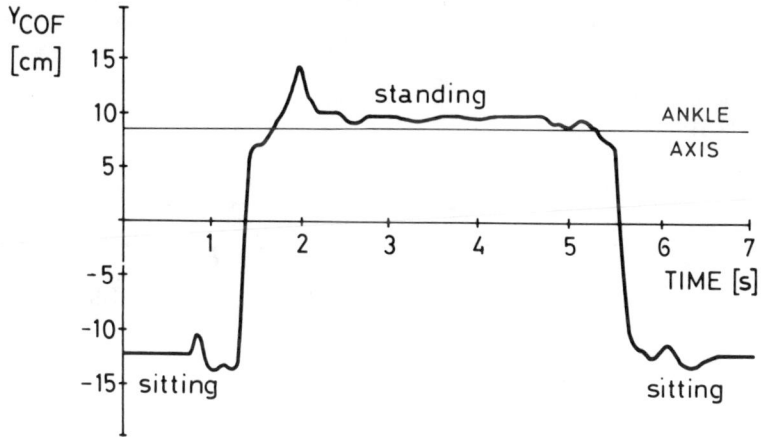

FIGURE 27. Kinematic and dynamic parameters during standing-up and sitting-down maneuver assisted by hand support (a, b, c, d, e, f).

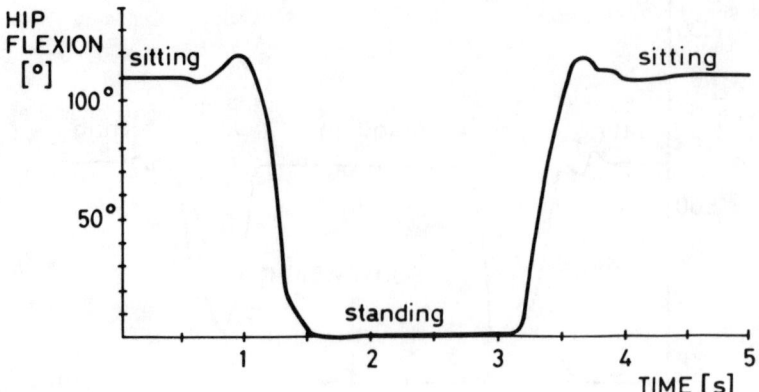

FIGURE 27d.

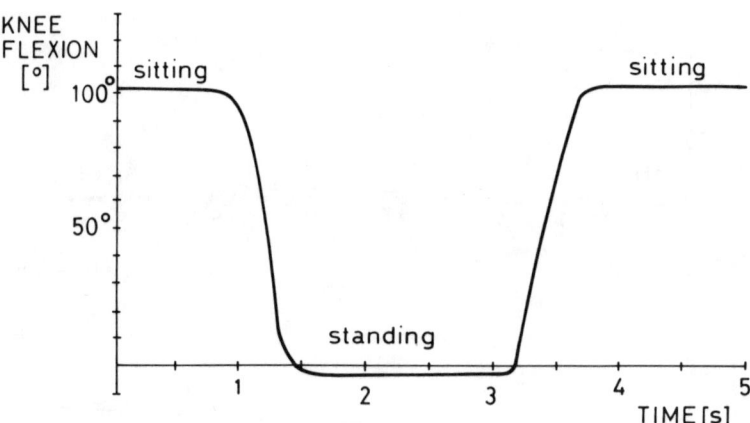

FIGURE 27e.

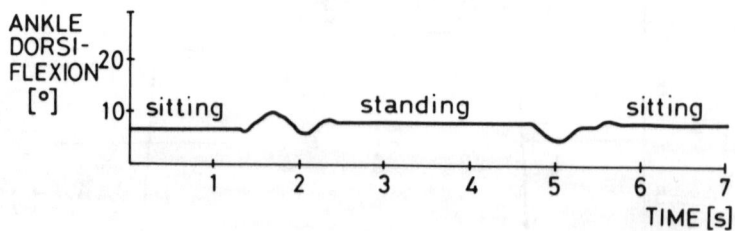

FIGURE 27f.

between the legs. No arm support was used during standing-up maneuver. The hip joint moment was found to increase rapidly to its maximal value, 80 Nm which was reached after 0.3 s (Figure 28). The whole standing-up maneuver was completed after 1.4 s. This moment must be compensated for by the hip extensors muscle group. The time course of the knee joint moment (maximal torque of 110 Nm) is similar and must be counterbalanced by both knee extensors. Much lower torque occurs in the ankle joints. The plantar flexors are responsible for this moment. In the next standing-up trial, the healthy subject was asked to rise from the sitting position with the trunk strongly leaned forward. The whole standing-up process was somewhat slower with the peak torques occuring at 0.5 s. Maximal value of the hip joint moment remained unchanged, while the maximum in knee torque was decreased from 110 to 80 Nm. No significant differences were observed in the time course of ankle joint.

Because of the lack of stability, a complete paraplegic patient (with his knees locked by FES) cannot stand without arm support. Therefore, the patient also will use his arms during standing-up. It can be expected that with the help of arms and partially preserved trunk muscles, he will be able to compensate for the torque occurring in the hip joints. As the values of ankle joint moment are rather small (up to 30 Nm), forces provided by arms counterbalance them easily and no stimulation is to be applied to the plantar flexors. FES must, therefore, provide sufficient force to knee extensors, so that knee joint torques will be compensated for. Taking into account the maximal isometric knee joint torques assessed after training program (Figure 13, Chapter 2) and the isometric moments obtained in eight standing paraplegic subjects (Figure 40a, see later), it can be observed that adequate knee joint torques provided by surface electrical stimulation can be encountered in about half of the paraplegic subjects tested. The rest of the patients will have to use a lesser or greater degree of arm support to assist their rising from sitting to the standing position. The torques during standing-up are 30 to 40 Nm in the ankle joints, 160 to 210 Nm in the knees, and about 160 Nm in the hip joints. For slow standing-up, the knee torques can be reduced to 160 Nm and, by arm support, lowered to half of the value. One knee extensor muscle group must provide, therefore, at least a torque of about 30 to 40 Nm,[91-94] depending on subject's body weight.

3. The Stand/Sit Trajectories

Comparing kinematic data for different trials of stand/sit maneuvers does not display appropriate changes and detailed differences in movement. The kinematic data, if displayed vs. time, are in a format convenient for kinematic calculations, but rather in an impractical format for evaluating patients performance. When using the same data to display the stick diagram postures vs. time during the stand/sit movement, more evidence about patients abilities is provided. Following the posture space mode (Figure 15) for displaying stand/sit data, we obtain a record which here will be named the stand/sit trajectory. Each point on this trajectory represents one particular posture during the movement. In the three-dimensional posture space, the trajectory is hard to be visualized. The projections of the posture space trajectory are therefore made. There are three projections possible (Figure 15): the projection to the hip-knee plane, to the ankle-knee plane, and to the hip-ankle plane. For the data presented in Figure 26, the corresponding projections are presented in Figure 29a, b, and c and for the Figure 27 in Figure 29d, e, and f, respectively. Utilizing the projection instead of joint goniograms, one can visualize the postures and, on these grounds, estimate the subject's standing performance. One can, for example, quantitatively estimate how close the erect standing is to the origin of the posture space, and by comparing several records belonging to the same subject, the posture trajectories repeatability can be demonstrated. One can also determine the symmetry of standing-up in comparison to sitting-down.

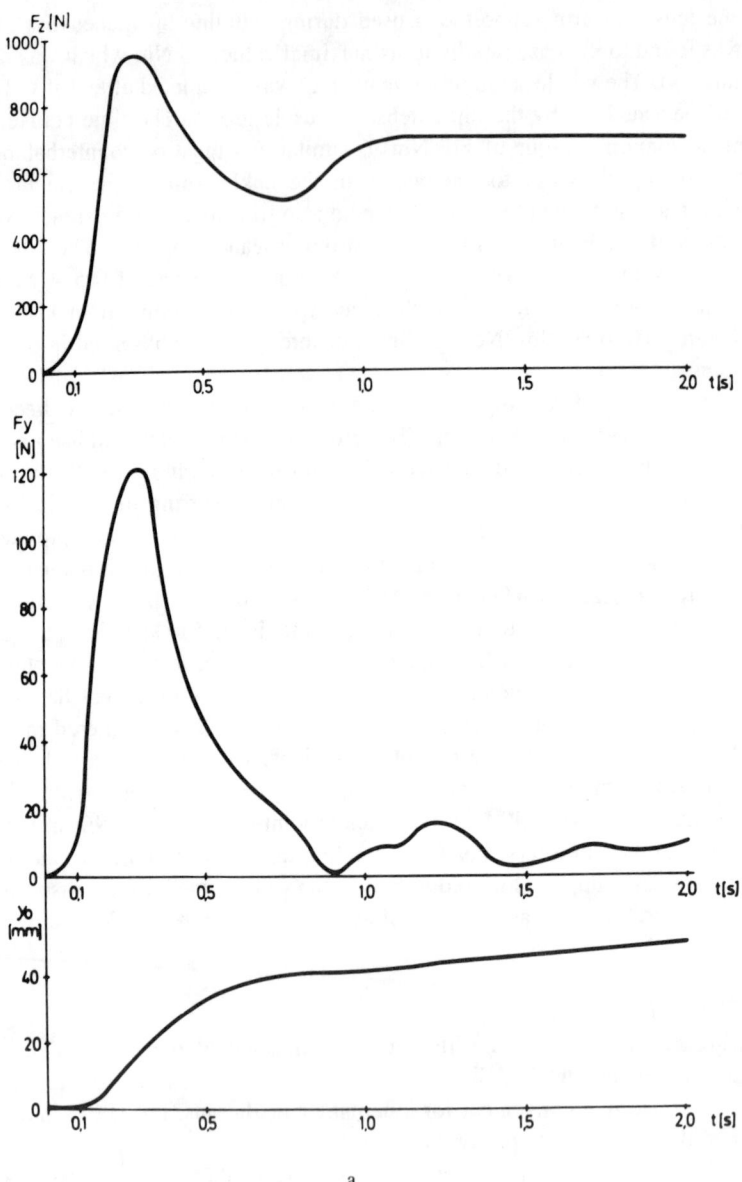

FIGURE 28. Measurement of standing-up of a healthy subject: force plate measurement including vertical and horizontal reaction force components, F_z and F_y, and the course of the point of resultant force application y_O (a) and the calculated joint torques in hips M_H, knees M_K, and ankles M_A (b).

In normal man, stand/sit trajectories have their origin somewhere in postural space (sitting position) and terminate close to the origin of the posture space. The trajectory runs diagonally in the postural space. All the projections also will display a diagonal course. Interesting differences in the projections can be noticed for arms-assisted stand/sit maneuver. Here, only the hip-knee projection has a diagonal form, while the ankle-knee projection is vertical, and hip-ankle projection is horizontal. Comparison of posture trajectories for FES-assisted stand/sit maneuver in patients, with respect to a normal subject, gives additional important differences. It seems that posture trajectories and their projections are rather sensitive when comparing and estimating even subtle differences which can be only hardly noticed by

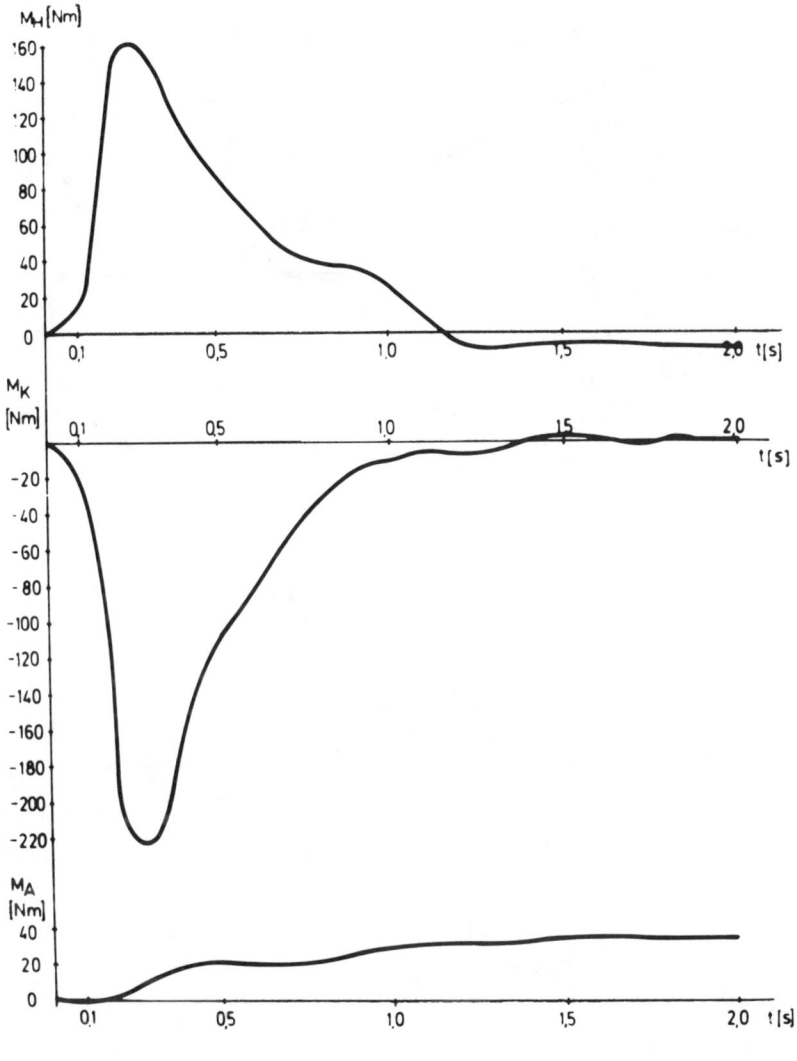

FIGURE 28b.

observing the joint angles vs. the time records. To illustrate the effectiveness of the stand/sit trajectories, two sets of data for a T-5 paraplegic patient are given. Figure 30a, b, and c present records of FES-assisted standing-up, while the patient was not instructed how to perform the maneuver and did not have practice for proper stand/sit transition. One can observe that because of improper initial feet placement and standing-up execution, the projections of stand/sit trajectory display unusual shapes indicating high energy expenditure and resulting in inadequate performance. After the patient was instructed how to assume the proper initial sitting position (feet placement, hand and trunk position) and practiced for only several times, the records in Figure 31a, b, and c were obtained. It is instructive to compare these records with those in Figure 29d, e, and f on one side and to compare them also with the records in Figure 30a, b, and c. We observe that the records of Figure 31 are much closer to the performance of a normal subject when using arm support. The projections of Figure 31 are also displaying on the first sight a more effective and smoother standing-up procedure.

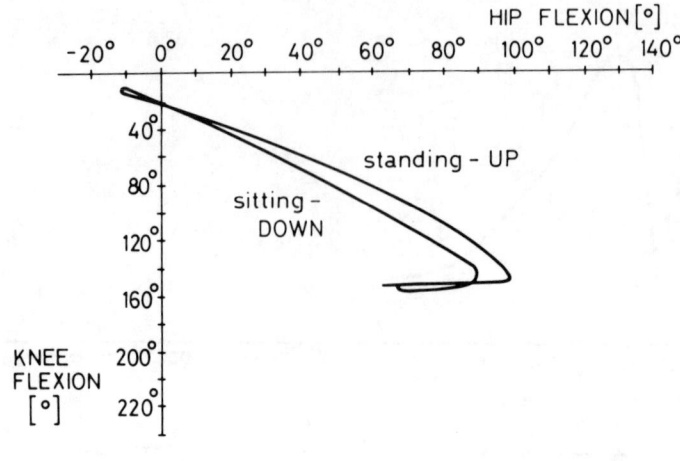
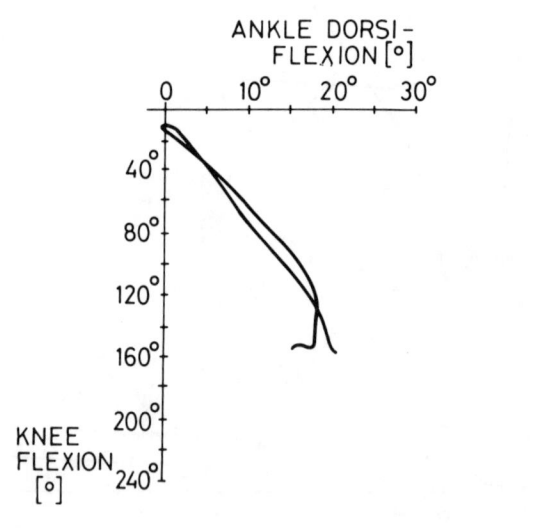
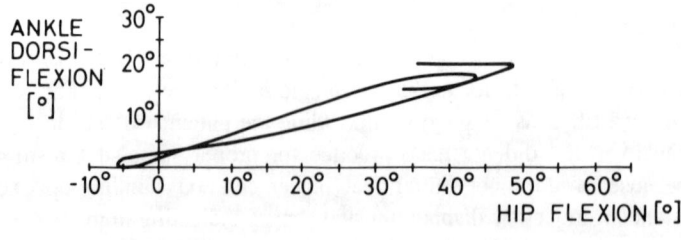

FIGURE 29. Stand/sit trajectories in hip/knee (a), ankle-knee (b), and hip-ankle (c) plane of the posture space during unassisted maneuver and while helping by arm support (d, e, f).

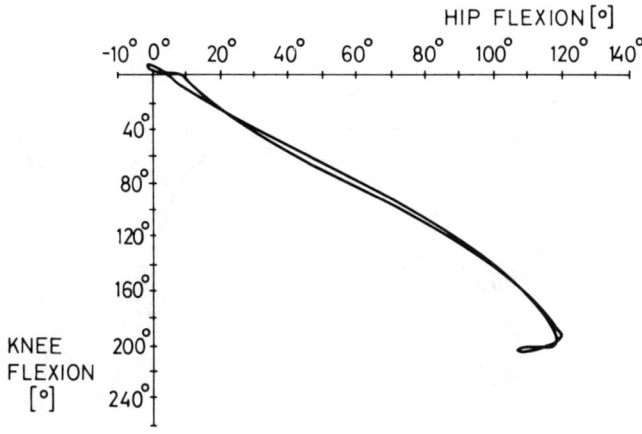

FIGURE 29d.

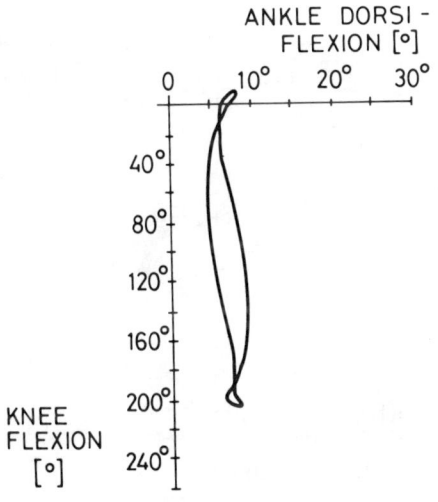

FIGURE 29e.

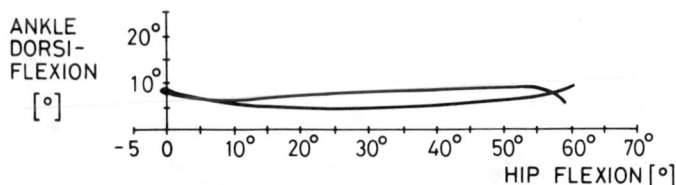

FIGURE 29f.

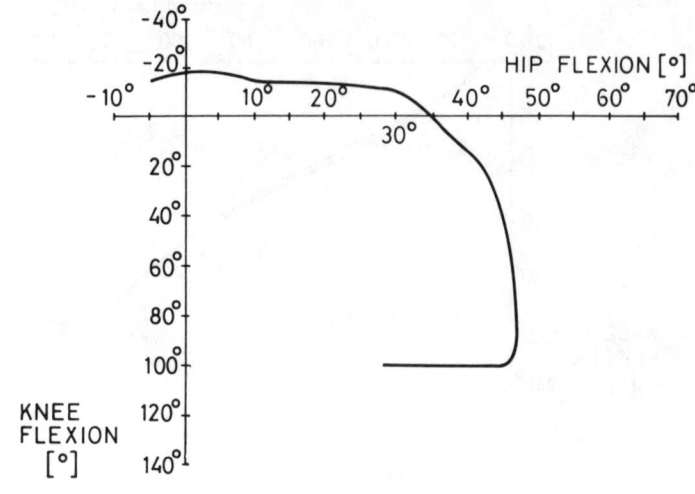

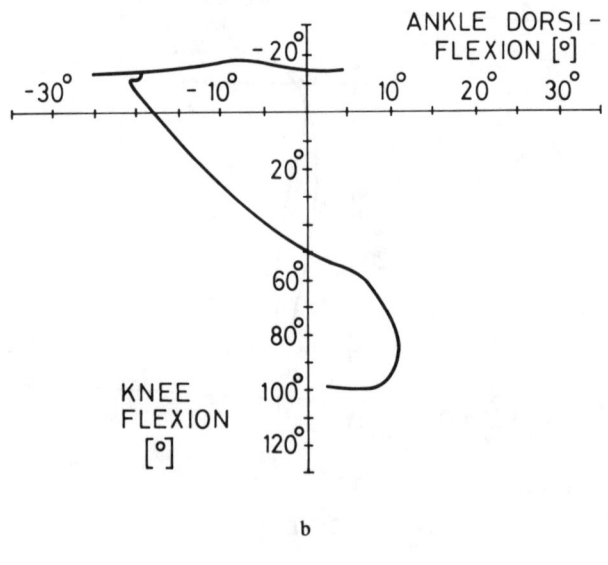

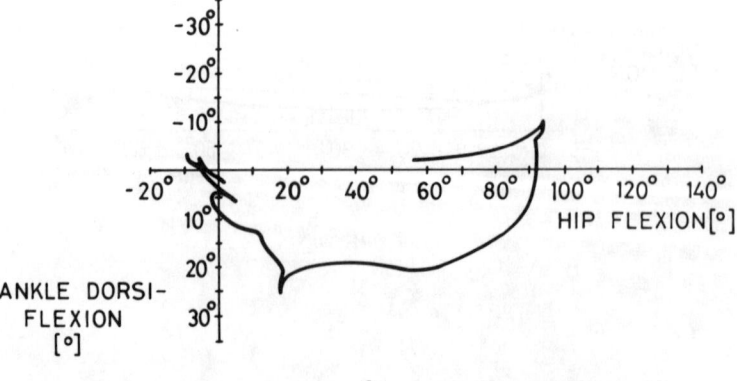

FIGURE 30. Stand/sit trajectories obtained in untrained paraplegic subject when using FES (a, b, c).

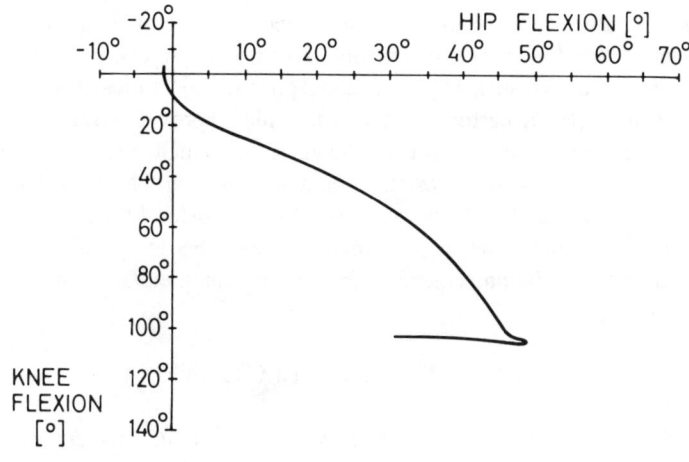

a

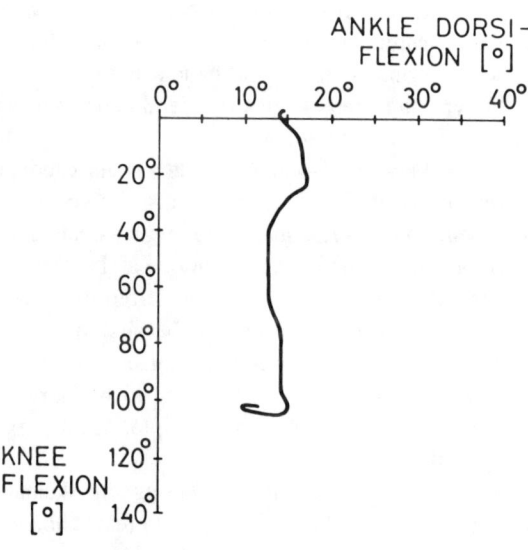

b

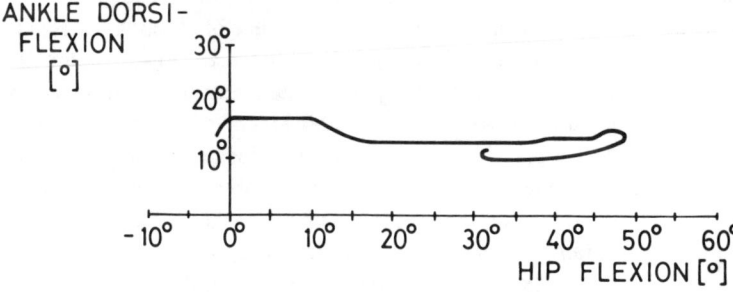

c

FIGURE 31. Stand/sit trajectories obtained in trained paraplegic subject when rising by the help of FES (a, b, c).

Summarizing the advantages of the presented stand/sit trajectories in the postural space, it can be concluded that trajectories of transitions and their projections can be utilized for diagnostic purposes. This is justified by the fact that posture trajectories of stand/sit transitions display subtle differences in performance and provide improved visualization of motion performed. The curves assessed in efficient stand/sit performance are simple and smooth. The domains of acceptable postures for standing and sitting can be easily determined. Any deviation in performance can be clearly recognized when postural trajectory projections are used. The evaluation of the stand/sit performance using FES in SCI patients can be successfully studied and stimulation sequences for an efficient stand/sit maneuver determined for each patient.

III. PATIENTS SELECTION

The rehabilitation possibilities and expectations for a particular patient should be determined as early as possible. After the life-saving procedures are administered, following SCI and multiple traumas, and the patient is in a stable condition with the spine stabilized, planning of further rehabilitation process may be started. Already, when the patient is still in the acute treatment phase and requires extensive decubiti protective bed positioning, deep venous thrombosis prevention care, etc., the physical examination for rehabilitation planning may be carried out. The functional status of the patient is examined and compared to the expectations given by the type and level of injury (general neurological examination, testing of the completeness of the lesion, and somatosensory evoked potential examination). At present, patients with lesions between T-4 and T-12 levels are candidates for realistic FES use and rehabilitation by means of FES.[46] It should also be stressed that FES is only an additional rehabilitation mean to the well-established regular treatments of SCI patients.[48,49] After the patient is conscious, the complete examination can be performed while the patient is still in the acute unit or immediately after he is transferred to the rehabilitation unit. The FES examination and treatment in the acute unit is, because of special care, condition of patient, and specific medical treatment procedures, not covered here. The procedures of patients selection described in this chapter are intended to be carried out after the patient was admitted to the rehabilitation unit, but, in principle, similar examinations could be started already in the acute unit.

The physical examination must be complete, covering the skeletal and neuromuscular system. It must include examination of before injury and present abnormalities of bones and joints, testing of the range of motion of all limb joints, eliciting normal and pathological reflexes, assessing sensory changes, spasticity, tremor, establishing the degree of voluntary control, muscular status of voluntary and reflex movements, as well as grading of muscular status produced by electrical excitation of muscles. During these examinations, the patient must be cooperative and, if possible, not under the influence of sedatives. It is very important to determine the muscles and body sites displaying upper vs. lower motor neuron lesion (UMNL/LMNL). The function of trunk and upper extremities muscles must also be examined in details. Examination directed toward the establishment of the general patient's status represents the next step incorporating personal, social, educational, and psychological data. Each category of the so far mentioned examination and obtained data results, according to logical reasons and criteria, in acceptance of the patient into the FES program or in excluding him because of the contraindications found. The indications and contraindications criteria for patient selection are mostly based upon the present state of the art in the field of FES and may be widened in the future so that larger patient populations will benefit from FES. In the proceeding sections, each category of examinations and data provided will be discussed in more detail.

Table 1
DIVISION OF SCI PATIENTS WITH REGARD TO POSSIBLE BRACING

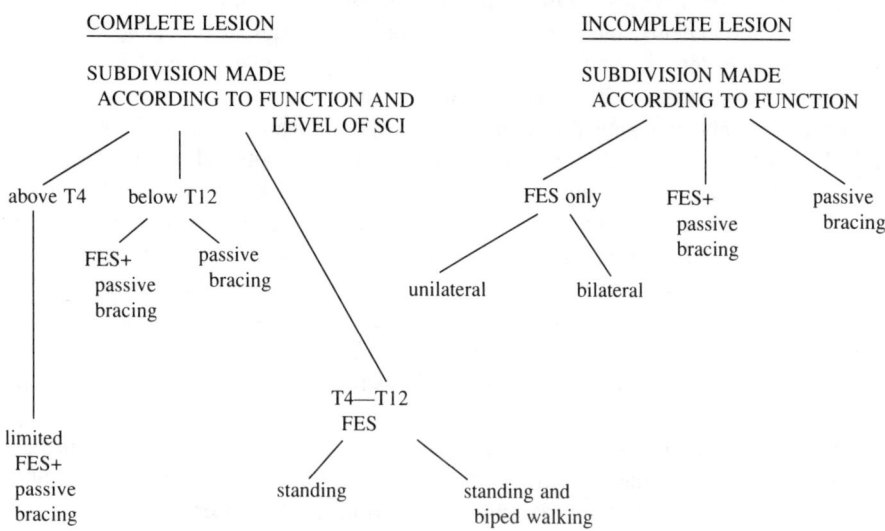

A. Patients Selection According to Level and Status of Lesion

The exact neurological level of lesion is best established by means of sensory evoked and centrally evoked potentials. According to the level and completeness of the spinal cord lesion, the patients may be, in respect to FES applicability, divided in the categories as indicated in Table 1.

In this rough division of patients into the categories with respect to possible use of orthotic equipment, an assumption was made that the lesions considered resulted predominantly in UMNL. Unfortunately, in practice this is far from being true. In many patients, because of blood supply occlusion, developed hemorrhages, hematoma, edema, mechanical factors, etc., the spinal cord below the lesion level is involved or substantially damaged. As a result, the involved sites develop partial or complete LMNL.

Consequently, the corresponding denervated muscles atrophy in a short time, hence, not allowing the use of FES. Therefore, also in T-4 to T-12 patients, many will be excluded and are to be treated in the same way as the below T-12 group of patients. This patient population can be divided, according to the UMNL of the main muscle groups of the lower extremity, into potential FES and mechanical orthoses users. In patients having lesions above T-4, the problem of unstable trunk and hence, very poor posture control, indicates passive mechanical bracing in addition to FES. The patients with higher lesions may also be limited in performance abilities because of associated autonomous disreflexia problems (temperature regulation, unstable blood pressure, etc.). Our experience indicates that patients with lesions above T-4 are very likely to develop pathological spine deformations. The continuous stressing, provoked by upper trunk and arm movements, of the highly susceptible spine results in pathologies because of destabilization caused by atrophied and paralyzed vertebral musculature. Paraplegics with T-4 and higher lesion levels are candidates for FES combined with mechanical orthotics (hybrid systems), and special care must be paid to spine stabilization in terms of chronic use of an orthotic system. In some patients (T-3 to T-4), re-strengthening of lower back muscles by means of FES also was found to be valuable. Patients with lesions below T-12, in most cases, develop substantial LMNL of below lesion innervated muscles. If m. quadriceps is also involved, FES cannot be used for knee stabilization and therefore, only FES combined with external bracing can provide acceptable solutions. In all hybrid applications, the mechanical means provide safety and support, while the FES muscle force is used for transitions from one state into another. Particularly, in high level paraplegics where trunk muscles are paralyzed, the propulsion moment generated by FES is very important. In contrast, paraplegics below T-12 have normal trunk stability and also the ability of limited pelvis movements, therefore, they are not to such an extent dependent on FES-generated propulsion forces. Nevertheless, they can make excellent use of knee and hip flexion obtained by means of FES. Patients, who fit within this group, may be good ambulators by using only mechanical bracing. The decision, when to use a hybrid or only mechanical system, must be made according to the general functional and physical status of the patient. In an almost identical way, similar decisions, are performed in incomplete patients. Here, the relevant criteria are looking for independent standing at least on one leg. For such patients, unilateral FES devices are indicated. In case we like to reduce the FES device complexity, external braces may also be applied in these patients. As a rule, FES should be applied for providing flexion and propulsion moment, while the mechanical system will provide stance phase support, balance, and safety. The mechanical bracing is indicated for incomplete patients only in cases where it is able to convert the patient from a wheelchair user into a limited range or, at least, into a home hold walker. If this is not the case, the bracing brings no important advantages to the patient. Mechanical bracing, providing only upright standing, is not a solution which will assure long time use, mainly because of the involvement and hassle associated in donning and doffing of the system.

In contrast, it is expected that FES systems will with the advancement of technology become extremely practical and not demanding for the user.

The T-4 to T-12 paraplegic patients are optimal FES users. In these patients, FES is used for antigravity support, propulsion, and, in the future, it also may provide short-time balance ability. According to the physical and general status of the patient, FES may be indicated for gait or standing. In patients with weak trunk muscles and poor strength of upper extremities associated with inadequate cardiopulmonary reserve, only FES-enabled standing is indicated. At present, all FES-based locomotion activities require a certain degree of arm assistance for balancing and propulsion. Finally, let us remark that with further FES application, refinements are expected in the coming years, and the arm involvement might be substantially reduced (FES will generate all the required propulsion and braking moments).

B. Patients Selection According to Their Neurological Status

The patients must be neurologically stable. First, the selection is made according to the completeness of the spinal cord lesion. Next, the sites of UMNL and LMNL are established and the level of sensation loss documented. At the same time, the reflexes are examined. Tendon tap testing with assessment of the stretch reflexes is performed in the lower extremities, spasticity and tremor are tested for, and presence of reflex synergistic pattern movements documented. In particular, extension and flexion type predominance of spasticity should be distinguished, as well as the ability for eliciting the flexion withdrawal reflex movement. Patients with an extension type of spasticity will often require shorter restrengthening programs for extensor muscles and usually, turn out to be good candidates for standing. Problems may occur in the swing phase of gait (scissoring is because of adduction type of spasticity often associated with extensor spasticity). Severe spasticity is an eliminating contraindiction for FES use, in particular if flexion type is displayed. Moderate spasticity, regardless of its type as well as moderate tremor, may, with daily FES use, improve and therefore, is not a contraindication. The presence of flexion withdrawal movement is advantageous because it can be utilized for substituting the swing phase in FES-induced gait. In contrast, multichannel stimulation of the main hip, knee, and ankle flexors must be applied for providing the swing phase. The UMNL vs. LMNL testing results, to a large extent, in conclusive patient selection, as well as gives measure to the application possibilities. When the main extensors (hip, knee extensor muscle groups) display LMNL, the patient is forced to use for transition activities, such as standing-up and sitting-down, his arms, while for ensuring upright locking of the joints external bracing must be provided. Such patients do not benefit much from FES because the latter can be applied only for swing phase assistance. In case that main flexors display LMNL, the patient will be able to stand successfully by FES, but unlikely able to perform adequate swing phase. In such cases, swing-to, swing-through, and four-point (low thoracic and lumbar lesions) gait is a possibility. Our experience indicates that if the m. quadriceps has LMNL, the decision about FES use must be carefully made and detailed screening for potential benefits of FES use precisely defined.

C. Patients Selection According to Physiological Status

In rehabilitation medicine, physical examination is an established and well-known procedure. Here, only the main elements relevant to FES application will be reviewed. The patient's functional status must be thoroughly documented. Physiological monitoring and examination are elaborated in great details, but on the other side not so extensively used in every day physical therapy practice. Here, let us repeat the basic principles of daily physical therapy practice, where owing to lack of equipment and partly also of time, the physiological monitoring of the patient must be performed "on the run". Any movement in man requires muscle work. The "metabolic fuel" is "burned" in muscular tissue in two ways: aerobically, using oxygen, or anaerobically in its absence. In most instances, the muscular mechanical work of the exercising body is associated with both modalities. Efforts lasting for less than 1 min and producing forces above 40 to 50% of maximal force use aerobic metabolism which is more efficient. In this mode, carbohydrates are "burned" using oxygen, and for each glucose molecule reaction, 36 molecules of ATP (adenosine triphosphate) are disintegrated to phosphate and adenosine diphosphate, resulting in accompanying mechanical energy necessary for movement. Anaerobic metabolism of one carbohydrate molecule will result in only two ATP molecules, but the additional difference in the reaction producing mechanical energy is in the byproduct of anaerobic reaction being the lactic acid, which must be converted into carbonic acid and from there into CO_2 and H_2O. Aerobic metabolism is directly followed by end products in the form of CO_2 and H_2O. Anaerobic metabolism is switched on in long lasting activities (more than 1 min) and for moderate efforts of up to 40 to 50% of maximal muscular force. In activities such as walking, wheelchair propulsion, etc., both modes of metabolism are utilized. All the described reactions occur in the mitochondria and cytoplasm of contracting muscle cells. Therefore, oxygen is brought from the lungs by the ventilation and cardiac action, while the same system is utilized also for transport and exclusion of the rest of CO_2 and H_2O. Obviously, any change in mechanical action must result and reflect in an accompanying reaction of the heart and lungs-cardiopulmonary system. The muscular effort is echoed in the heart activity by increasing the rate of contractions (HR — heart rate) and the volume of blood ejected per beat (SV — stroke volume). The total increase of the circulated blood is therefore given by the product $HR \cdot SV = CO$ — called the cardiac output. For an increase of CO, the lungs must supply more oxygen and transport more CO_2 back into the air. Human neural control of cardiopulmonary function will, in case of increased content of CO_2 in blood, facilitate the lung function by increasing the rate and tidal volume of ventilation (minute ventilation = rate of breathing × tidal volume).

If muscular effort is gradually increased, soon a limit is reached when the body no longer has the ability to increase CO or the minute ventilation. In this state, the subject tested will stop performing the current activity because of exhaustion. There are numerous symptoms signalling exhaustion: feeling of fatigue and heaviness in the exercised muscles, breathlessness, an uncomfortable feeling, etc. Because of waste products built-up in muscle tissue (lactic acid), the muscles feel stiff and painful. Any weak link in the mechanical energy producing chain may disable and limit the human performance. Pathologies or present diseases may be the causes of disfunction in the mechanical work generation chain. The main sources of disfunctions can be situated in muscle, peripheral blood circulation, heart, pulmonary circulation, and lungs. Any disfunction or pathology of these elements may result in low patient's tolerance to mechanical effort. In patients, the locomotion system is, because of pathology (contractures, spasticity, etc.), very inefficient and demands high power and muscle work. In addition, other elements in the energy chain may be involved as well, resulting in very low effort tolerance and fast onset of exhaustion. Emotional stress and anxiety are also limiting factors, substantially reducing exercise tolerance. Physiological fitness may be built-up by carefully planned exercising. The physiological assessment is performed by monitoring five important quantities: (1) heart rate (pulse), (2) blood pressure, (3) signs and symptoms of exhaustion, (4) electrocardiography, and (5) ergonometry (work quantification). It is out of the scope of this paragraph to review in detail all these monitorings. Instead, we will give border values which are indicative for the correct patient selection and admittance to the FES therapeutic program. In principle, the same limits and methodology as established in physiotherapy apply also to the FES approach. First, patient's resting heart rate is monitored, normally being between 50 to 95 beats/min. Any resting heart rate above 100 is abnormal and the patient should not be exercised. As it is well known, the heart rate increases with exercising. When values of 160 beats/min or higher are expected during the exercise, then the heart rate should be monitored. When the heart rate starts to rise abruptly, patient's tolerance to physical stress is reached and physical effort should be decreased or stopped. Also, any arrhythmias and other irregularities of the heart function are contraindications for FES. If the systolic blood pressure is rising because of exercise, up to 26 kPa (200 mmHg), this is also a contraindication. Normally, the systolic pressure must be in the range of 12 to 18 kPa (90 to 140 mmHg) and the diastolic 5.5 to 12 kPa (40 to 90 mmHg). Systolic hypotension (under 12 kPa or 90 mmHg) and diastolic hypertension (above 13.3 kPa or 100 mmHg) are also contraindicating parameters. If in systolic hypotension, the systolic pressure is decreased for more than 2.6 kPa or 20 mmHg at increased effort, it is a contraindication for further therapy. Only patients with systolic/diastolic pressure adapting to exercising efforts are suitable for the FES rehabilitation approach. With exercise effort, the systolic pressure is gradually increasing, while the diastolic pressure remains at the same level or it is slightly decreased.

If cardiac and blood pressure assessments indicate application of FES therapy, the dysfunctions of circulation or lung may still prevent it because of low effort tolerance. Usual exhaustion signs and symptoms are: balance problems and unusual unsteadiness, pallor or cyanosis, chest discomfort, dizziness or room spinning, etc. These signs are indicating the occurrence of hypoventilation and cerebral ischaemia. All these signs with dyspnea — difficulty in breathing — are contraindications for further exercise and are signalling that the exercise effort should be decreased or diminished. A simple test may be used for dyspnea evaluation. If the patient is able to count loudly for 7 to 8 s from 1 up to 15 in one breath, his dyspnea level is estimated by number 1. In case, the patient must break counting for taking a breath (grade 2), it is a sign that he has reached the border line of dyspnea. For grade 3, more than one break is necessary to finish counting. It is generally adopted that exercise effort should not be increased beyond the dyspnea grade 2. For all limiting cases with respect to physiological examinations, it is suggested that quantitative and specialized medical examinations are performed.[47-49]

D. Physical Evaluation and Indications for FES

Physical examination is focused on upper and lower extremities and trunk in general. The elements of these examinations are given in Table 2.

This examination is intended to establish the initial patient's status before rehabilitation

Table 2
PHYSICAL EXAMINATION NECESSARY BEFORE INTRODUCEMENT OF FES

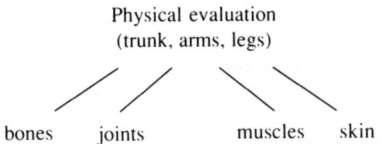

and FES application is started. In respect to the bones status, patients with osteoporosis must be eliminated, as well as those with other bone problems not allowing adequate bone loading and hence, locomotion activities. FES is indicated when a patient is found by generally accepted physical medicine criteria suitable for ambulation training program with long leg braces.[48,49,80] Next, the joints are evaluated for stability and range of motion. Unstable joints with distended ligaments present contraindications for FES. Any limit in the range of motion of the ankle joint for more than 5° in plantar flexion is also a contraindication for standing preventing adequate posture and trunk weight acceptance and leading also to secondary deformities like hyperextended knees. Lordosis is developed because of hip flexion contractures.

Limited hip extension (for 5 to 10°) and limited knee range of motion[50] preventing complete extension are also severely reducing FES application unless it is expected that the range of motion (ROM) of the affected joints could be improved with exercise. For successful FES standing and ambulation, at least neutral or better of up to 5° or more of dorsiflexion in ankle joint is required and full extension of the knee with at least 5° of hyperextension in the hip joint are considered as satisfactory requirements. Muscle tests[51,52] are performed for voluntary and FES-activated muscles. Note, if muscle forces (see Chapter 2) obtained by FES are below given limits, it is very likely that FES muscle restrengthening may not result in a sufficient muscle force required for functional activities. In respect to muscle force evaluation, quantitative approaches are preferred in comparison with manual testing because of excluding subjective factors. According to our experiments, when the maximal isometric knee joint torque provided by FES attains 30 to 40 Nm (depending on patient's posture and body weight), a standing training program can be started.

Skin problems like ulcers, decubiti, skin rash, etc. are contraindicating the use of FES on a temporary basis. After the skin problem is removed, FES may be employed. Because of electrode jell or ingredients contained in the moisturizing media of electrodes, fixating adhesive tapes, or the electrodes themselves, skin rash may develop. Our experience showed that the skin rash disappears after the irritating substances are removed, indicating the use of a different type of electrodes or fixation means. Therefore, in most cases, skin rash produced by FES did not appear to be a serious contraindication. The patient selection process is not complete without considering the patient's general status including age, general physical condition, vision, nutritional status (obesity is often a contraindication for FES), patient's cooperativeness, and social and educational level. Low mental and educational level are contraindicating FES application because daily home use at the present state of art is rather demanding. Similar problems may occur in patients not being sufficiently cooperative or having hearing or vision problems.

The application of FES and patient selection is performed by a multidisciplinary team task requiring careful and good cooperation of the involved disciplines. In Table 3, a review of indications for FES is given, while in Table 4, the contraindications are summarized.

IV. FES STANDING

First, patient's tolerance of vertical positioning must be established according to the

Table 3
PATIENTS INDICATIONS FOR FES

1. Lesion level T-4 to T-12
2. Upper motor neuron lesion
3. Positive results of FES restrengthening program
4. No joint contractures or other involvements (e.g., ossification, osteoporosis)
5. No major skin problems
6. Normal balance and orientation sensation
7. Satisfactory mental and emotional condition
8. Motivated and cooperative
9. Adequate upper extremities and trunk function
10. Nearly normal physiological status (heart, lung, blood circulation, metabolism, etc.)

Table 4
CONTRAINDICATIONS FOR FES

1. Heart, lung, or blood circulation pathologies
2. Metabolism and other involvements resulting from damage to autonomous system
3. Osteoporosis
4. Ossification of joints
5. Lower motor neuron lesion of main leg muscles
6. Pressure sores or other skin problems
7. Hypersensitivity to electrical currents
8. Obesity
9. Very severe spasticity
10. Inadequate sitting balance
11. Poor vision or hearing
12. Inadequate mental and/or educational level

standard procedures[48,49,77] by using a tilt table. When the patient can tolerate upright position of the tilt table, he is ready for standing sessions in the standing frame. In patients having a plaster cast, the cast is replaced by polyethylene braces or collars. Physiotherapists must be sure that patient protective extension reactions are present, together with equilibrium reactions and sense of balance. These prerequisites, together with patient's adequate sitting balance, awareness of standing posture, orientation in space, and fulfillment of general health criteria, with appropriate physical status provide a good basis for efficient upright standing. In particular, the tilt table upright training must be completed already at this stage, and initial prolonged standing in the standing frame using knee and pelvic fixations already must be well under way. We must also ensure, while the patient is upright, that he is not experiencing cerebral ischaemia, high blood pressure, dizziness, and room spinning. It is further convenient to start FES standing training after the patient is already familiar with

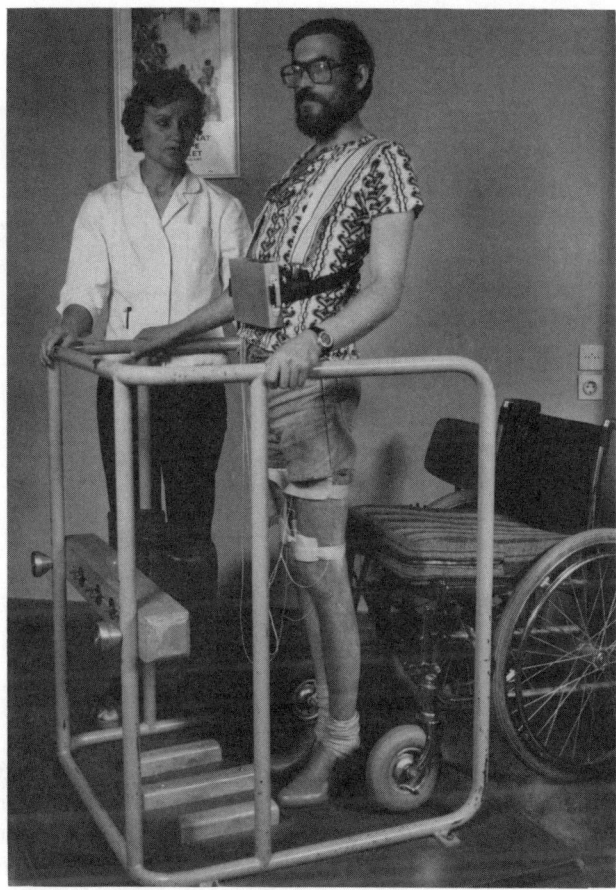

FIGURE 32. First trial of paraplegic patient standing in special frame.

the stimulator and electrodes after using FES for 1 to 2 weeks for muscle restrengthening. In patients with adequate initial force of m. quadriceps (for standing a minimal value of 30 to 50 Nm of knee joint torque) where substantial restrengthening is not a prerequisite for ensuring functional joint locking torques, FES standing training may be started immediately.

For the initial trials of FES-assisted standing-up and upright standing, it is suggested to utilize a standing frame similar to the one shown in Figure 32. The patient is using the frame for balance and during the act of standing-up and sitting-down to assist the transition by arm forces. Because of rather fast m. quadriceps fatiguing while stimulated, the standing-up trials should at beginning last not more than 1 to 2 min and thereafter, the patient is seated again. Between several standing trials, the patient should be allowed to rest for several minutes and his reactions to the standing exercise should be, at that time, observed by palpation and visual observation. Also it is advised to document blood pressure and perform pulmonary measurements. If patient is pale and breathless and high pulse rate is assessed, then the standing trials should be stopped or at least more rest given between them. Such standing training can be performed twice a day for 10 to 15 min. After 1 to 2 weeks, the patient will master the procedure and become secure in standing-up, standing, and sitting-down. At that time, prolonged standing training is initiated, and the patient is instructed to shift his body weight by the help of trunk and arms movements in order to achieve necessary balance by the help of one arm support only. The starting position for standing-up, as proven

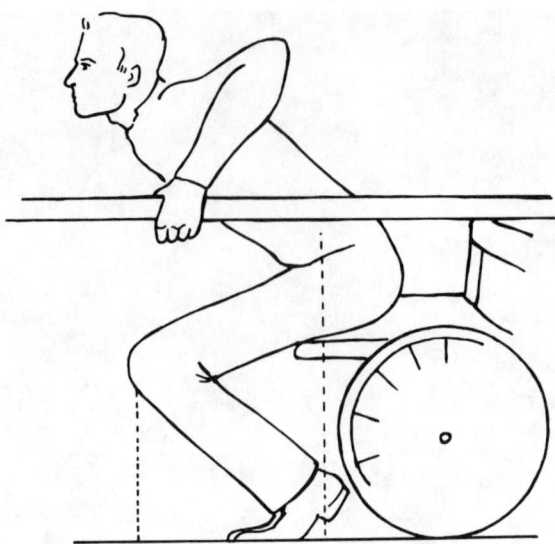

FIGURE 33. The starting position for standing-up from the wheelchair with the help of electrical stimulation of knee extensors.

by our experiences, is a substantial influence on the effectiveness of the standing-up maneuver and also on assuming the appropriate upright standing (see posture C in Figure 12). The starting position to be assumed before standing-up is displayed in Figure 33. Note that the arm supports must be provided at adequate height. The patient must be leaned forward with his trunk. The C.G. line should pass close to the ankle joint center, and the knees should be in front of the toes. As standing-up using FES substantially differs from standing-up using long leg braces, the patient must be carefully taught to understand the differences in case he is also in a training program for long leg braces use. While standing-up, the arm assisting forces should only add the difference which is not provided by stimulated m. quadriceps activity. In this maneuver, the arms are also providing necessary trunk and hip extension moments. Once the patient is upright, he is instructed to use as much as possible of his preserved dorsal trunk muscles together with his arms to force the hip joints into hyperextension and to maintain the proper standing position. In some patients when stimulating the knee extensor, m. rectus femoris is exerting a too strong hip flexion moment which must be overcome during the standing-up maneuver. Once the hips are in hyperextension, the action of m. rectus femoris should be balanced by trunk hyperextension. To decrease the action of m. rectus femoris, it is helpful to position the stimulation electrodes more distally so that less m. rectus femoris activation is achieved. The most effective location of electrodes for m. quadriceps stimulation is to place one electrode approximately 7 to 10 cm above the patella and the second one 7 to 10 cm higher in the proximal direction. For eliminating the m. rectus femoris stimulation, one electrode is placed medially on the m. quadriceps medialis and the second one laterally a few centimeters from the motor point of m. quadriceps lateralis in the proximal direction. In most patients, the standing-up and standing are easily mastered, while problems often arise with the sitting-down procedure. For sitting-down, the patient must position the hands slightly backwards with respect to body position, be aware where the sitting area is, and then synchronously with the diminishing FES take over the body weight by the arms. At the same time, he must bend the upper body forward, while exerting with the arms the forces to push the whole body backwards toward the chair. In the beginning, the patient is often missing the right moment for picking up the

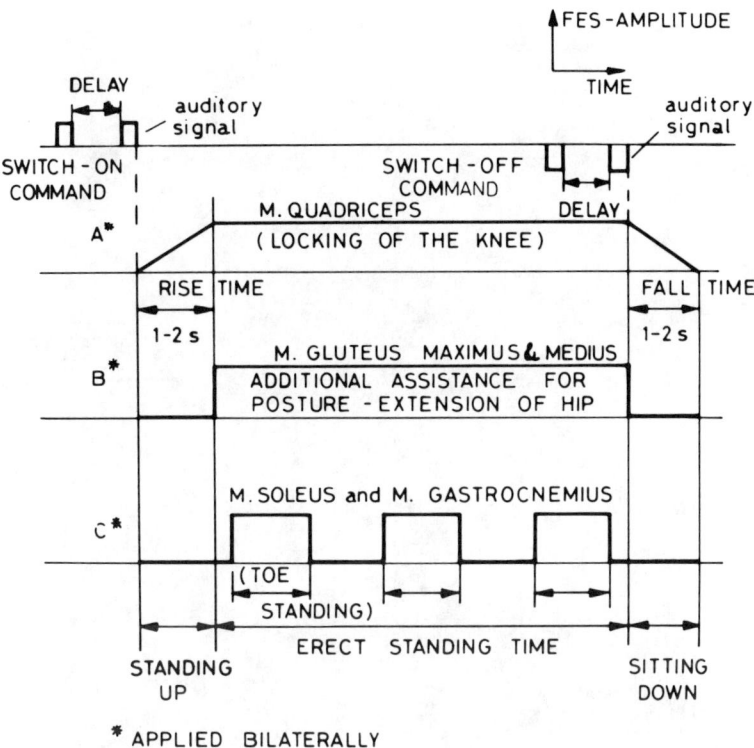

FIGURE 34. The FES sequence for standing-up and erect standing, with or without toe lifting and sitting-down.

body weight by the arms, and because FES is already off and no m. quadriceps action is present, he descends abruptly into sitting position. During the initial training trials in the first weeks, the physiotherapist must assist the sitting-down maneuvers very carefully. Once the patient has mastered smooth and soft standing-up with sitting-down, the help provided by physiotherapist is gradually reduced and finally not provided or practiced any more. The maximal FES standing time depends on the posture assumed, m. quadriceps strength, and fatiguing time. It should be practiced using the lowest, yet still functional, stimulation amplitude (strength of m. quadriceps) providing adequate safety of standing. When fatiguing is taking place, the physiotherapist or, later, the patient himself must gradually increase the stimulation amplitude and, in this way, compensate for the fatiguing effect. Such a procedure ensures only minimal overstimulation of the m. quadriceps and reduces the stress to the knee joint. The patient and physiotherapist must be aware of the longest possible standing time for a particular patient. Standing must be terminated before jackknifing may occur. For allowing to the patient to handle the switch of the stimulator and to provide sufficient time for hands placement before standing-up, the FES is not switched on immediately, but rather, after a short delay and through gradual rising. The timing of FES switching on and off is shown in Figure 34. According to the stimulation sequence given in Figure 34, the auditory signal reminds the patient to start the movement. In Figure 34, the stimulation of m. soleus together with m. gastrocnemius is displayed also, as it can be applied for providing intermittent toe standing (Figure 35). The latter mode of standing is beneficial for muscle restrengthening.

The fatiguing process considerably limits the total standing time. Therefore, it should be determined how long the patient is able to stand safely. Once the knee joint torques are

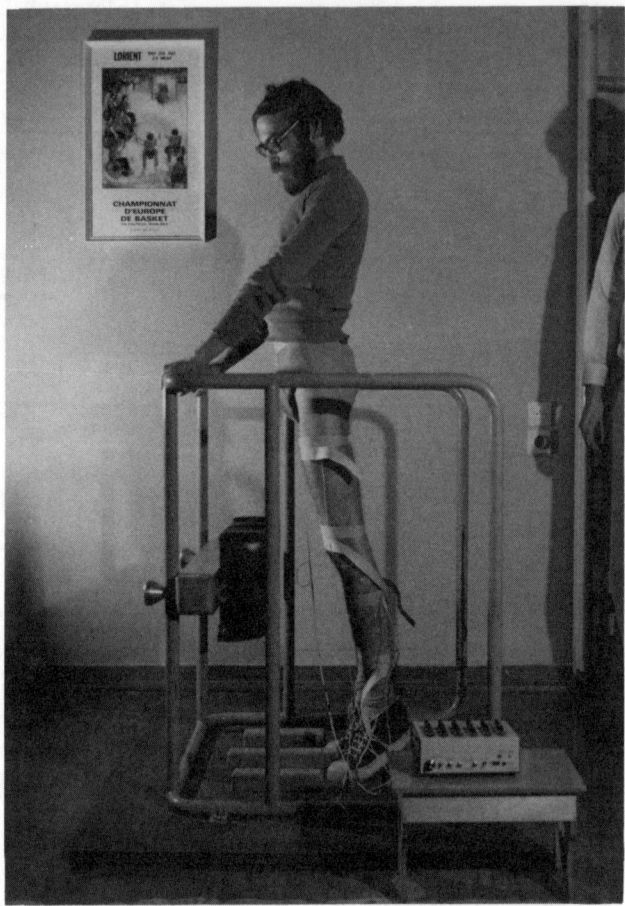

FIGURE 35. Paraplegic patient, while standing on his toes, with the stimulated plantar flexors.

reduced because of fatigue, knee buckling results. In most patients, one leg fatigues faster, the knee bending starts at this side first being a sign that the patient must sit-down. During the first few weeks of standing training, the patient should be placed in front of a body size mirror providing visual feedback of posture during standing. Attempts have also been made to use continuous feedback of patient's pelvis vertical position and also of the location of ground reaction vector. These preliminary investigations rose the hopes that in the future, the patient's ability of standing may be, because of feedback and other refinements in stimulation control, further improved.[53]

A. Supporting Frames for FES Standing

Most patients achieve standing times of up to 30 to 60 min and more. For incorporating FES standing into patient's daily life activities, in 1981, we proposed a design of a wheelchair-attached folding frame.[54] The hardware is allowing the patient to propel himself in the wheelchair without hindrance to the desired location (Figure 36). Once there, he is able to stand-up by means of FES and, during standing, to perform some manipulation tasks using one hand, while the other is utilized for maintaining the balance. In Figure 37a and b, the patient is shown prepared for standing-up and finally, while standing with the help of one arm support only. The benefits of standing and possible functional daily use of FES standing

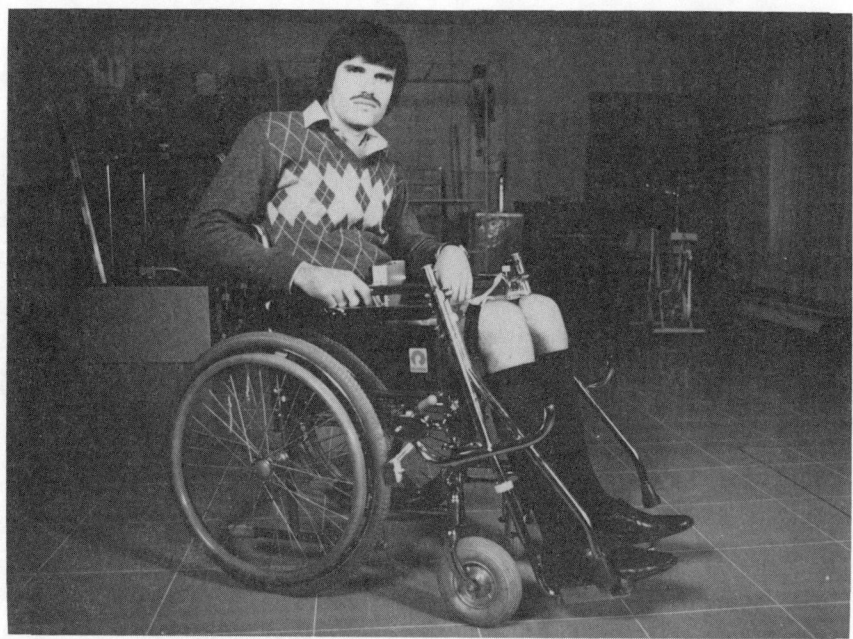

FIGURE 36. Wheelchair attached supporting frame while folded.

are described in the following chapter. There are numerous possible designs for the wheelchair-attached frame. The challenge of the search for the most appropriate design is still not completed. The most important requirements for such frame are simplicity, lightweight, simple use, fast setting and folding, and safe support. The wheelchair-attached folding frame should be attached in a simple way to the wheelchair.

In our case, it is inserted into the hand rest holes and therefore, built around the hand rest sides. In the latter case, the frame does not interfere with the wheelchair's regular use and storing. The patient himself can, for example, without any help, fold the wheelchair and store it on the back seat of the car.

B. Posture Dependence of Standing Performance

Considering the explanations and finding of the section describing the mechanics of standing, it is more than evident that the standing ability of a patient depends on two main factors: posture and muscle force with associated fatiguing. Here, we are going to elaborate in more detail the performance of patient's standing. The abilities of eight patients were compared and the quantitative results studied.[55] In Table 5, patients' general data are presented. Two standing patients, one with adequate and the other with unsatisfactory posture are presented in Figure 38a and b. Maximal standing times for the patients studied are presented in Figure 39. One may expect, after considering Figure 38, that patients being able to perform long-lasting standing would have the highest muscle strength, displaying also some extension spasticity providing additional support. The patients' muscle strength was assessed through maximal isometric knee joint torques measurements. For the evaluation of the knee extensor spasticity, relaxation indices were measured (Figure 40a, b). The patients 1, 2, 3, and 7 had the strongest m. quadriceps muscles, while the patients 2 and 5 demonstrated substantial spasticity. In contrast, patients 7 and 8 had almost no spasticity and patients 3 and 6 only moderate spasticity as depicted in Figure 40b. It is also interesting to note that the knee bending joint torque measured was, in all the patients, relatively low,

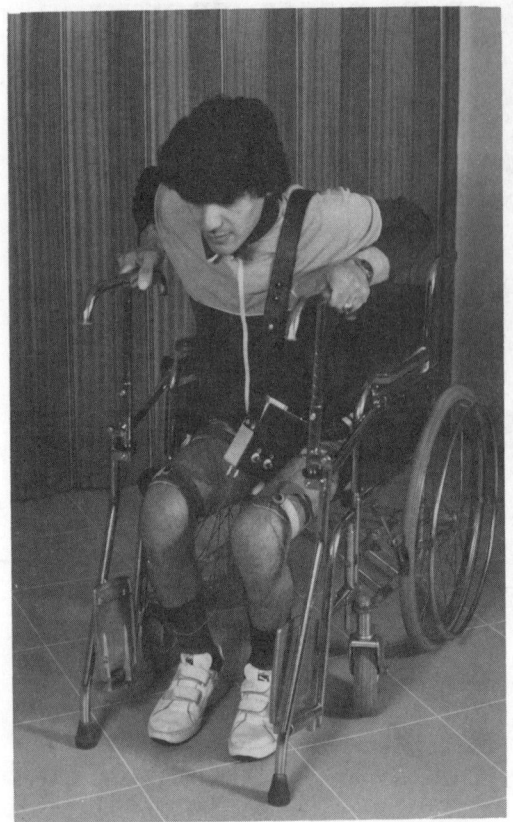 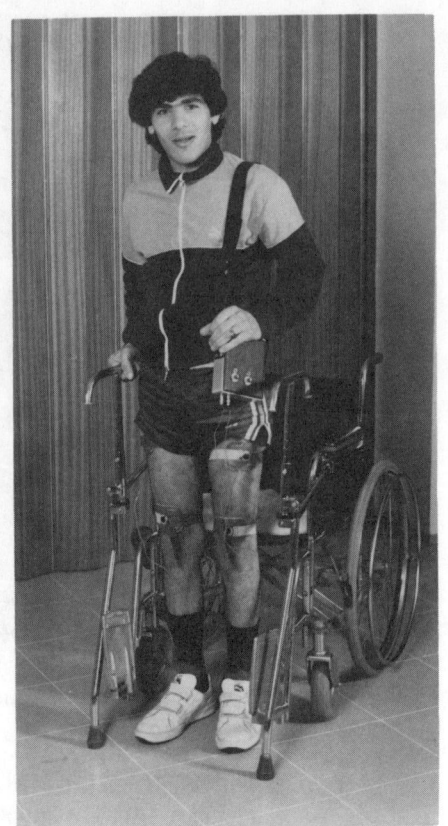

a   b

FIGURE 37. Complete paraplegic patient while standing-up (a) and while standing with the help of the two-channel electrical stimulator (b).

Table 5
GENERAL DATA ON PARAPLEGIC SUBJECTS PARTICIPATING IN FES STANDING ASSESSMENT

No.	Sex	Age	SCI level	Time past injury (months)	Accident	Time of FES training (months)
1	M	19	T-3	29	MVA[a]	21
2	M	31	T-11	118	MVA	3
3	M	20	T-11	11	Fall	9
4	M	50	T-5	39	GSW[b]	5
5	M	46	C-6	53	Fall	12
6	M	26	T-8	65	MVA	17
7	M	20	T-5	19	MVA	17
8	M	26	T-5,6	29	MVA	24

[a] MVA — motor vehicle accident.
[b] GSW — gun shot wound.

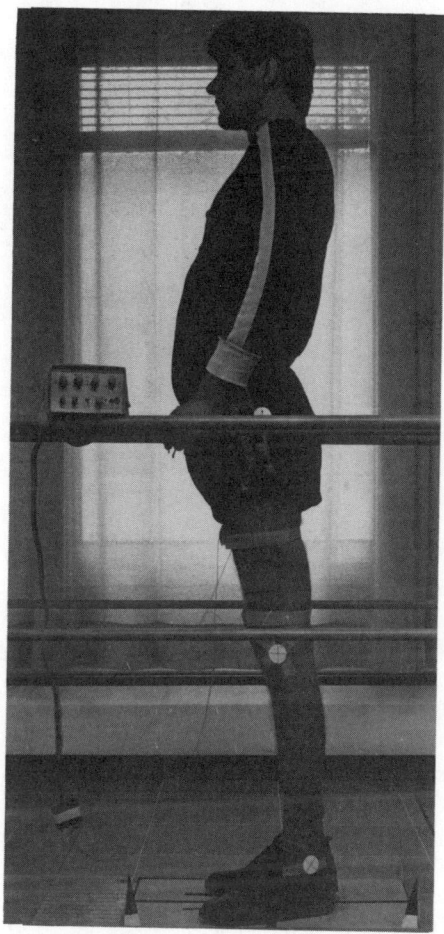 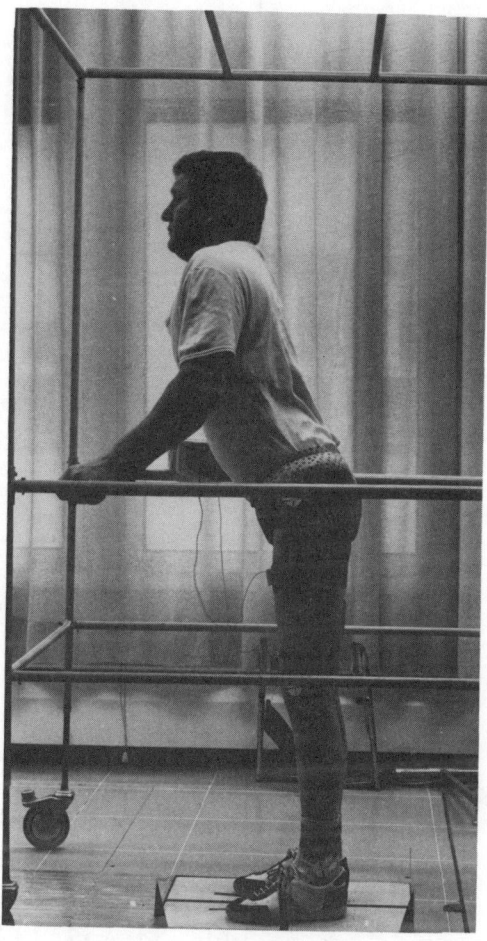

FIGURE 38. Adequate standing posture (a) and unsatisfactory aligned standing (b).

while standing did not exceed 10 Nm, except in patient 7 where the torque of 20 Nm was measured. There was no correlation found between the measured knee bending torque and maximal standing time. Also, the amount of the body weight supported by the legs does not correlate with the standing time performance. Patients 4 to 8 were able to support nearly 100% of their body weight by their legs only, nevertheless only patients 7 and 8 were performing standing successfully. Considering the results in Figure 41a and b, it seems that only patients with low horizontal reaction forces ranging around 10 N and having low ankle joint torques are good candidates for standing. These are patients 7 and 8. Comparing the standing performance in Figure 39 and the results of Figure 41, good correlation is evident. It appears that the biomechanical parameters of posture are most important for the long standing time achievement. Well-aligned standing with low values of the torques in all three joints is a prerequisite for good standing in paraplegic patients. It was found that the ankle joint torque is the most significant parameter in evaluation of paraplegic patient's standing, as this joint represents the contact of standing body with the ground. It is therefore not difficult to realize that any ankle joint stabilization by mechanical bracing may significantly prolong the maximal standing time. Here, we have further evidence that ankle joint stabi-

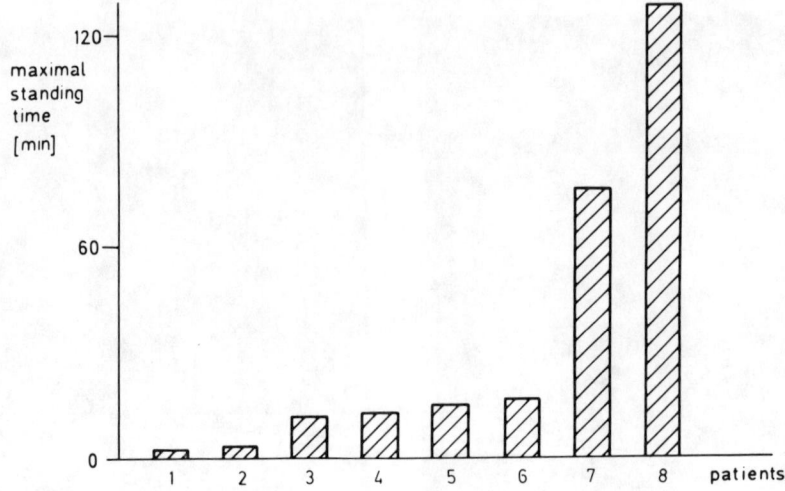

FIGURE 39. Maximal standing times as measured in a group of eight patients.

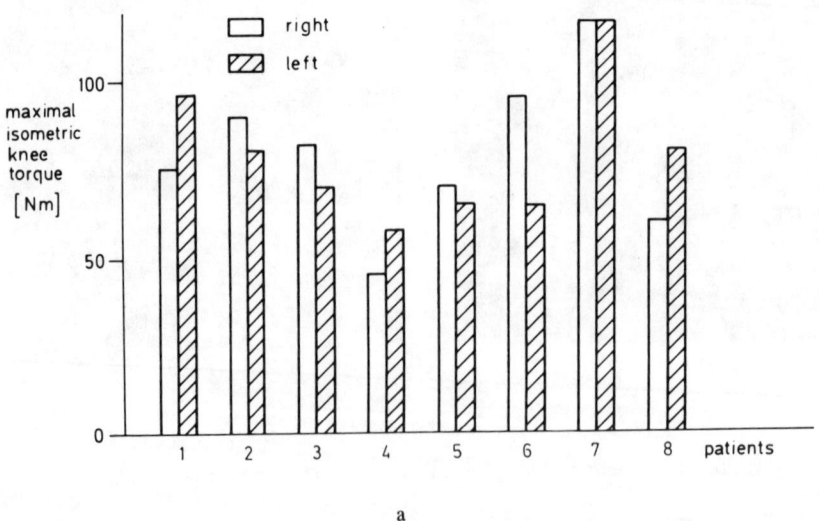

FIGURE 40. Maximal isometric knee joint torques (a) and relaxation indices (b) in a group of eight patients in whom standing performance was evaluated.

lization by means of FES of m. soleus may improve standing performance and increase the standing time.

C. Posture Switching

Utilizing the principles of upright standing with different postures as discussed in Section II, one may wonder whether these biomechanical findings may improve performance if introduced into FES standing. In 1982,[7,56] it was proposed to use the posture switching principle for prolonging standing in paraplegic patients using FES. By employing this principle, the standing times can be prolonged three to five times because the stimulated muscles are cyclically activated in a pattern displaying low fatiguing. The postures given in Figure 12 are utilized. An adequate sequence of postures is provided by cyclical stimulation of

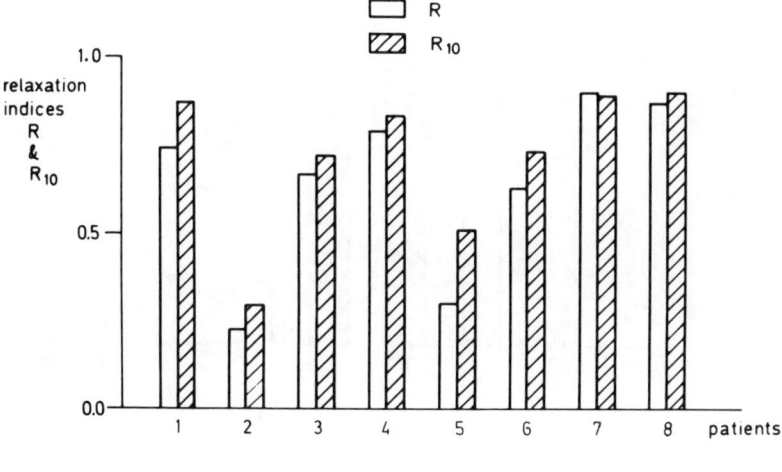

FIGURE 40b.

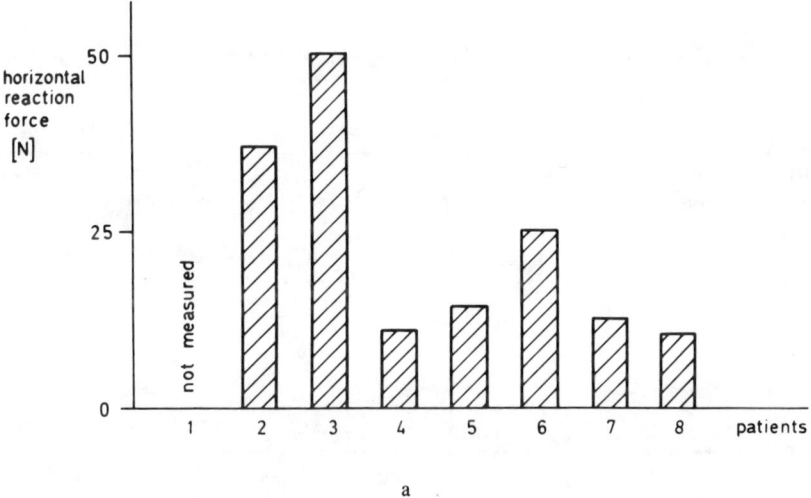

FIGURE 41. Horizontal reaction forces (a) and ankle joint torques (b) in a group of eight paraplegic patients.

muscles with prolonged resting times in between the stimulation sequences. Taking into account the findings from muscle restrengthening, it is evident that considerably decreased fatiguing is taking place. In Figure 42, a record of posture switching obtained by exchanging intermittently the postures of Figure 12a and b is presented. The upper trace in Figure 42 is presenting the on-time stimulation of plantar flexors and knee extensors. The F_z and F_y traces are showing the vertical and horizontal (sagittal plane) ground reaction forces for a 70 kg body weight patient with complete T-5,6 car accident lesion. The F_z record displays that almost 60 N of body weight was supported by the help of arms. During and shortly after the switching transitions, the arms supported about 12 kg of the body mass. All the transitions are clearly displayed also in the magnitude of the horizontal F_y shear force, changing from 40 N during m. soleus and m. gastrocnemius stimulation to an average of about 5 N for m. quadriceps standing. The F_y force is counterbalanced by the arm forces. At the exchange of postures, the point of ground reaction vector application was displaced

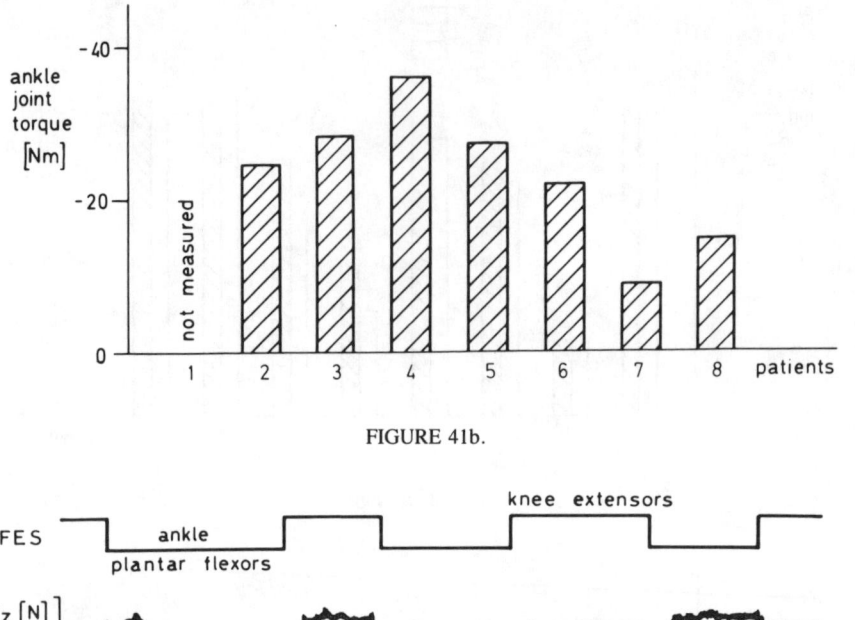

FIGURE 41b.

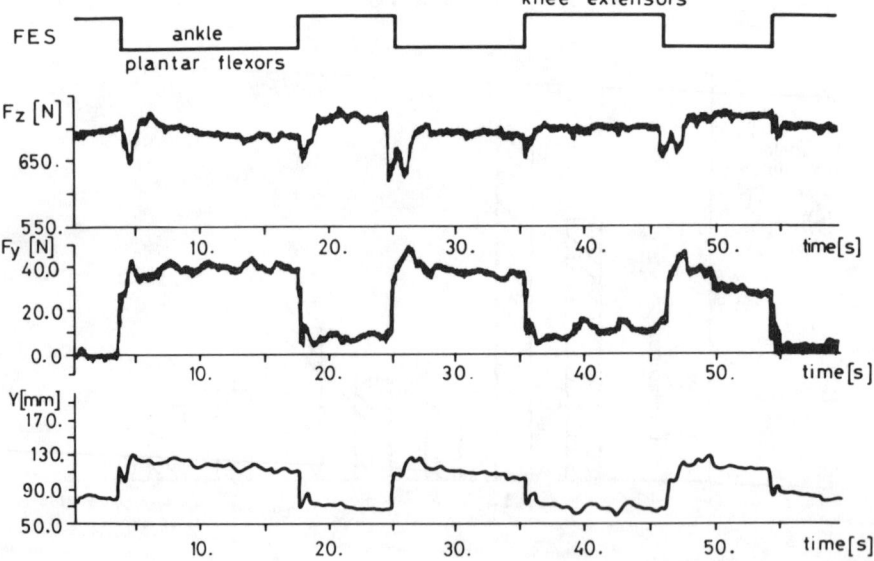

FIGURE 42. Force plate record of posture switching when patient was, by himself, controlling the switching of stimulation from knee extensors to ankle joint plantar flexors.

for about 40 mm. The latter is nicely seen from the bottom trace Y. During posture switching, FES was controlled by the patient himself. He had a switch in his hand. When pressed, m. soleus and m. gastrocnemius FES was on and while released, the m. quadriceps stimulation was switched on bilaterally. Studies of automatic posture switching were also performed.[56] Namely, the improvements of FES systems toward less involvement of patient or even toward nearly subconscious use are the ultimate goal. The main question related to automatic posture switching was whether the patient will be able to maintain his upright posture in case FES switching will take place randomly and without his knowledge. In Figure 43, posture switching is demonstrated where FES was switched randomly and the patient was not aware when the switching was going to take place. Comparison of Figures 42 and 43 strikes for similarity. All the traces show comparable time courses. The most noticeable difference is in trace Y. Here, the oscillation of the application of the ground reaction vector in the posterior-anterior direction occurred after each transition during random posture switch-

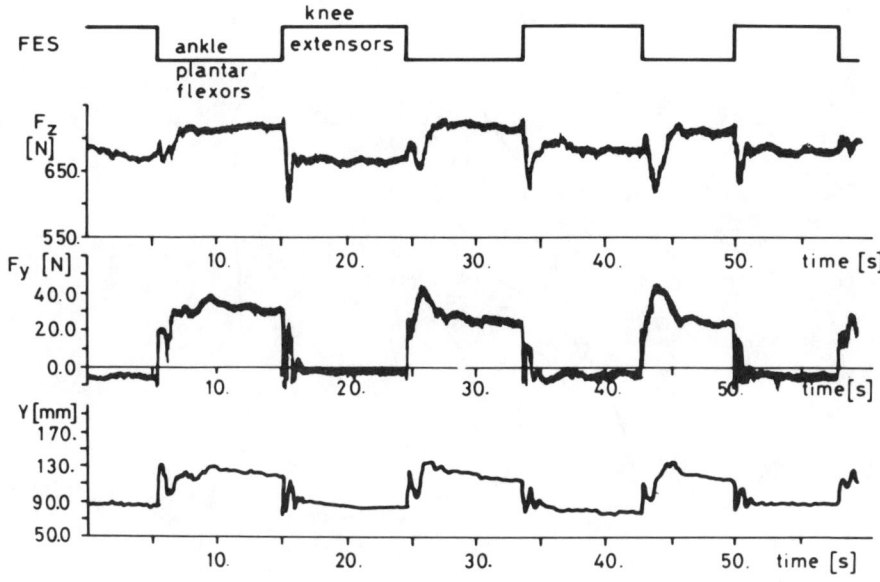

FIGURE 43. Force plate record of randomly performed posture switching.

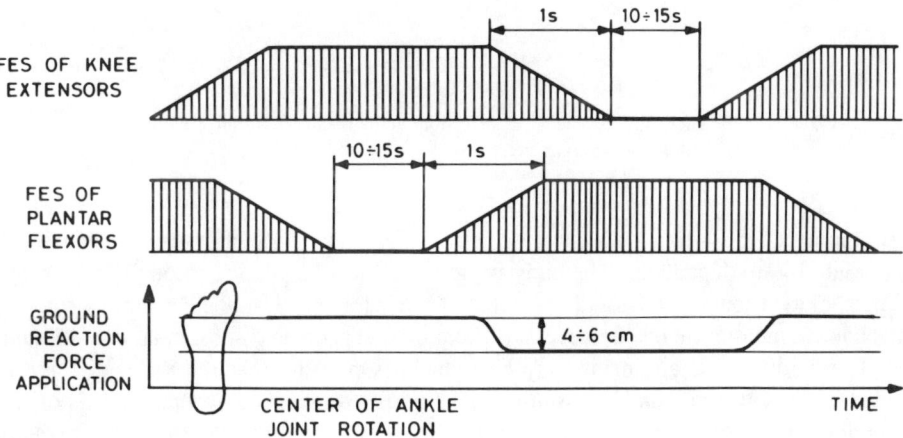

FIGURE 44. Ramped switching between knee extensors and ankle plantar flexors during exchange of postures.

ing. This represents an evidence of the stabilization efforts carried out by the patient through trunk shifting and arm forces.

When standing postures are exchanged, at the very instance of transition from one posture into another, it is necessary to exchange gradually also the electrical stimulation between the muscle groups. Here, the timing is important, because if, e.g., the m. quadriceps stimulation is switched off, instantly collapsing of the subject may occur. Obviously, the FES transition must be carried out smoothly, by ramped stimulation sequences belonging to the appropriate muscles as shown in Figure 44. Correct overlapping of stimulation sequences must be ensured. The m. quadriceps activity must remain present until the new posture is assumed and the m. soleus and gastrocnemius stimulation reach a safe level. At this time, falling of the m. quadriceps stimulation starts. Rising of m. soleus and m. gastrocnemius electrical stimulation is not critical (assuming knees extended), while the

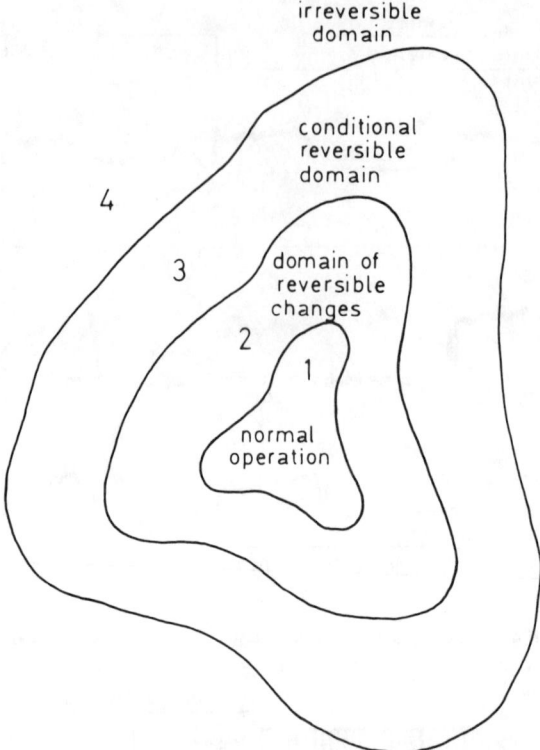

FIGURE 45. Domains of reversible and irreversible conditions in living systems.

precise moment for starting with decrease of m. quadriceps stimulation is biomechanically critical and posture dependent. The body weight line must be passing through or in front of the knee joint instantaneous rotation center. To ensure the described posture switching, biomechanical measurements are necessary, requiring sensors and substantial control equipment. The hardware requirements may be reduced supposing that the knee joint is fully extended. In the latter case and by assuming the hip joint is in locked hyperextended position, the standing model of a man can be simplified by an inverted pendulum.[57,58,61] It was our aim to determine minimal hardware and simplest control circuitry necessary for control of posture switching. McGuinness et al.[59] have shown that for an inverted pendulum model the knowledge of the time history of ankle angle can be used to determine the shear force and also (because of relatively low dynamics during standing) the point of ground reaction force application. We can therefore conclude that for controlling the FES sequences for posture exchanging as proposed in Figure 12a and b, one may measure the ankle angle or the point of ground reaction force application. The FES control of posture transitions when hip and knee joints are not locked is more complex and requires additional sensors and decision making.[60] This control knowledge will be in future FES devices stored in the memory of the microprocessor-based controller.

V. BENEFITS OF FES STANDING

Living systems have adopted different autodiagnosing and self-repair properties into their functional schemes. It is not difficult to realize that for autodiagnosing functions different body sensors are providing various forms of information. In general, the domain (Figure 45) of safe or normal operation for a living system can be described as being surrounded by a second outer domain where operation, while exerted over a longer time period, may cause a damage. After sufficient time, the self-repair mechanisms in most cases may completely restore the damage. In this region of operation, reversible changes are caused to the system. When the living system is operating under longer-lasting and stronger stress, the operation takes place in the conditional reversible domain and irreversible or pathological damages are provoked. Living systems when operating in this third domain still have the ability to readapt and often recover to a certain degree, so that the operation after damage is still as close as possible to the normal operation. The latter can happen when favourable restoration process is started and necessary boundary conditions are fulfilled, for example, like in cardiac arrest, if sufficient fluid and oxygen are administered, the damage to the heart muscle may be minimized and the short term operation in the third domain may not be fatal. This conditional reversible domain is encompassed by the irreversible domain of the system operation, where, once operation sets in, the system will not recover under any circumstances.

In an injury and, particularly, after spinal cord damage, because of multiple trauma, sensory loss, disturbances in autonomous nervous system, and malfunctioning of different organs, the regions of safe and reversible operations are reduced. For each particular state of body operation, one can envisage a given point in the domain of operation. This point can be described by a multidimensional vector with the components which are variables of time and are representing numerous parameters influencing the homeostatic regulation in a living system, e.g., blood pressure, pCO_2, pO_2, glucose in blood, body liquid equilibrium, pressure to skin, etc.). The question raised in medicine is which components of vector should be changed in order that a good prognosis and fast recovery may take place. One can also influence the size of the domain and thus, create a situation where even a very prolonged operation in the domain of reversible changes or in the conditional reversible domain may not cause severe damage.

In SCI, the latter possibility seems to be important immediately after the injury during the acute treatment. Any changes, reducing the environmental stress, which are at the same time also favourable with regard to the components of the vector in order to increase the region of the reversible domain are beneficial from the recovery point of view. Let us, in this aspect, critically consider the standing exercise and its benefits to spinal cord injured patients. The human system is built predominantly for upright posture and therefore, prolonged sitting or supine position are, in the long run, not preferable positions. Prolonged sitting is therefore degrading all the mechanisms responsible for physiological benefits associated with upright standing. Prolonged sitting is, for instance, forcing the bladder and kidney in a position where drainage, urine flow, and voiding are rendered difficult. Continuous sitting for years, like many SCI patients are forced to, does with time lead to physiological changes and pathological degradation of the body functions which are in normals maintained and reinforced by the upright position. Before we shall in detail describe some of these functions, it is essential to note that standing by any assistive means is beneficial to break this pathological degradation when the upright posture is maintained for a given minimal time period daily. At present, exact quantitative data for determining this minimal time for each patient are not yet available. Also to note is that active (FES-assisted) upright standing seems to be, at least subjectively, more beneficial as passive standing (calipers). We believe that FES-enabled standing-up and standing has physiological advantages in comparison with passive standing in long leg braces. In addition, there are psychological factors to be considered as well. For a SCI patient, it is very important to maintain his physical fitness and the integrity of all physiological body structures. Therefore, any factors influencing pathological developments must be minimized (in order to provide safe operation in domain 2 or even 3). All this requires from the patient considerable self-discipline and

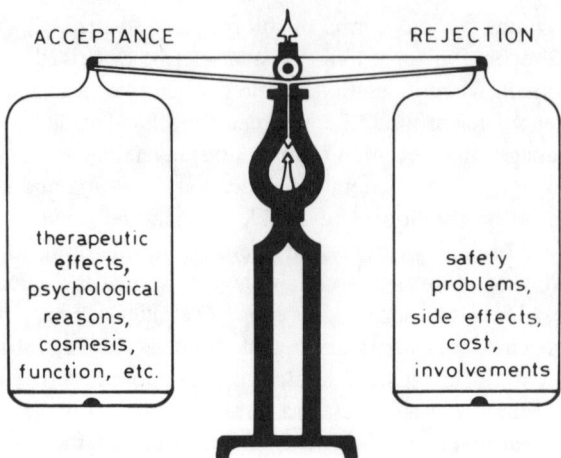

FIGURE 46. The "scale" presentation of the acceptance/rejection problem for assistive devices.

Table 6
PHYSIOLOGICAL ADVANTAGES OF FES ENABLED STANDING

Maintains muscle trophic properties
Utilizes active power from paralyzed muscles, improves blood flow, and activates cardiopulmonary system
Prevents disuse atrophy and contractures
Prevents losses of bone calcium
Prevents hypercalciuria
Prevents urinary system calculi
Maintains bone and joints functions
Provides daily exercising for maintaining adequate joints ROM
Augments blood circulation and hence, prevents blood pooling in the venous system
Favourably assists skin integrity
Prevents pressure sores development
Maintains and reinforces upright balance reflexes
Augments bladder and bowel function (decreased residual volume)
Maintains fitness of body without additional training for possible future FES use in gait
Reduces exaggerated muscular tone and extreme spasticity
Promotes in a natural way activation of most trunk muscles

starts, with time, to be a burden so that daily standing exercise is disliked by many patients. Consequently, after the discharge from the rehabilitation institution, the patients do not practice standing regularly.

Placement of feet on the wheelchair foot rests is rather sloppy and inadequate. Some paraplegic patients are using shoes with high heels, some are changing their wheelchairs and do not pay attention to the foot-rest adjustment. In a short time, under the described circumstances, irreversible pathological changes take place, such as plantar flexion contractures, hip flexion contractures, and, in the worst case, also pressure sores. Joints with limited ROM are very prone to ossification because of absent movement, contracted muscles, and spasms. The patient's physiological and physical status is degrading. On the other side, we must be aware that any exercising or use of assistive devices which requires time-consuming daily involvement is soon disliked by the patients. Patients tolerance with respect to devices varies. The decision about patient's acceptance of a device in the long run is a difficult task. Figure 46 illustrates simply the acceptance problem. Note that the final judging about a rehabilitation device is performed by the patient himself. Therefore, the FES system must be designed functionally so that major functions are provided to the patient without

Table 7
PSYCHOLOGICAL FACTORS ASSOCIATED TO FES STANDING

Paralyzed muscles are reactivated changing patient's image of paralysis
No external mechanical bracing is required
Cosmetic appearance
Almost normal standing as in healthy subject
Standing-up procedure is very similar to healthy subjects' standing-up
Possible standing at any time and any place
Possible socializing with healthy subjects in equal standing position
Permanently on disposal for functional use

time-consuming donning, adjusting, and doffing procedures. In addition, the system should be cosmetic and should provide to the patient a feeling of being with the rehabilitative system more like a nonparalyzed subject.

Any rehabilitation or training modality being able to minimize the cost, patient's involvement, and, at the same time, improving cosmesis and functional issues is very likely to be accepted by the patients. FES standing, in particular when considering the application of the implanted stimulation systems, has no comparable device in respect to its function and cosmesis. In the next few paragraphs, the benefits of FES standing will be described and brief comments with regard to comparison with other assistive devices will be made. The most significant difference between FES and KAFO standing is active use of paralyzed muscles during FES standing. Standing in KAFO is more stable because of the locked ankle joints and sometimes also locked hip joints. FES standing is demanding for the patient because of constant balancing in ankle joints, maintaining of stable trunk position in space, and keeping the hips in hyperextension. Therefore, the low back musculature must be activated. The obvious disadvantage of KAFOs is difficult donning and doffing, standing-up, and constant danger for developing pressure sores. KAFOs are also custom made and require adjustments to changes in body weight. The FES donning and doffing is simpler and will be further simplified in the future with the implanted devices. Table 6 lists the main physiological advantages of FES standing while Table 7 lists the main psychological factors playing an important role in the patient's acceptance of the orthotic means. For instance, a n. femoralis implant, providing also stimulation of hip extensors, can decrease patient's efforts for maintaining the upright posture. The described physiological advantages of FES standing and the improved functionality in the patient's daily life provoke also beneficial psychological changes. The latter is an important issue which should not be neglected. Particularly, FES-implanted system for standing may even further increase the psychological advantages listed in Tables 6 and 7. Only functional, physiological, and psychological integration may efficiently rehabilitate the patient and provide a solid start for his independent life. A wheelchair-attached folding frame is effectively utilized for balance and support. The described standing function provided by FES may be functionally utilized in daily life for executing simple tasks such as opening of a window, taking or storing an object to a high shelf in the kitchen, taking books from shelves in libraries, and for assisting transfers and other functions of daily life.[62] With abductors stimulated, the patient's stability will be further improved. Such systems are very likely to be accepted by the paraplegic subjects. For keeping balance, the patients have to depend on external means. The increased functionality by adding posture switching has not been, up to now, taken into account. Posture switching may further increase the functional use because of prolonged time of standing. In addition, FES standing increases the natural appearance of standing in man by adding the possibility of dynamic transitions like toe standing, left-right leg standing, more or less forward leaned standing, and standing-up provided by synergistic action of all three main antigravity extensor muscle groups.

Regular use of standing and standing-up with preserved voluntary controlled and FES-activated muscles is beneficial for conditioning and maintaining of the general fitness in the patient and, in particular, of his cardiopulmonary system.[63,64]

Issekutz et al.[65] performed experiments in normal subjects to document the effects of passive standing. They have demonstrated that up to 4 h of daily exercise in bed does not reduce the urine calcium which is increased because of bed resting. Also, quiet sitting for 8 h/d has no effect upon reducing the urinary levels of calcium. In contrast, 3 h of quiet standing per day are sufficient to induce a slow decline of the elevated calcium level in urine. These data illustrate how important bone loading is which can be most efficiently accomplished by weight bearing during standing. Prolonged bed rest and absent bone loading are the main causes for bone degradation in SCI patients and consequently, hypercalciuria. The calculi removed from SCI patients show both calcium and phosphorus ingredients as the principal constituents. Claus-Walker et al.[66] have shown a 46% increase in calciuria in normal men after only 3 d of bed rest. Donaldson et al.[67] have found even higher degradation of bone and have reported 83% increase of calcium in urine after 2 weeks of bed rest. Heaney,[68] Kaplan et al.,[69] and Abramson and Delagi[70] have proven the interrelation between hypercalciuria and bone loss in immobilized patients. Bone density loss and hypercalciuria are also associated with soft-tissue ossification, pathological fractures, bone osteoporoses, and urinary system calculi.[71,72] The presence of urinary calculi increases the risk of urinary and renal disfunction with possible infections. Compressive axial bone loading is beneficial and effective in reducing bone demineralization when applied in adequate extent with respect to the body weight of the subject. NASA, after discovering abnormally high losses of calcium during the Gemini space flights,[73] introduced axial loading for reducing the rate of bone loss in all later space flights.[74]

Claus-Walker et al.[66] demonstrated high increase of calcium in urine of normal subjects following only 3 d of bed rest. The same functional dependence of bed rest and hypercalciuria was proven also by other researchers (Abramson and Delagi,[70] Abramson,[71] Odeen and Knutsson,[75] Heaney,[68] Kaplan et al.,[76] Albright and Keifenstein,[77] Comar,[78] Freeman,[72] and Hattner and McMillan.[73]). In addition, the importance of standing, with respect to bladder function, was also described. Gould et al.,[79] has shown that standing increases bladder pressure which helps in training of the automatic bladder and also reduces the residual volume in the hypotonic bladder.[81-83]

In summary, FES standing is maintaining ROM[84] in all joints of lower extremities, reduces muscle spasticity because of regular stretching and afferent FES influence, further it can reduce bone calcium losses[88] hence, reducing hypercalciuria and urinary calculi, it may improve orthostatic circulatory regulation[86,87] and bladder pressure, and facilitate other beneficial physiological effects, such as maintaining upright reflex mechanisms and improved position of internal organs together with better posture of the body.

VI. FUNCTIONAL USE OF FES STANDING

If standing is to be a useful functional activity, a person must be able to rise from sitting to the standing position independently. In our investigation,[90] it has been demonstrated that successful standing-up can be achieved by using only bilateral stimulation of both knee extensor muscles. In this way, the same two-channel stimulator[89] can be applied for both prolonged standing and standing-up. Because of the lack of stability, a complete paraplegic patient (with his knees locked by FES) cannot stand without arm support. The patient will therefore use his arms also during standing-up. It can be expected that with the help of arms and preserved trunk muscles, he will be able to compensate for the torque occurring in the hip joints. As the values of ankle joint moment during standing-up of a normal subject were found very small, no stimulation is applied to plantar flexors. FES must, therefore, provide sufficient force to knee extensors so that knee joint torques will be compensated for.

The starting position for standing-up can be such as displayed in Figure 33. Here, it is

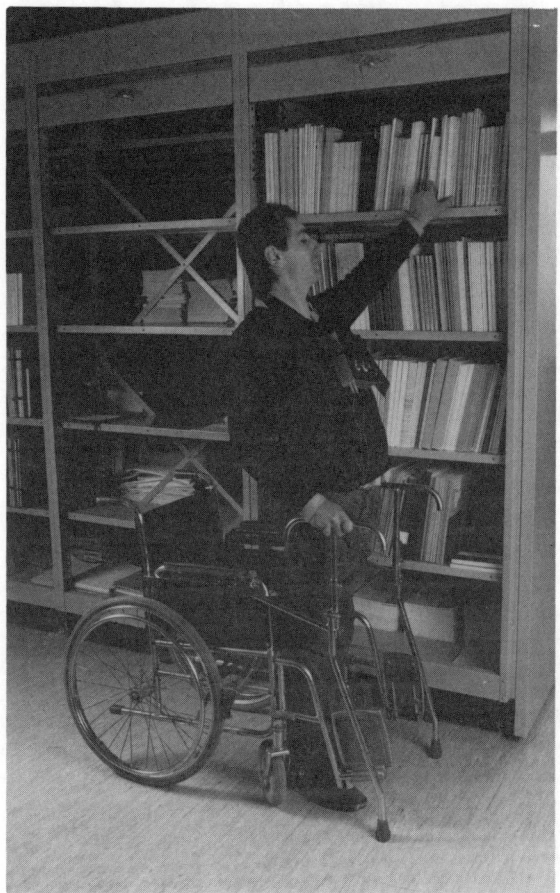

FIGURE 47. Paraplegic patient reaching a book in the library.

important that the feet are positioned backwards and the knees are pushed as much as possible forward, while the paraplegic subject is sitting on the very edge of the wheelchair. The trunk is to be leaned strongly forward which results in lesser knee joint torques which have to be compensated for by the help of two-channel knee extensors stimulation.

For rising from the wheelchair, the complete paraplegic patient can use the wheelchair-attached supporting frame. Standing-up can be performed also by the help of a solid support (a piece of furniture) for one hand and by the help of a crutch in the other hand. Paraplegic patients are usually very strong in their arms. They can often easily lift the whole body weight by their arm support only. There is, therefore, another standing-up maneuver possible for the completely paralyzed paraplegic subjects. Here, the knees are first locked by the help of bilateral stimulation of knee extensors. A paraplegic patient starts standing-up with both legs fully extended. He must then lift the body to the erect position by the help of arms only. With preserved trunk and pelvic muscles, he must bring the feet somewhat backwards (aligned with the hand support). This standing-up maneuver can be performed in parallel bars or by the help of two crutches and is similar to KAFO standing-up.

The tasks, that can be carried out by the help of the described rehabilitation system (stimulator and supporting frame) can be divided into two major groups: reaching objects out of reach from the wheelchair and different transfers from the wheelchair.[62,85] In Figure 47, a paraplegic patients is shown using the rehabilitation system in a library. Similar situations occur in kitchen (Figure 48), self-service markets, at the high counters in banks

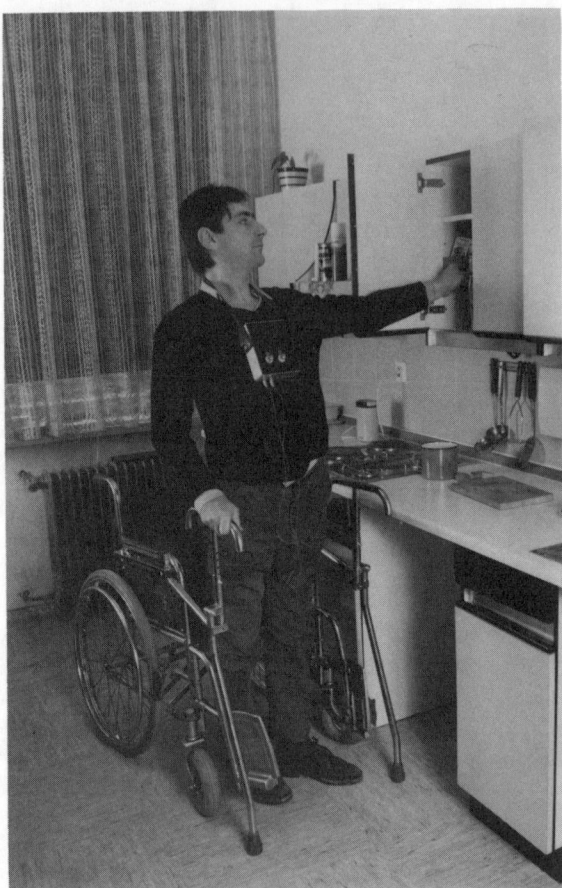

FIGURE 48. Paraplegic patient performing a simple task in the kitchen.

(Figure 49) and post offices, while opening or closing the windows, while trying to reach the doorbell, light or lift switches, or when attempting to perform other simple tasks.

In Figure 50, transfer from wheelchair to the toilet is shown. Paraplegic patient is often caught in a bathroom which is narrow and not adapted for wheelchair users. Patient can enter through the door and stand-up by the help of the two-channel stimulator and supporting frame. Next, the patient can turn around himself in a similar way as in parallel bars. By switching off the stimulator paraplegic can sit-down on the toilet. Similarly, transfers to the chair in theater or cinema, to the car, and to the crutches can be accomplished.

When sitting-down, the paraplegic patients are using three different maneuvers. The paraplegic subject can switch off the stimulator and assist sitting-down by the help of arm support. In another type of sitting-down, the patient makes a rapid sway of the trunk backwards, while the stimulation remains switched on. When the center of gravity of the body is suddenly transferred from the central line, the knee joint torque is increased. The stimulation of knee extensors can no more counterbalance this external torque and the subject is seated. When he is already sitting, the legs go into extended position. The patient must switch off the stimulator and place the legs in normal sitting position. Some patients make the transition from the standing to the sitting position with the legs fully extended in the same way as when using calipers. This sitting-down procedure requires more arm activity than the previously described maneuvers.

Paraplegic subjects find standing by the help of FES and wheelchair-attached supporting

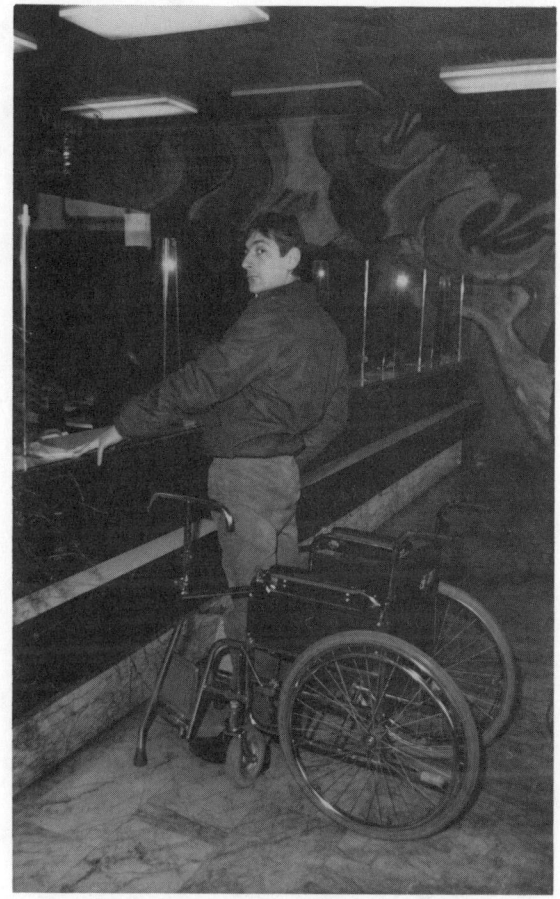

FIGURE 49. Paraplegic patient at a high counter in the bank.

frame useful in many other simple tasks and activities associated with their employment and recreation, not the least important is standing in the barroom as presented in Figure 51.

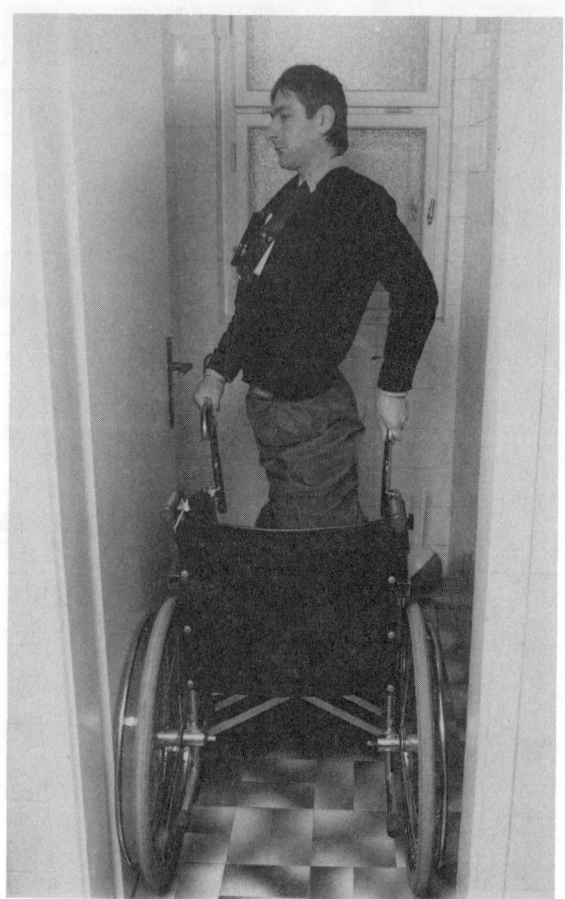

FIGURE 50. Transfer from wheelchair to the toilet.

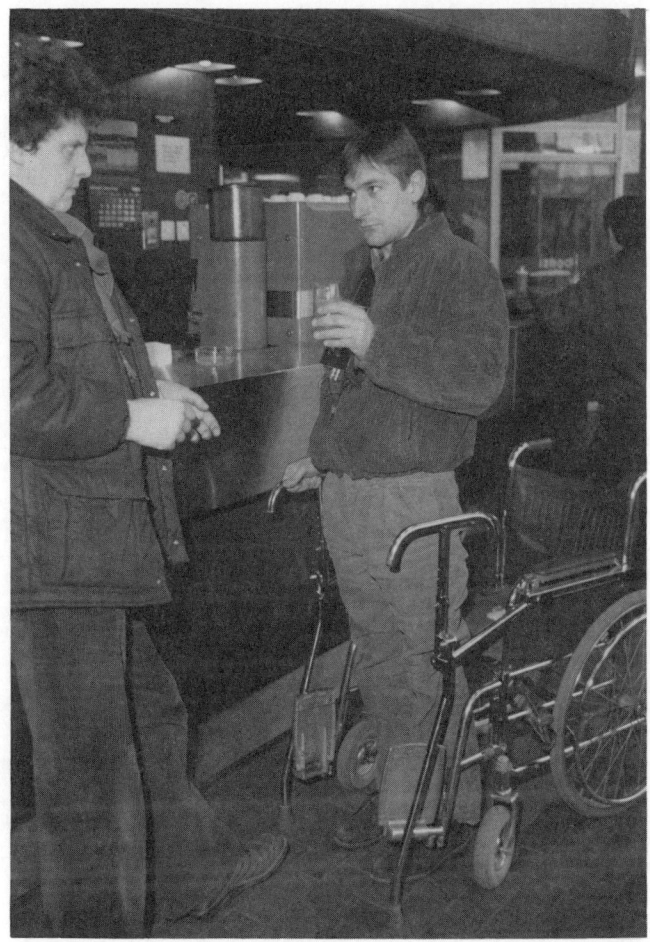

FIGURE 51. Paraplegic subject standing in a barroom.

REFERENCES

1. **Sears, F., Zemansky, M., and Young, M.,** *College Physics,* Addison-Wesley, Reading, Mass., 1980.
2. **Frankel, V. and Burstein, A.,** *Orthopaedic Biomechanics,* Lea & Febiger, Philadelphia, 1971.
3. **Winter, D.,** *Biomechanics of Human Movement,* John Wiley & Sons, New York, 1979.
4. **Stallard, J.,** Mechanics allied to orthoses, *Physiotherapy,* 63, 84, 1977.
5. **Rose, G. K.,** Orthoses for the severely handicapped — rational for empirical choice, *Physiotherapy,* 66, 76, 1980.
6. **Rodgers, M. and Cavanagh, P.,** Glossary of biomechanical terms, concepts, and units, *Phys. Ther.,* 64, 1886, 1984.
7. **Kralj, A., Jaeger, R., and Bajd, T.,** Posture switching enables prolonged standing in paraplegic patient functionally electrically stimulated, in *Proc. 5th Annu. RESNA Conf.,* RESNA Association for the Advancement of Rehabilitation Technology, Washington, D.C., 1982, 60.
8. **Perry, J.,** Cerebral palsy gait, in *Orthopaedic Aspects of Cerebral Palsy,* Samilson, R. L., Ed., J. B. Lippincott, Co., NY, 1975, chap. 4B.
9. **Powell, G. and Dzendolet, E.,** Power spectral density analysis of lateral human standing sway, *J. Motor Behav.,* 16, 424, 1984.
10. **Dietz, V., Mauritz, K., and Dichgaus, J.,** Body oscillations in balancing due to segmental stretch reflex activity, *Exp. Brain Res.,* 40, 89, 1980.

11. **Watanabe, I. and Okubo, J.**, The role of the plantar mechanoreceptor in equilibrium control, *Ann. N.Y. Acad. Sci.*, 81, 855, 1981.
12. **Paulus, W., Straube, A., and Brandt, T.**, Visual stabilization of posture, *Brain*, 107, 1143, 1984.
13. **Nashner, L.**, Strategies for organization of human posture, in *Vestibular and Visual Control on Posture and Locomotor Equilibrium*, Igarashi, M. and Black, F., Eds., S. Karger, Basel, 1983, 1.
14. **Kralj, A.**, Electrical stimulation of lower extremities in spinal cord injury, in *Spinal Cord Injury Medical Engineering*, Ghista, D. and Frankel, H., Eds., Charles C Thomas, Springfield, Illinois, 1986, chap. 21.
15. **Nashner, L. and McCollum, G.**, The organization of human postural movements: a formal basis and experimental synthesis, *Int. J. Behav. Brain Sci.*, 8, 135, 1985.
16. **Fick, R.**, *Handbuch der Anatomie und Mechanik der Gelenke*, Jena Verlag von Gustav Fischer, Jena, 1910.
17. **Forssberg, H. and Nashner, L.**, Ontogenetic development of postural control in man: adaptation to altered support and visual conditions during stance, *J. Neurosci.*, 2, 545, 1982.
18. **Stockwell, C.**, Conceptual model of human postural control, in *Vestibular and Visual Control on Posture and Locomotor Equilibrium*, Igarashi, M. and Black, F., Eds., S. Karger, Basel, 1983, 22.
19. **Kralj, A. and Jaeger, R.**, Analysis of standing-up and sitting-down in human subjects: establishment of standard technology, *J. Biomech.*, 1988, submitted.
20. **Kralj, A. and Grobelnik, S.**, Functional electrical stimulation — a new hope for paraplegic patients, *Bul. Prosthet. Res.*, BPR-10-20, Fall, 75, 1973.
21. **Seireg, A. and Arvikar, R.**, A mathematical model for evaluation of forces in lower extremities of the musculo-skeletal system, *J. Biomech.*, 6, 313, 1973.
22. **Crouninshield, R. and Brand, R.**, A physiologically based criterion of muscle force prediction in locomotion, *J. Biomech.*, 14, 793, 1981.
23. **Perry, J.**, Rehabilitation of spasticity, in *Spasticity, Disordered Motor Control*, Feldman, R. G., Young, R. R., and Koella, W. P., Eds., New Book Medical Publishers, Chicago, 1981, 87.
24. **Lukert, B.**, Osteoporosis — a review and update, *Arch. Phys. Med. Rehabil.*, 63, 480, 1982.
25. **Orzel, J. and Rudd, T.**, Heterotopic bone formation: clinical laboratory, and imaging correlation, *J. Nucl. Med.*, 26, 125, 1985.
26. **Rafii, M., Firoosnia, M., Golimbu, C., and Sokolow, J.**, Bilateral acetabular stress fractures in a paraplegic patient, *Arch. Phys. Med. Rehabil.*, 63, 240, 1982.
27. **Hemami, H. and Jaswa, V.**, On a three link model of the dynamics of standing up and sitting down, *IEEE Trans. Syst. Man Cybernet.*, 8, 115, 1978.
28. **Koozekanani, S., Barin, K., McGhee, R., and Chang, H.**, A recursive free-body approach to computer simulation of human postural dynamics, *IEEE Trans. Biomed. Eng.*, 30, 787, 1983.
29. **Pauwels, F.**, *Biomechanics of the Locomotor Apparatus*, Springer-Verlag, Berlin, 1980.
30. **Roux, W.**, *Gesammelte Abhandlungen über Entwicklungsmechanik der Organismen*, Leipzig, Wilhelm Engelmann, 1895.
31. **Burstein, A., Currey, J., Frankel, H., and Reilly, D.**, The ultimate properties of bone tissue: the effects of yielding, *J. Biomech.*, 5, 35, 1972.
32. **Chamay, A.**, Mechanical and morphological aspects of experimental overload and fatigue in bone, *J. Biomech.*, 3, 263, 1970.
33. **Carter, D.**, Bone compressive strength: the influence of density and strain rate, *Science*, 194, 1174, 1976.
34. **Alle, W., Piotrowski, G., Burstein, A., and Frankel, V.**, Biomechanical principles of intramedullary fixation, *Clin. Orthop. Relat. Res.*, 60, 13, 1986.
35. **Bertolini, R. and Leutert, G.**, Atlas der Anatomie des Menschen — nach systematischen und topographischen Gesichtspunkten, *Band I: Arm und Bein*, VEB Georg Thieme, Leipzig, 1978.
36. **James, H., Vincent, L., and Blair, C.**, Functional muscle partitioning during voluntary movement: fascial muscle activity for speech, *Exp. Neurol.*, 85, 469, 1984.
37. **Russel, C. J., Dunbar, D. C., Ruchmer, D. A., Macpherson, I. M., and Philips, J. O.**, Differential activity of innervation subcompartments of cat lateral gastrocnemius during natural movements, *Soc. Neurosci. Abstr.*, 8, 948, 1982.
38. **Mauritz, K., Dietz, V., and Haller, M.**, Balancing as a clinical test in the differential diagnosis of sensorymotor disorders, *J. Neurol. Neurosurg. Psychiatry*, 43, 407, 1980.
39. **Mauritz, K., Dichgaus, J., and Hufschmidt, A.**, Quantitative analysis of stance in late cortical cerebellar atrophy of the anterior lobe and other forms of cerebellar ataxia, *Brain*, 102, 461, 1979.
40. **Prost, J.**, Varieties of human posture, *Hum. Biol.*, 46, 1, 1974.
41. **Baron, J.**, History of posturography, in *Vestibular and Visual Control on Posture and Locomotor Equilibrium*, Igarashi, M. and Black, F., Eds., S. Karger, Basel, 1983, 54.
42. **Kralj, A.**, Optimum coordination and selection of muscles for functional electrical stimulation, in Proc. 8th Int. Conf. Med. Biol. Eng., Chicago, 1969, 7-7.
43. **Patriarco, A., Mann, R., Simon, S., and Mansour, J.**, An evaluation of the approaches of optimisation models in the prediction of muscle forces during human gait, *J. Biomech.*, 14, 513, 1981.

44. **Dul, J., Townsend, M., Shiari, R., and Johnson, G.**, Muscular synergism I. On criteria for load sharing between synergistic muscles, *J. Biomech.*, 17, 663, 1984.
45. **Dul, J., Johnson, G., Shiari, R., and Townsend, M.**, Muscular synergism II. A minimum-fatigue criterion for load sharing between synergistic muscles, *J. Biomech.*, 17, 675, 1984.
46. **Kralj, A., Bajd, T., Turk, R., Krajnik, J., and Benko, H.**, Gait restoration in paraplegic patients: a feasibility demonstration using multichannel surface electrode FES, *J. Rehabil., R & D*, 20, 3, 1983.
47. **Schoneberger, W.**, *Guidelines for Physiological Monitoring in Physical Therapy*, Rancho Los Amigos Hospital, Univ. of Southern California, Los Angeles, 1981.
48. **Guttman, L.**, *Spinal Cord Injuries — Comprehensive Management and Research*, Blackwell Scientific Publications, Oxford, 1973.
49. **Bedbrook, G. M.**, *The Care and Management of Spinal Cord Injuries*, Springer-Verlag, Berlin, 1981.
50. **Ford, W. R.**, Analysis of knee joint forces during flexed knee stance, in *Resident Papers*, Univ. of Southern California, Rancho Los Amigos Hospital, Los Angeles, 5, 135, 1972.
51. **Beasley, W. C.**, Quantitative muscle testing: principles and applications to research and clinical services, *Arch. Phys. Med.*, 42, 398, 1981.
52. **Bick, E. M.**, *Source Book of Orthopedics*, Hofer Publishing Co., New York, 1968.
53. Annual Progress Report, Use of biofeedback at standing of paraplegic patient, Ljubljana Rehabilitation Engineering Center, (project director A. Kralj), Lubljana, Yugoslavia, 1981, 33.
54. Annual Progress Report, Standing of paraplegic patient, Ljubljana Rehabilitation Engineering Center (project director A. Kralj), Ljubljana, Yugoslavia, 1980, 34.
55. **Bajd, T., Kralj, A., Krajnik, J., Turk, R., Benko, H., and Šega, J.**, Standing by FES in paraplegic patients, in Proc. 8th Int. Symp. Ext. Contr. Human Extremities, Dubrovnik, Yugoslavia, September 3 to 7, 1984, 51.
56. **Kralj, A., Bajd, T., Turk, R., and Benko, H.**, Posture switching for prolonging functional electrical stimulation standing in paraplegic patients, *Paraplegia*, 24, 221, 1986.
57. **Guersen, J., Altena, D., Massen, C., and Verdnin, M.**, A model of the standing man for the description of his dynamic behaviour, *Agressologie*, 17, 63, 1976.
58. **Jaeger, R.**, Stimulation of quiet standing by a hypothetical closed-loop electrical stimulation orthosis, in Proc. 8th Int. Symp. Ext. Contr. of Human Extremities, Dubrovnik, Yugoslavia, September 3 to 7, 1984, 67.
59. **McGuinness, K., Meade, M., and Jaeger, R.**, Prediction of ground reaction vector using a single-link model, in Proc. 38th Annu. Conf. Med. Biol. Eng., Chicago, IL, September 30 to October 2, 1985, 61.
60. **Cybulski, G., Jaeger, R., and Troyk, P.**, Quantitative analysis of standing balance in paraplegic individuals, in Proc. Annu. RESNA Conf., RESNA Association for the Advancement of Rehabilitation Technology, Washington, D.C., Ottawa, 1984, 553.
61. **Jaeger, R.**, Design and simulation of closed-loop electrical stimulation orthoses for restoration of quiet standing in paraplegia, *J. Biomech.*, 19, 825, 1986.
62. **Turk, R., Benko, H., Bajd, T., Kralj, A., and Šega, J.**, Functional electrical stimulation as a help in activities of daily living, *Annu. Meet. Int. Soc. Paraplegia*, Edinburgh, Scotland, September, 1985.
63. **Phillips, C. A., Petrofsky, J. S., Hendershot, D. M., and Stafford, D.**, Functional electrical exercise — a comprehensive approach for physical conditioning of the spinal cord injured patient, *Orthopedics*, 7, 1112, 1984.
64. **Cybulski, G., Penn, R., and Jaeger, R.**, Lower extremity functional neuromuscular stimulation in cases of spinal cord injury, *Neurosurgery*, 15, 132, 1984.
65. **Issekutz, B., Blizzard, N. C., and Rodahl, K.**, Effects of prolonged bed rest and urinary calcium output, *J. Appl. Physiol.*, 21, 1013, 1966.
66. **Claus-Walker, J., Campos, R. J., Carter, R. E., Vallbona, C., and Lipscomb, H.**, Calcium excretion in quadriplegia, *Arch. Phys. Med. Rehabil.*, 53, 14, 1972.
67. **Donaldson, C. L., Hulley, S. B., Vogel, J. M., Battner, R. S., Bayers, J. H., and McMillan, D. E.**, Effects of prolonged bed rest on bone mineral, *Metabolism*, 19, 1071, 1970.
68. **Heaney, R. P.**, Radiocalcium metabolism in disuse osteoporosis in man, *Am. J. Med.*, 33, 188, 1962.
69. **Kaplan, P. E., Roden, W., Gilbert, E., Richard, L., and Goldschmidt, J. W.**, Reduction of hypercalciuria in tetraplegia after weight-bearing and strengthening exercises, *Paraplegia*, 19, 289, 1981.
70. **Abramson, A. S. and Delagi, E. F.**, Influence of weight bearing and muscle contraction on disuse osteoporosis, *Arch. Phys. Med. Rehabil.*, 42, 147, 1961.
71. **Abramson, A. S.**, Bone disturbance in injuries to the spinal cord and cauda equina (paraplegia), *J. Bone Jt. Surg.*, 30A, 982, 1948.
72. **Freeman, L. W.**, The metabolism of calcium in patients with spinal cord injuries, *Ann. Surg.*, 129, 177, 1949.
73. **Hattner, R. S. and McMillan, D. E.**, Influence of weightlessness upon the skeleton: a review, *Aerosp. Med.*, 39, 849, 1968.

74. **Birge, S. J. and Whedon, G. D.**, *Hypodynamics and Hypogravics: Physiology of Inactivity and Weightlessness in Bone,* Academic Press, New York, 1968.
75. **Odeen, I. and Knutsson, E.**, Evaluation of the effects of muscle stretch and weight load in patients with spastic paraplegia, *Scand. J. Rehabil. Med.,* 13, 171, 1981.
76. **Kaplan, P. E., Gandharadi, B., Richards, L., and Goldschmidt, J.**, Calcium balance in paraplegic patients: influence of injury duration and ambulation, *Arch. Phys. Med. Rehabil.,* 59, 447, 1978.
77. **Albright, F. and Keifenstein, E. C.**, *The Parathyroid Metabolic Bone Disease, Selected Studies,* Williams & Wilkins, Baltimore, 1948.
78. **Comar, A. E.**, A long-term survey of the incidence of renal calculosis in paraplegia, *J. Urol.,* 74, 447, 1955.
79. **Gould, D. W., Hsieh, A. C., and Tickler, L. F.**, The effect of posture on bladder pressure, *J. Physiol.,* 129, 448, 1955.
80. **Sutton, N.**, *Injuries of the Spinal Cord, The Management of Paraplegia and Tetraplegia,* Butterworths, London, 1973.
81. **Ragnarsson, K. T., Krebs, M., Naftchi, N. E., Demeny, M., Sell, G. H., Lowman, E. W., and Tuckman, J.**, Head-up tilt effect on glomerular filtration rate, renal plasma flow and mean arterial pressure in spinal man, *Arch. Phys. Med. Rehabil.,* 62, 306, 1981.
82. **Machek, O. and Cohen, F.**, A new standing table, *Am. J. Occup. Ther.,* 9, 158, 1955.
83. **Krebs, M., Ragnarsson, K., and Tuckman, J.**, Orthostatic vasomotor response in spinal man, *Paraplegia,* 21, 72, 1983.
84. **Leo, K.**, The effects of passive standing, *Paraplegia News,* November, 45, 1985.
85. **Kralj, A.**, Restoration of locomotion for paraplegic patients by the help of functional electrical stimulation, EEC COMAC/BME Workshop "Restoration of Walking for Paralysed Persons", The Robert Jones and Agnes Hunt Orthopaedic Hospital, Oswestry, Shropshire, England, March, 26 to 27, 1985, 13.
86. **Figoni, S. F.**, Cardiovascular and haemodynamic responses to tilting and to standing in tetraplegic patients: a review, *Paraplegia,* 22, 99, 1984.
87. **Petrofsky, J. S. and Phillips, C. A.**, Active physical therapy: a modern approach to rehabilitation therapy, *J. Neurol. Orthop. Surg.,* 4, 165, 1983.
88. **Geiser, M. and Trnota, J.**, Muscle action, bone rarefaction and bone formation, *J. Bone Jt. Surg.,* 40, 282, 1958.
89. **Bajd, T., Kralj, A., Šega, J., Turk, R., Benko, H., and Strojnik, P.**, Two channel electrical stimulator providing standing of paraplegic patients, *Phys. Ther.,* 61, 526, 1981.
90. **Bajd, T., Kralj, A., and Turk, R.**, Standing-up of a healthy subject and a paraplegic patient, *J. Biomech.,* 15, 1, 1982.
91. **Ellis, M. I., Seedhom, B. B., Amis, A. A., Dowson, D., and Wright, V.**, Forces in the knee joint whilst rising from normal and motorized chairs, *Eng. Med.,* 8, 33, 1979.
92. **Ellis, M. I., Seedhom, B. B., and Wright, V.**, Forces in the knee joint whilst rising from a seated position, *J. Biomech. Eng.,* 6, 113, 1984.
93. **Murray, M. P., Seireg, A., and Scholtz, R. C.**, Center of gravity, center of pressure, and supportive forces during human activities, *J. Appl. Physiol.,* 23, 831, 1967.
94. **Yoshida, K., Iwakura, H., and Inone, F.**, Motion analysis in the movements of standing-up from and sitting down on a chair, *Scand. J. Rehabil. Med.,* 15, 133, 1983.
95. **Quintern, J. and Jaeger, R.**, Analysis of modes of quiet standing in neurologically intact human subjects, in Proc. Symp. Adv. External Control of Human Extremities, Dubrovnik, Yugoslavia, August 31 to September 5, 1987, 167.

Chapter 5

FES AMBULATION PROGRAM IN INCOMPLETE SCI PATIENTS

I. GENERAL CHARACTERISTICS OF INCOMPLETE SCI LESIONS

There is considerable variation with respect to the incidence of incomplete spinal cord injuries in different parts of the world. Nevertheless, there are some common observations which will help to understand the importance of the special FES rehabilitation approach to this group of patients. One of such characteristic property is the greater number of incomplete patients among tetraplegic than paraplegic patients. According to Guttmann,[1] there was 72% of incomplete lesions in a group of 466 cervical traumatic lesions, while there was only 26% of incomplete cases out of 1036 thoracic lesions. Also, it has been observed in the past decades[2] that the number of cervical injuries has gradually been increasing compared to thoracolumbar injuries. The majority of the incomplete injuries are traumatic lesions caused by road, sport, and industrial accidents. Among the sport injuries, diving represents the major reason for incomplete cervical lesions. As an incidence of incomplete spinal cord injury, also to mention are knife and gunshot wounds. A significant number of incomplete paraplegic and tetraplegic patients arises from different falls. On the basis of the statistical results, it can be concluded that incomplete tetraplegics represent an interesting group of paralyzed patients suitable for FES treatment.

In the last decades, different preventive measures have been reducing the number of complete paraplegic and tetraplegic patients. The seat belt legislation certainly resulted in a reduction in death rate from motor vehicle accidents. At the same time, the introduction of seat belts caused an increase in cases of tetraplegia due to cervical injuries. Improved motor vehicle engineering has also helped to decrease the number of disastrous traffic accidents. An increase of incomplete lesions accompanied by a decrease of complete spinal cord injuries is present also due to more efficient first aid and improved transport to the hospital. By simply educating the people, before getting their drivers license, to not allow any rotary movement to occur at the cervicodorsal and lumbodorsal junction when giving first aid to the patients with possible fractures of the vertebral column may effectively reduce the incidence of complete cases. All such preventive measures together with an advanced treatment in an emergency center result in an increasing number of incomplete cases in spinal units.[3]

The problem of regeneration of the spinal cord following transaction in man and animals has for many years been the subject of intensive clinical and experimental research. Some promising experiments with transplanted embryonic neurons establishing functional connections in the adult brain and spinal cord[30] have been conducted in different mammals. Unfortunately, the experimental results regarding regeneration of the nervous system in other vertebrates cannot be taken as valid for man. There is, namely, the ability of the spinal cord in some lower animals to take on an independent role after it has become detached from brain. Functional recovery through regeneration of the severed spinal cord is still unproven. Nevertheless, some limited repair of the spinal cord can occur.[4] The dura and pia mater are regenerated easily after trauma. Spinal vessels, connective tissue and neuroglia are also capable of repair after injury. Spinal motor neurons regenerate their peripheral processes, but not their central processes. Nevertheless, within the spinal cord, the regeneration of motoneurons also occurs, but the fibers are more likely to be directed wrongly. Long intraspinal neurons are not regenerated, while nothing is known of regeneration of the smaller internuncial neurons of the spinal cord. On the basis of this data, it can be expected that further research will probably result not in conversion of complete spinal cord injured patients

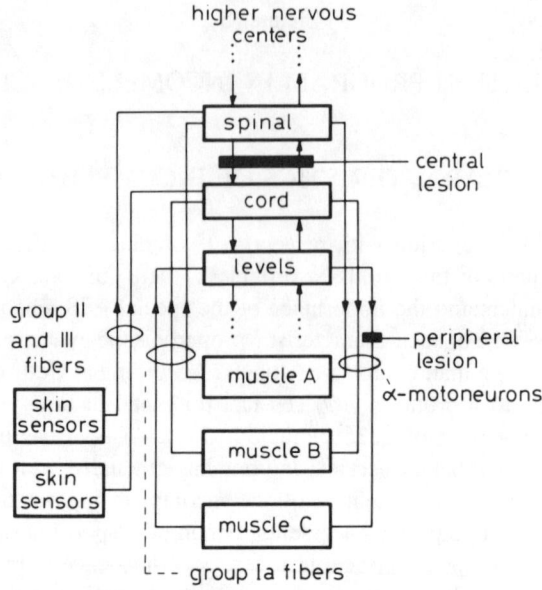

FIGURE 1. Schematic representation of spinal cord connection for normal (A), centrally denervated (B), and peripherally denervated (C) muscle.

into normals, but rather in conversion of some complete lesions into incomplete cases which may further increase the population of incomplete paraplegics and tetraplegics.

II. NEUROPHYSIOLOGICAL CHARACTERISTICS OF INCOMPLETE SCI LESIONS RELEVANT TO FES APPLICATION

Incomplete lesions of the spinal cord can be divided into two main groups.[1] There are lesions affecting more or less all the efferent and afferent neurons at a certain level, but not resulting in complete interruption of their functions. The second group consists of lesions where distinct parts of the cord are completely damaged while the others are preserved. Both types of lesions result in three kinds of muscles (Figure 1): normal (muscle A), centrally denervated (muscle B), and peripherally denervated (muscle C). While there is fully preserved efferent and afferent neural information flow between muscle A and spinal cord with the higher nervous centers, there are two spinal reflexes characteristic for the muscle B where corresponding spinal cord level is detached from the higher nervous centers. These reflexes are monosynaptic stretch reflex and polysynaptic flexion reflex which are both schematically represented in Figure 1.

Stretch reflex is the simplest spinal reflex with an afferent and an efferent neuron and a single intervening synapse (monosynaptic). The receptors for the stretch reflex are the annulospinal endings of the muscle spindle, which detect the length of the muscle. The neural information is conducted centrally in large-diameter, fast-conducting afferent fibers (group Ia fibers). These fibers are in direct contact with the α-motoneurons carrying efferent impulses to the extrafusal muscle fibers. The pathological stretch reflex (detached from the higher nervous centers) is to a great extent responsible for the occurrence of spasticity, being an important property of thoracic and cervical spinal cord injuries. In many incomplete paraplegic and tetraplegic patients, exaggerated extensor tone can be observed providing more or less safe standing to some of those patients. Placing the paralyzed limbs during spinal shock in abduction and extension at hips and knees and keeping feet and toes in dorsiflexion while the patient lies in supine position or placing the patient in prone position further promotes the extension reflex activity. Activation of ankle flexor and extensor muscles was studied during the stretch reflex, volitional activity, and posture in 21 ambulatory incomplete SCI patients.[5] Segmental stretch reflex was assessed by passive dorsal and plantar flexions with patients lying supine. Tibialis anterior responded to stretch in 48% of muscles, while the reflex response was present in 90% of triceps surae muscles. Volitional descending control was well preserved both in the tibialis anterior and triceps surae. During standing, all triceps surae and 90% of tibialis anterior muscles were activated. Frequent coactivation of both antagonist muscles was observed in all three experimental conditions. This study further demonstrates the preponderance of extensor activity in incomplete SCI patients.

Many patients are unable to break this exaggerated extensor tone during standing and hence, they are unable to achieve adequate flexion for gait and initiate a step. It has been shown that in thoracic and cervical complete and incomplete patients electrical stimulation of a afferent nerve augments dorsiflexion, knee, and hip flexion in a total lower limb flexion reflex pattern. The flexion reflex is a protective response that allows withdrawal of a limb from a noxious stimulus. The flexion reflex is polysynaptic (6 to 10 neurons constituting the reflex arc) and is evoked by an afferent input through skin sensors, cutaneous nerve endings, or group II or III muscle or cutaneous afferents. The afferent neuron is connected onto interneurons and they onto α-motoneurons at a number of spinal cord segments, since the withdrawal reflex of the entire extremity implies a simultaneous and coordinated activity of several muscle groups.

Considerable research efforts have been devoted to the neurophysiological studies of flexion reflex responses in the patients with the disorders of the central nervous system (CNS). Different stimulation sites and various stimulation parameters were applied in numerous investigations. The nociceptive reflexes of the lower limb were studied by Kugelberg et al.[6] The reflexes were elicited by painful electrical stimuli delivered to the skin and deep tissues of the balls of the toes, the ball and hollow of the foot, the plantar surface of the heel, the dorsum of the foot, and the buttock. Square wave pulses of 1.5 ms duration, 500 Hz frequency, and amplitude up to 20 mA were used. The stimulus consisted of a series of pulses delivered over a period of 30 to 40 ms. The needle electrodes were used in the experiments. Spinal withdrawal reflexes in the human lower limbs are also described by Hagbarth.[7] Different skin areas of the lower limb were electrically stimulated. The withdrawal reaction was obtained by current stimuli of 500 to 1000 Hz frequency, 5 to 10 mA amplitude, and 10 to 30 ms pulse train duration passed through bipolar needle electrodes held in the contact with the skin. The stimulation threshold of the flexor reflex afferent nerve fibers was investigated by Shahani.[8] The tibial nerve was stimulated at the level of ankle and knee. Electrical shocks, consisting of 20 ms trains of 1 ms square wave pulses, were delivered with surface bipolar stimulating electrodes. The stimulus amplitude ranged from 10 to 50 V. The stimulation frequency was 500 Hz. Extensive studies of flexion reflex in spinal man were performed by Dimitrijević and Nathan.[9-10] The surface electrodes were fixed onto the skin, usually on the medial aspect of the plantar surface of the foot. Each stimulus consisted of a train of rectangular pulses with pulse duration 0.2 to 0.3 ms, frequency 2 kHz, and train duration 20 ms. The stimulation voltage was varied between 5 and 100 V. Changes in reflex response evoked by rhythmically and stochastically delivered trains of electrical pulses were studied by Faganel.[12] The plantar surface was stimulated by rectangular pulses of 0.2 ms pulse duration, 2 kHz frequency, 20 ms train duration, and stimulation amplitudes of 40, 50, and 80 V. The electrical induction of the flexion reflex during the ambulation of hemiplegic patients was proposed by Lee and Johnston.[13] The sole of the foot, the dorsal surface of the foot, and lower posterior thigh were separately stimulated by two surface electrodes. With a frequency of 30 Hz, pulse duration of 30 ms, and stimulus current sufficient to produce the reflex (up to 20 mA), the duration of the reflex was adjusted for each patient

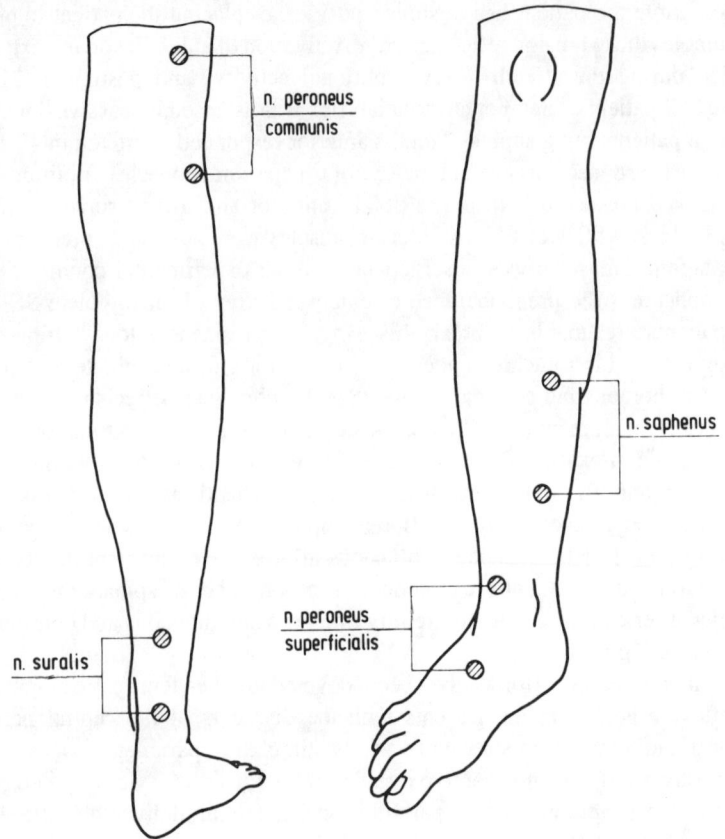

FIGURE 2. Approximate stimulation points for eliciting the flexion response by electrical stimulation.

by varying the train duration from 100 to 700 ms. It is characteristic for most of the investigations described that biomechanical responses have been not assessed along with the neurophysiological data.

In the FES ambulation program of complete and incomplete SCI patients, the flexion response is implemented into the simple reciprocal gait pattern. It is of interest, therefore, to determine the influence of stimulation amplitude, pulse duration, stimulation frequency, pulse train duration, and stimulation site on the dynamic properties of the functional flexion response.[14] In the study, the electrodes were placed over one of the following nerves: superficial peroneal, common peroneal, sural, and saphenous (Figure 2). Two small (diameter 2.5 cm) round electrodes made of stainless steel sheet metal and covered by gauze saturated with water were used. Patient under the test was placed upright on the tilt table. Electrogoniometric system[16] was mounted to all three joints of one extremity. Hip, knee, and ankle angles were recorded together with the start of the stimulation train. The influence of stimulation amplitude (U_{st}), frequency (f), and the duration of train of pulses (T) on the maximal joint angle angle were observed (Figure 3). During all the experiments, the duration of stimulation pulse was kept at 0.3 ms. The stimulation with larger pulse durations was often found painful to the patients with preserved skin sensations. In Figure 3, the dependence of hip peak angle on stimulation amplitude, frequency, and duration of the train of stimuli is shown. The response is increased when increasing any of the three parameters. The measurement was performed in T-3, 4 incomplete paraplegic patient when stimulating n. cutaneous femoris. Similar diagrams were obtained also in the knee and ankle of all patients measured.

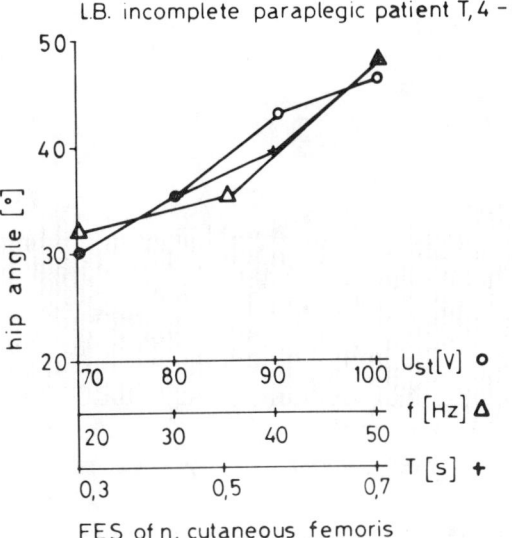

FIGURE 3. The influence of stimulation amplitude (U_{st}), frequency (f), and the duration of the train of pulses (T) on the maximal hip joint angle.

As the hip flexion during normal walking ranges from 30 to 36°, it can be seen from the Figure 3 that such hip angles can be easily obtained with the afferent stimulation. When changing one of the three parameters from Figure 3, the two others were kept at the following values: U_{st} = 80 V, f = 30 Hz, and T = 0.5 s. The duration of the flexion response depends on pulse train duration, but is relatively independent when changing stimulation amplitude and frequency. When using, e.g., 0.5 s pulse train duration, the flexion response lasted for about 1.5 s. Another important property of the flexion response is its habituation. The trains of electrical stimuli were repeated a hundred times every 2 s for what corresponds to very slow walking. In almost all of the patients tested, the responses were stronger at the beginning and they diminished after the first five to ten trains of stimuli. Thereafter, the maximal flexion remained fairly constant (Figure 4).

The incomplete SCI patient's muscle, described as muscle B (Figure 1), becomes in a short period of time disuse atrophied. It can be easily restrengthened by the electrical stimulation where the following approximate parameters are to be selected: 20 to 50 Hz stimulation frequency, 0.1 to 0.5 ms pulse duration, and 50 to 140 V stimulation amplitude. As long as the peripheral nerve with the motor endplate is intact, we are dealing with the nerve stimulation even if the electrodes are placed over the belly muscle. Direct muscle stimulation is applied only in peripherally denervated muscles (muscle C). Here, paralysis is caused by a disturbance of the α-motoneuron starting a degenerative atrophy in the affected muscle. Any reflex activities, as well as any tonus, are missing. In the case of muscle B, electrical stimulation provokes muscle contraction through depolarization of the appropriate motoneuron membrane, while it is supposed in the case of muscle C that the calcium ions which are indispensable for contractions, are directly released by the electrical field.[17] The pulse duration is distinctly longer than in spastic paralysis, but it can be shortened by daily training from several 100 ms, applied in the case of most severe degeneration, to about 20 ms. The necessary current intensity is between 20 and 50 mA. Bidirectional stimulation pulses were found more effective as the fatigue is significantly lower when compared with stimulation by monodirectional currents. It has been shown[18] that with training by using appropriate stimulation currents, the excitability and controllability of denervated muscle

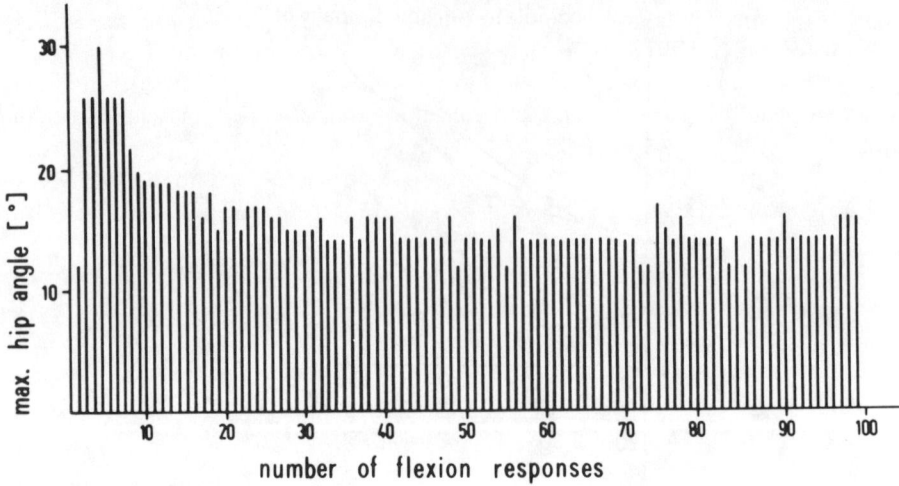

FIGURE 4. Flexion reflex passing through phases of build-up, gradual decrease, and habituation when elicited repetitively.

can be increased to functional levels. A patient with complete paralysis of the peroneal nerve, 4 months after the injury, was stimulated twice daily for 30 min for 3 weeks. His dorsiflexors were excited by monodirectional square pulses of 20 ms pulse duration, 25 Hz frequency, and 30 mA stimulation intensity. Stimulation trains of 3 s and 3 s pause were used. After one week of training, the maximum ankle angle (dorsiflexion) increased from 12 to 20° and continued to increase for the following 2 weeks up to about 30°. The improvements within the stimulation program were of such an extent that useful functional movement could be elicited. Experiments of denervated muscle stimulation were undertaken on rabbits by Guttmann.[1] It was found that daily application of electrical stimulation of 20 to 30 min duration, with a current strength sufficient to elicit powerful contractions delayed and diminished atrophy in denervated muscles. The earlier the treatment was started following denervation, the greater was the effect. After a treatment of 1 h daily, beginning the day after denervation, it was found that the muscles lost only 17% in weight in 60 d, compared with a loss of 59% of the untreated muscle. On the basis of the described animal experiments, Guttmann suggests the following therapy for lower motoneuron lesions: "Daily electrical exercise is started as early as possible, following lower motor neuron lesion in paraplegics and tetraplegics (about 5 days after injury), and is applied in gradually increasing number of contractions, starting with 50—100 per session of 15 min. In due course, as many as 600—800 and more contractions are applied to paralysed muscle groups during one session of about 30—45 min. This treatment is given at least once a day, if possible twice daily. Care is taken to elicit powerful muscle contractions, separated by rest periods of a few seconds." In more recent research efforts, it has been found that computerized tomography appears to be an excellent research and perhaps also clinical tool to monitor muscle atrophy and to assess the effectiveness of the electrical therapy of denervated muscles.[19]

In more clinical terms the muscle named in this text as muscle B is called spastic muscle, while muscle C is flaccid muscle. In this way, we are talking also about spastic and flaccid incomplete neurological spinal cord lesions. On the cervical and T-1 to T-5 thoracic level, only spastic lesions are encountered, while below T-6 level, both incomplete spastic and incomplete flaccid injuries may occur. An incomplete spinal cord lesion may also initially reveal a complete sensory loss below the level of the lesion, but sooner or later certain, if not all, modalities of sensibility may recover. Disturbances of sensibility in the later stages of particular incomplete cervical lesions are often irregular and dissociated.[1] Nevertheless, it must be stressed that very rarely were abnormal unpleasant sensations accompanying surface electrical stimulation noticed while using short durations of stimuli (0.1 to 0.5 ms).

It is not difficult to realize that all three kinds of muscles: normal (muscle A), centrally lesioned (muscle B), and peripherally lesioned (muscle C) may be found not only in the lower extremity of an incomplete paraplegic or tetraplegic patient, but also in a single muscle group. This makes the FES rehabilitation approach extremely complex. Nevertheless, some patterns of incomplete lesions can be recognized.[20]

There are four such patterns defined and generally recognized although the mixed patterns may also occur. The first one is acute anterior cervical cord syndrome. It is found mainly with compression fractures and anterior dislocations of the cervical spine. The patient will have bilateral motor loss below the lesion, and bilateral loss or impairment of pain and temperature sensibility. Light touch, proprioception, and vibration sense will be relatively unimpaired or normal. The second pattern is acute central cervical cord syndrome. A central cord lesion usually results from hyperextension injuries of the cervical spine, particularly when the spinal cord has been narrowed by preexisting degenerative changes. The effect of such a lesion is to cause greater motor and sensory impairment of the arms and hands than the legs, which sometimes may even be normal. This pattern of incomplete spinal cord lesions is therefore not interesting for introducing FES ambulation program. The third type, Brown-Sequard lesion, is due to hemisection of the spinal cord. It results in complete motor loss below the lesion on the same side, and loss of pain and temperature sensation on the opposite side. Partial Brown-Sequard lesions are quite common, and are often present in combination with partial anterior or central cord lesions. Injuries to the cauda equina present very variable neurological patterns with mixed motor and sensory loss. The traumatic lesions are usually due to fracture dislocations of the lumbar vertebrae resulting in lower motoneuron lesion. This fourth type of incomplete paraplegic patients are therefore candidates for stimulation of peripherally denervated muscles only.

III. FES THERAPEUTIC PROGRAM

Because of the complex neurophysiological state of incomplete SCI patients, it is impossible to predict the outcome of the FES rehabilitation process when the patients are after the accident examined and admitted to the spinal unit. Similarly, it is not possible to decide what rehabilitation aid the patient will need after stabilization of the spinal cord injury. The first step in the FES program is, therefore, application of therapeutic electrical stimulation. At first sight, the therapeutic electrical stimulation does not essentially differ from the usual exercising of single joints. Nevertheless, the electrical stimulation influences not only the muscle on which electrodes have been positioned, but via afferent nervous pathways, also higher nervous centers and thereby, supposedly also the reorganization of the neuromuscular activity. Following the application of electrical stimulation in incomplete SCI patients, there can be noticed an increase of the voluntary movement, strengthening of atrophied muscles, reduction of contractures, increased range of motion, and lesser spasticity. The sooner the therapy is begun after the injury, the better the success of therapeutic electrical stimulation. Therapeutic effects also depend on the period of time during which a paralyzed extremity is stimulated each day and through how many days the therapy is performed.

Therapeutic electrical stimulation is considered an effective complement of the standard rehabilitation program for incomplete paraplegic and tetraplegic patients. Of the utmost importance is the fact that the physiotherapists need not be with the patients all the time. It suffices to adjust the electrodes and preset stimulation parameters. The physiotherapist can devote the attention to another patient, as many commercially available therapeutic stimulators switch themselves off after the preset therapy has been completed. In case of certain stimulator types, patients can perform the therapy by themselves by manual triggering of the stimulation trains.

The therapeutic electrical stimulation consists of cyclic stimulation of partially paralyzed knee extensor muscles where stimulation trains of 4 s and pauses of equally 4 s alternately follow one another. The electrical stimulation is applied through large (6 × 4 cm) electrodes covered with water-soaked gauze. If the upper electrode is placed in a more proximal position, there also results some flexion in the hip. The positioning of electrodes in view of achieving an effective and strong movement is not critical. The hip flexion is prevented also by placing the proximal electrode more laterally, thus stimulating mainly m. vastus lateralis and not the two-joint attached rectus femoris. The exercise results in isotonic contractions. The electrical pulses used are rectangular and monophasic. A stimulation frequency of 20 Hz, a pulse duration of 0.3 ms, and a stimulation amplitude of sufficient intensity to bring the legs into full extension are used. During the training, the patients are positioned supine with both lower extremities semiflexed to approximately 30° by a pillow under the knees. The FES session lasts 30 min/d.

It is quite common that at the beginning of the therapy the patients may be afraid of electrical stimulation and even feel pain at its application. In such a case, the first day's therapy should be started at a lower amplitude although we obtain neither movement nor contraction. Thus, the patients will grow used to this new sensation, so that on the following day, the amplitude can already be increased. An unpleasant sensation is rather frequently experienced by patients with whom adipose tissue covers the muscle to be stimulated. Adipose tissue is a bad conductor, and to achieve an appropriate muscle contraction, higher amplitudes should be used. Skin receptors register them as a sensation of pain.

The first benefit of the therapeutic electrical stimulation for the incomplete SCI patients is facilitation of a voluntary movement. This facilitation implies relearning of the lost movement by means of electrical stimulation in order that a patient might regain voluntary control of a certain muscle group. Although electrical stimulation itself exerts an influence upon the afferent nervous system, better effects are achieved if a patient takes an active part in the therapy. In the simplest case, the patient watches a movement and triggers it by himself by means of a special hand switch. New possibilities are offered by a biofeedback which usually by means of acoustic and visual signals informs the patient on his efforts.[21]

Another important advantage of cyclic therapeutic stimulation in incomplete SCI patients is lessening of contractures. This anomaly usually results from shortening, thickness, and fibrosis of muscle fibers and appears after prolonged immobilization or else from a permanent unbalance between the antagonistic and the agonistic muscle. In case of contractures, we do not stimulate a muscle group with which the contracture has been observed, but its antagonist. The stimulation program should last no more than 1 h/d; it may, however, be divided into a number of portions, e.g., three times 20 to 30 min. Muscle contraction provoked by electrical stimulation has to be strong enough to have a joint move throughout the entire range of motion. We should take care, however, that too strong a stimulation might not cause an excessive movement and consequently pain.

Cyclical electrical stimulation also moderates the state of spasticity.[22] Quantitative measurements of spasticity performed on a group of patients with a spinal cord injury have shown that with approximately one half of patients, electrical stimulation considerably decreases spasticity and that the influence of electrical stimulation remains at least 30 min after stimulation. Due to short-term effects of electrical stimulation on spasticity, cyclical stimulation can be applied to spastic knee extensors immediately before starting the training of gait. There suffices already 30 min of stimulation therapy.

The main profit of the cyclic electrical stimulation of knee extensors with incomplete paraplegic and tetraplegic patients is strengthening of the disuse-atrophied muscle, which is highly advisable also due to the fact that the provoked muscle contraction promotes better

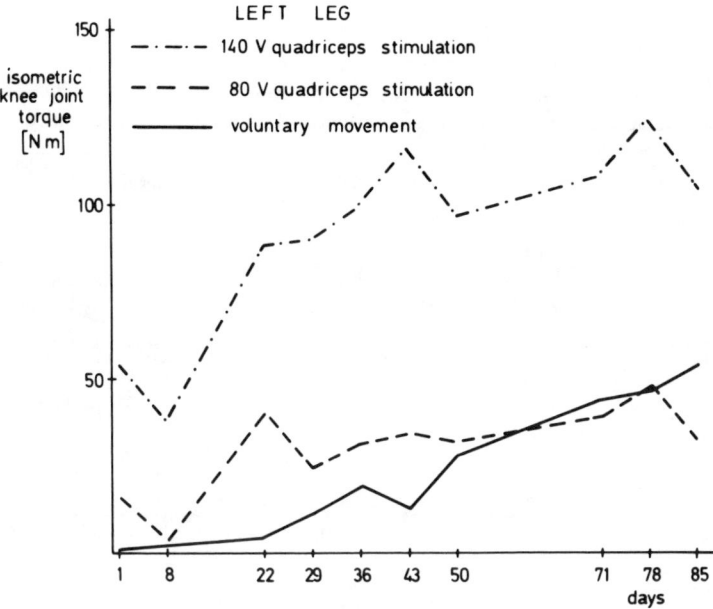

FIGURE 5. The results of electrical stimulation muscle strengthening program in C-7 incomplete tetraplegic patient 2 months postinjury.

blood circulation and indirectly leads to improved skin condition and may also prevent pressure sores. The strengthening of atrophied muscles can be combined with various classical rehabilitation aids such as exercises with weights, pulleys, and other mechanical systems offering resistance to an electrically induced torque. As a result of the described FES training program, the muscle force is increased. The effects of the muscle strengthening program can be tested and assessed through isometric knee joint torque measurement, namely, the torque at a firmly fixed joint. In our investigations, the patients were seated during the measurement on a special chair to which the electronic force transducer was attached. The device provided measurement of the right or left knee torque at different joint angles. The fixation of extremity was simple and fast to perform. The isometric knee joint torque was assessed once every week in each incomplete SCI patient. The training program lasted for about 2 months.

Both voluntary and electrically provoked knee joint torques were assessed in a group of incomplete SCI patients. After 2 to 3 months of training, three different groups of incomplete patients were found. In the first group, there were patients where both voluntary and electrically stimulated muscle force were improved. In the second group, there were patients where stimulated muscle force only was increased. Finally, some cases were encountered where neither voluntary or stimulated response were augmented. Three case studies belonging to three different groups of patients are described in further text.

The results of strengthening of the right knee extensors in incomplete tetraplegic patient are presented in Figure 5.[23] The 21-year-old patient (B. C.) had incomplete C-7 spinal cord lesion after a fall. When the electrical stimulation training program started, he was 2 months postinjury. During 85 d of the muscle strengthening program, his isometric knee joint torque was measured once every week at 80 V and 140 V of m. quadriceps stimulation. The isometric torque achieved during the maximal voluntary knee extension was also assessed. The muscle exercise resulted in a rather regular increase of the torque measured. An increase of about 50 Nm was observed when comparing the initial and final results obtained, both during electrically stimulated and voluntary muscle contraction. Another important fact is

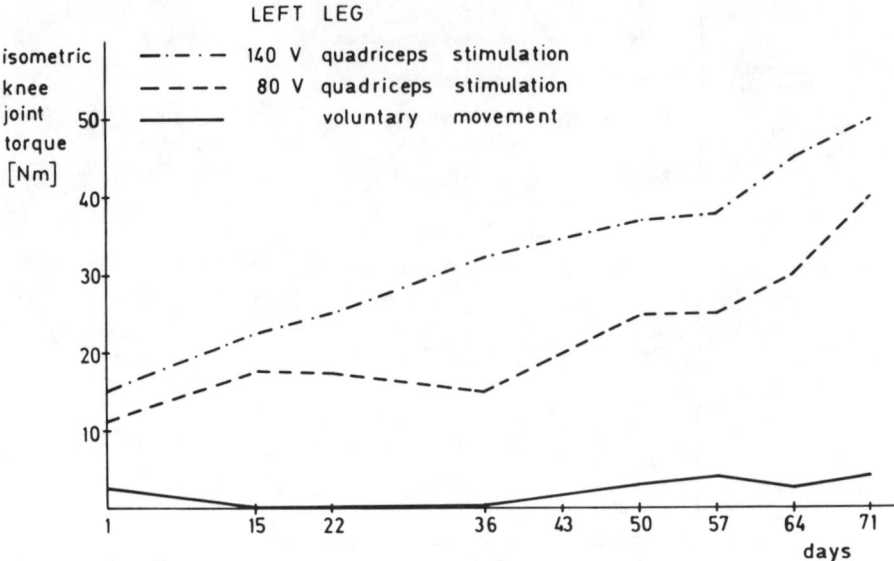

FIGURE 6. The results of electrical stimulation muscle stregthening program in C-3,4 incomplete tetraplegic patient 8 months postinjury.

revealed by comparison of the electrical stimulation and voluntary responses. When comparing the rates of increase of response during quadriceps stimulation and voluntary movement, it can be noticed that both values are quite similar. This means that all the voluntary movements gained during the patient's stay in the rehabilitation center resulted only from strengthening of the disuse-atrophied muscles and cannot be ascribed to an improved neurological status of the patient. The patient was included also in regular rehabilitation program of the spinal unit. The described observation is not in accordance with the general belief of the physiotherapists who often attribute the increased muscle force to improved neural control over paralyzed muscle. Nevertheless, the voluntary knee joint torque increased from almost 0 to about 50 Nm, which was found sufficient for unassisted walking with the help of two crutches. The patient was not using a wheelchair after leaving rehabilitation center.

Another patient (R. A., 42 years) suffered C-3,4 cervical incomplete spinal cord lesion from a vehicle accident 8 months before being admitted to the rehabilitation center from neurological clinic. The success of training program is shown in Figure 6. Both stimulated and voluntary joint torque had quite low values at the beginning of the program. The voluntary isometric torque remained at this initial value for the rest of the program. In contrast, the stimulated isometric knee joint torque was constantly increasing. After the rehabilitation program, the patient was able to walk by the help of a walker and electrical stimulation on a short distances only. The patient was using bilateral m. quadriceps stimulation during the stance phase of walking, while the swinging of both legs had to be triggered by peroneal stimulation. The patient was using a wheelchair to a considerable extent.

The C-6,7 incomplete SCI patient (D. A., 43 years) had a car accident. He came to the spinal unit for the electrical stimulation purposes 2 years after the accident. It is evident from the Figure 7 that no effect was achieved by the daily stimulation of his knee extensors. The patient remained confined to the wheelchair.

It is known from animal experiments[24] that intermittent stimulation affects the ability of the muscle to develop tension, while continuous stimulation results in decreased fatiguability of the muscle. The application of chronic, low frequency (10 Hz) stimulation results in decreased muscle fatigue.[25] In our clinical applications of FES, the problem of stimulated

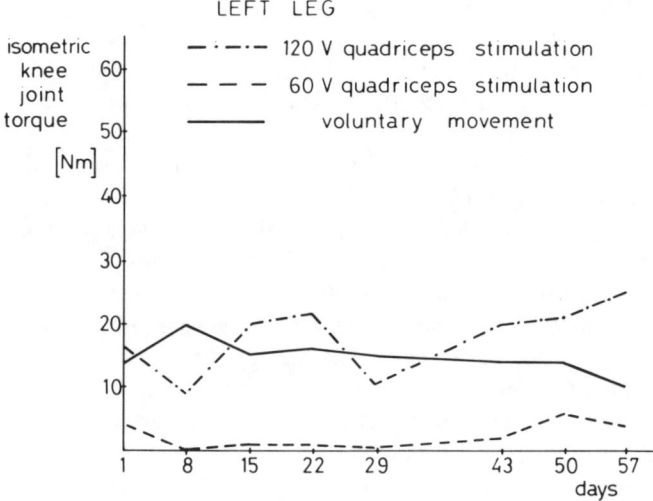

FIGURE 7. The results of electrical stimulation muscle strengthening program in C-6,7 incomplete tetraplegic patient 2 years postinjury.

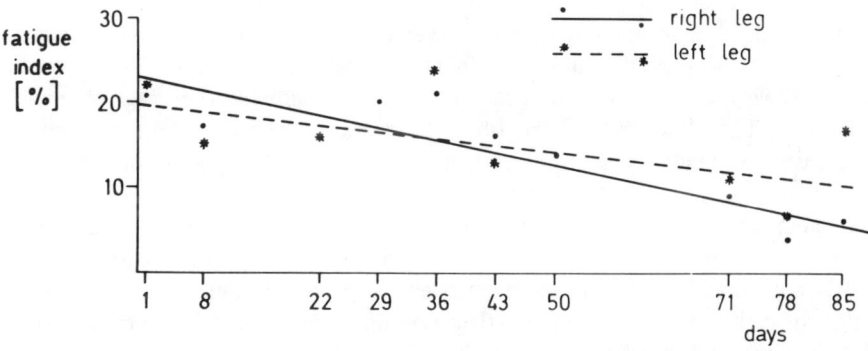

FIGURE 8. Muscle fatiguing decrease provoked by electrical stimulation training.

muscle fatigue is, to a great extent, minimized by choosing a low stimulation frequency of 20 Hz. Nevertheless, there was a decrease in muscle fatiguing observed also in our investigation. It is presented for the patient (B. C.) in Figure 8 by the help of the fatigue index defined in Chapter 2. Muscle fatiguing was decreased for approximately 10% in both the right and left leg.

IV. FES-ASSISTED WALKING

Some of the incomplete SCI patients are able to walk with the help of various short leg or long leg orthoses fixing the knee and ankle joints. Support of the foot is often provided by the addition of a toe spring. Some severe incomplete lesions result in severe weakness of the flexors of the limb, along with increased extensor muscle tone. These problems greatly inhibit the ability to initiate a step. The majority of these patients with incomplete thoracic or cervical lesions are candidates for functional so-called household and community ambulation.[26] Locomotion of other incomplete SCI patients is mostly performed with the help of a wheelchair. They can walk only for very short distances, usually in their homes. Some incomplete tetraplegic patients are totally confined to the wheelchair. The reason is often very strong spasticity or developed contractures. In incomplete tetraplegic patients, the upper extremities are also partially paralyzed. Nevertheless, the arms and hands are usually strong enough to provide support on the crutches. Wrist and finger movements are often limited and the grip is rather weak. However, the patients are in most cases able to hold the handle of the crutch.

It was observed that in a great number of the incomplete tetraplegic patients, one leg was almost completely paralyzed, while the other leg was under voluntary control and sufficiently strong to provide safe standing for short periods with only crutches. Unilateral stimulation of knee extensors and peroneal nerve was helpful in these patients. Stimulation over common peroneal nerve resulted in simultaneous flexion of the hip and the knee and dorsiflexion of the ankle and thus provided swinging of the leg. Somewhat less frequently, it was found that the patients can stand, but cannot make a step with one or both legs. Unilateral or bilateral stimulation of peroneal nerve proved helpful for them. There are also the patients whose voluntary extension and flexion activities in both lower extremities are so poor that they need three or even four channels of stimulation.

The gait of most of the incomplete SCI patients can be restored by the two-channel stimulator only. Stimulator parameters must be adjusted close to the following values: 0.3 ms pulse duration, 20 Hz pulse repetition frequency, and an amplitude up to 120 V (measured with a 1 kohm resistive load). Surface electrical stimulation of knee extensors is delivered to the muscles through large (6 × 4 cm) electrodes covered with water-soaked layers of gauze. When stimulating the common peroneal nerve, two small round electrodes (diameter 2.5 cm) are used. The positioning of the large electrodes over knee extensors is not critical and is identical to the procedure described in therapeutical FES program. The peroneal nerve is stimulated with the first electrode near fossa poplitea medially to m. biceps femoris and with the second electrode behind the fibula head above the trunk of n. peroneus ramus superficialis or profundis. The positioning and the polarity of the electrodes are critical to the effectiveness of the obtained movement.

It is sometimes difficult to correctly position the electrodes to avoid obtaining plantar flexion instead of dorsiflexion. Placement of electrodes with respect to hip and knee flexion usually is not difficult. Initially, the electrodes are placed on the approximate positions, regardless of their polarity, while the patient is sitting in a wheelchair. They are connected to the stimulator, and the stimulator is switched on. One of the electrodes is then slightly shifted to find satisfactory dorsiflexion. If appropriate movement is not achieved, the search is repeated by changing the position of the other electrode. If the dorsiflexion still is not appropriate, the polarity of the electrodes is reversed. A somewhat higher stimulation intensity than one needed for dorsiflexion results in synergistic hip, knee, and ankle movement. The flexion response is altered by increasing or decreasing the stimulation amplitude.

From the patient's control point of view, the gait cycle was divided into stance and swing phase. The transition from one phase into another was achieved by pressing a hand switch mounted on the handle of the crutch. When the switch was not pressed, knee extensors were stimulated. When the switch was pressed the peroneal nerve was excited, resulting in swing phase of walking. The duration of the swing phase was regulated by the time of pressing the switch. When applying unilateral or bilateral peroneal stimulation, a switch inserted under the heel of one or both legs has proven a sufficiently effective artificial "sensory organ" in gait control. A microswitch or a tape switch is usually embedded into the shoe insole and connected with the stimulator by a wire. The heel switch should neither be too little nor too sensitive. In the former case, it does not switch on if the patient's gait is uncertain, whereas in the latter it remains switched on all the time if the patient's shoe is too tight. As a control or a triggering signal, either the heel-on or heel-off event is used. Each stimulation train must be synchronized with respect to the control signal. A delay between heel-switch control signal and the beginning of the train of stimuli can be internally preset. The duration of the stimulation train must be predetermined as well.

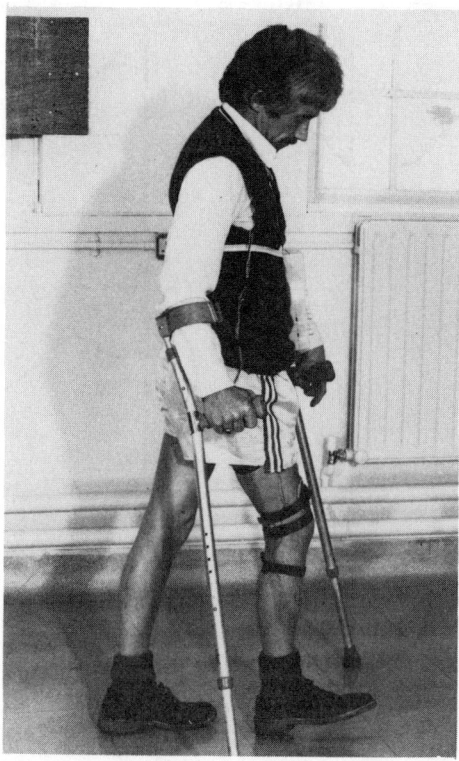

FIGURE 9. Incomplete paraplegic patient with T-6,7 lesion walking on level ground. Somewhat exaggerated flexion response can be clearly seen.

Because of largely preserved sensation and proprioception, the learning program of walking is extremely fast and simple in incomplete SCI patients.[27] After the first few days, the patients are able to go from mobile parallel bars to crutches (Figure 9). The subject shown in Figure 9 has an incomplete lesion at the T-6,7 level and was 7 years postinjury when joining the FES training program. In his case, one leg was paralyzed, while the other had sufficient voluntary control to maintain safe standing with crutches without stimulation. The difference between walking with and without FES was evident. The patient was not able to take a single step with his severely paralyzed extremity when the two-channel stimulator providing knee extensors stimulation and flexion reflex triggering was switched off. After a few days of training, the patients are, in general, able to rise from the sitting to the standing position independently with the help of the crutch support and knee extensor stimulation only. Soon they are able to walk also on uneven ground and go up and down steps.

The FES assisted walking requires less energy from the SCI patients with incomplete lesions than walking with passive mechanical knee and ankle orthoses because no hip hiking is necessary with active FES systems. Finally, FES-assisted walking is much more aesthetic than orthoses-assisted for the observer and is preferred by the patients. There may be a number of therapeutic benefits to be gained from the use of such orthoses. These may include prevention of pressure sores, contractures, muscle atrophy, and bone demineralization.

To be able to determine quantitatively the efficiency of an electrical stimulator during walking, gait measurements and analyses have to be performed. When optimizing the time courses of a multichannel stimulator, the results of the measurement have to be available instantly following the experiment. The readjustment of the multichannel FES orthosis

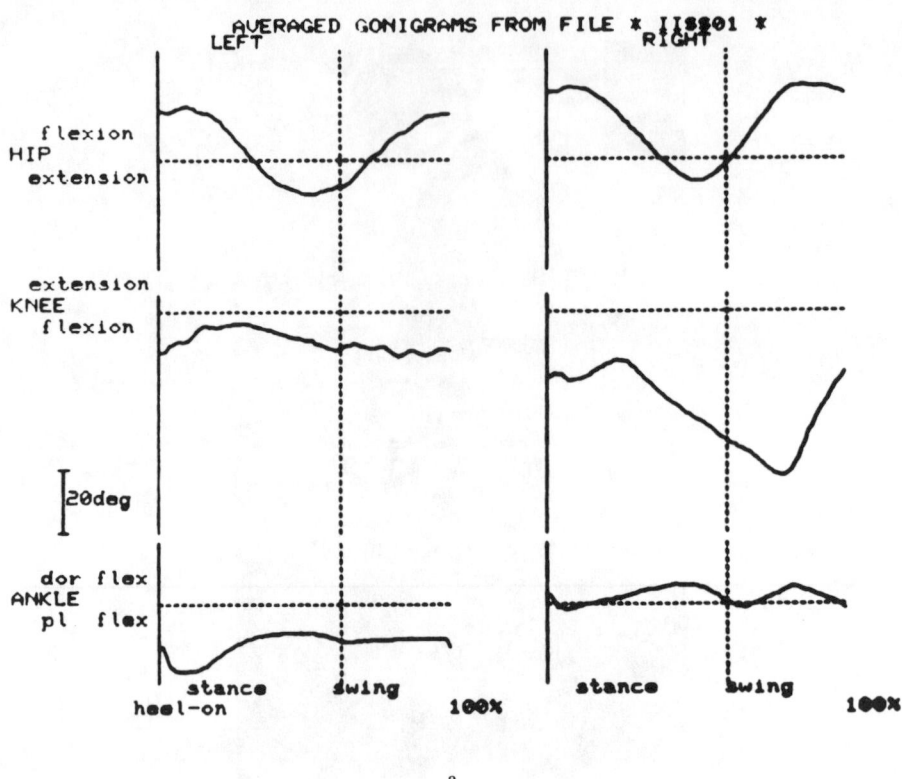

FIGURE 10. Hip, knee, and ankle averaged angles in the sagittal plane measured in an incomplete paraplegic patient before and after unilateral stimulation (a, b).

parameters is based on results of the previous measurement. Processing the great number of measured gait data with a computer is therefore, advantageous.[16] Among several methods for measuring gait parameters, the electrogoniometric system is appropriate because of the following properties: suitability for on-line processing of measured data, simplicity and reliability, low cost, simultaneous measurement of right and left leg movements, and possible consideration of a great number of steps. The last statement is of particular interest for FES-assisted walking. Due to a continuous "man-machine" interface, gait is less repeatable than that with passive aids. This applies particularly to the initial phase of the therapy when the patient is still adapting himself to the stimulator. When applying FES, gait should be measured by methods assessing a sufficiently high number of steps. The electrogoniometric method is based on an analog measurement of joint angles by means of potentiometers. The potentiometer is fixed onto the extremity segment proximally and distally to the joint where the angle is being measured. Throughout the measurement, the voltage at the potentiometer is proportional to the joint angle. Averaged hip, knee, and ankle goniograms in the sagittal plane measured in a T-12 incomplete paraplegic patient 1 year postinjury are presented in Figure 10 before and after application of unilateral peroneal stimulation. The major improvement can be observed in the left knee angle time course. A normalization of gait can be noticed also in left hip and ankle goniograms.[28] The patient was using a one-channel peroneal stimulator permanently for 2 years when his walking pattern improved to such an extent that he could abandon FES.

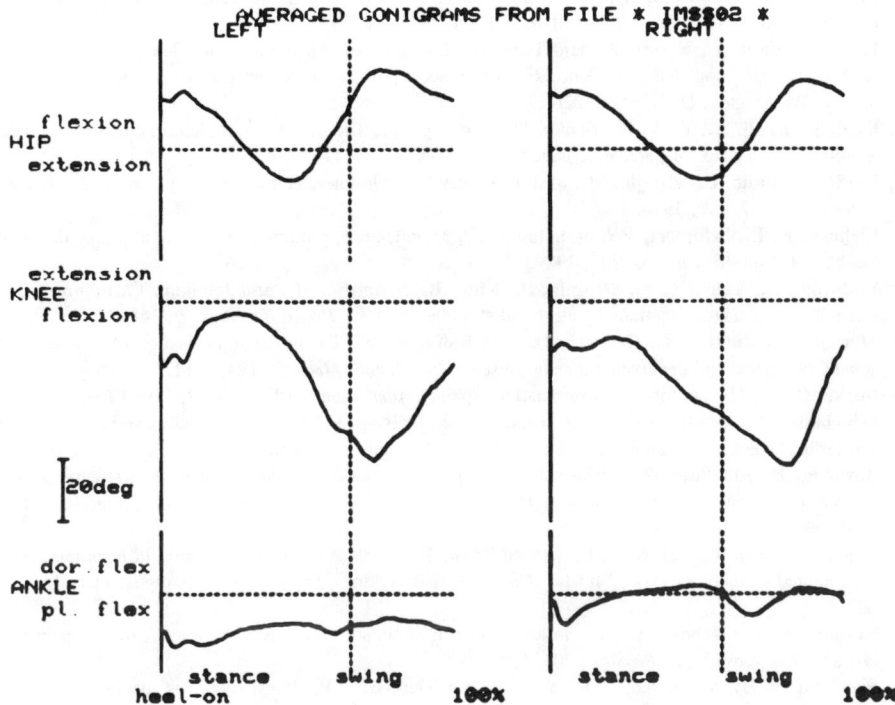

FIGURE 10b.

REFERENCES

1. **Guttmann, L.**, *Spinal Cord Injuries — Comprehensive Management and Research,* Blackwell Scientific Publications, Oxford, 1973.
2. **Sutton, N. G.**, *Injuries of the Spinal Cord — the Management of Paraplegia and Tetraplegia,* Butterworths, London, 1973.
3. **Bedbrook, G. M.**, *The Care and Management of Spinal Cord Injuries,* Springer-Verlag, Berlin, 1981.
4. **Hughes, J. T.**, Regeneration in the human spinal cord: a review of the response to injury of the various constituents of the human spinal cord, *Paraplegia,* 22, 131, 1984.
5. **Maležič, M., Dimitrijević, M. R., Dimitrijević, M. M., and Faganel, J.**, Activation of ankle flexor and extensor muscles during stretch reflex, volitional activity and posture in ambulatory spinal cord injury patients, in Proc. Eight Int. Symp. External Control of Human Extremities, Dubrovnik, Yugoslavia, September 3 to 7, 1984, 421.
6. **Kugelberg, E., Eklung, K., and Grimby, L.**, An electromyographic study of the nociceptive reflexes of the lower limb — mechanism of the plantar responses, *Brain,* 82, 394, 1960.
7. **Hagbarth, K. E.**, Spinal withdrawal reflexes in the human lower limbs, *J. Neurol. Neurosurg. Psychiat.,* 23, 222, 1960.
8. **Shahani, B.**, Flexor reflex afferent nerve fibers in man, *J. Neurol. Neurosurg. Psychiat.,* 33, 786, 1970.
9. **Dimitrijević, M. R. and Nathan, P. W.**, Studies of spasticity in man. 3. Analysis of reflex activity evoked by noxious cutaneous stimulation, *Brain,* 91, 349, 1968.
10. **Dimitrijević, M. R. and Nathan, P. W.**, Studies of spasticity in man. 4. Changes in flexion reflex with repetitive cutaneous stimulation in spinal man, *Brain,* 93, 743, 1970.
11. **Dimitrijević, M. R. and Nathan, P. W.**, Studies of spasticity in man. 5. Dishabituation of the flexion reflex in spinal man, *Brain,* 94, 77, 1971.
12. **Faganel, J.**, An analysis of flexor reflex elicited by rhythmic and stochastic stimulation in normal man, *Yugoslav Physiol. Pharmacol. Acta,* 6, 145, 1970.

13. **Lee, K. H. and Johnston, R.**, Electrically induced flexion reflex in gait training of hemiplegic patients: induction of the reflex, *Arch. Phys. Med. Rehabil.*, 57, 311, 1976.
14. **Kralj, A., Bajd, T., Kvesić, Z., and Turk, R.**, Electrical stimulating of incomplete paraplegic patients, in Proc. Fourth Annu. RESNA Conf. RESNA Association for the Advancement of Rehabilitation Technology, Washington, D.C., 1981, 226.
15. **Bajd, T., Kralj, A., Turk, R., Benko, H., and Šega, J.**, The use of a four-channel electrical stimulator as an ambulatory aid for paraplegic patients, *Phys. Ther.*, 63, 116, 1983.
16. **Bajd, T., Stanič, U., Kljajić, M., and Trnkoczy, A.**, On-line electrogoniometric gait analysis, *Comp. Biomed. Res.*, 9, 439, 1976.
17. **Eichhorn, K. F., Schubert, W., and David, E.**, Maintenance, training and functional use of denervated muscles, *J. Biomed. Eng.*, 6, 205, 1984.
18. **Vodovnik, L., Valenčič, V., Strojnik, P., Klun, B., Štefančič, M., and Jelnikar, T.**, Improvement of some abnormal motor functions by electrical stimulation, *Med. Progr. Technol.*, 9, 141, 1982.
19. **Merletti, R., Burzio, M., Granero, L., and Rolfo, M. F.**, Tomographic evaluation of size and X-ray density of normal and denervated human muscles, *Int. Rehab. Med.*, 3, 193, 1981.
20. **Burke, D. C.**, The neurological examination (spinal), *Aust. Family Physician*, 8, 119, 1979.
21. **Winchester, P., Montgomery, J., Bowman, B., and Hislop, H.**, Effects of feedback stimulation training and cyclical electrical stimulation on knee extension in hemiparetic patients, *Phys. Ther.*, 63, 1096, 1983.
22. **Bowman, B. and Bajd, T.**, Influence of electrical stimulation on skeletal muscle spasticity, in Proc. Seventh Int. Symp. External Control of Human Extremities, Dubrovnik, Yugoslavia, September 7 to 12, 1981, 567.
23. **Bajd, T., Kralj, A., Andrews, B. J., and Turk, R.**, Use of electrical stimulation in incomplete spinal cord injured patients, in Proc. 14th Int. Conf. Med. Biol. Eng., Espoo, Finland, August 11 to 16, 1985, 400.
24. **Salmons, S. and Vrbova, G.**, The influence of activity in some contractile characteristics of mammalian fast and slow muscles, *J. Physiol.*, 201, 535, 1969.
25. **Peckham, P. H., Mortimer, J. T., and Van der Meulen, J. P.**, Physiologic and metabolic changes in white muscles of cat following induced exercise, *Brain Res.*, 50, 424, 1973.
26. **Stauffer, E. S., Hoffer, M. M., and Nickel, V. L.**, Ambulation in thoracic paraplegia, *J. Bone Jt. Surg.*, 60-A, 823, 1978.
27. **Bajd, T., Andrews, B. J., Kralj, A., and Katakis, J.**, Restoration of walking in incomplete spinal cord injured patients by use of surface electrical stimulation — preliminary results, *Prosthetics Orthotics Int.*, 9, 109, 1985.
28. **Valenčič, V., Marinček, Č., and Bajd, T.**, The pattern recognition based analysis of paraparetic patient's gait, in Proc. Sixth Int. Symp. External Control of Human Extremities, Dubrovnik, Yugoslavia, August 28 to September 1, 1978, 351.
29. **Fine, A.**, Transplantation in the central nervous system, *Sci. Am.*, 255, 42, 1986.

Chapter 6

FES-ASSISTED WALKING IN COMPLETE SCI PATIENTS

I. PATIENT SELECTION

This chapter is focused onto principles, fundamentals, control, and synthesis of walking by means of FES to restore simple reciprocal walking in complete SCI patients. Most of the presented experiences and knowledge were obtained while employing surface electrical stimulation. Also, it is fair to state that in spite of more than a dozen SCI patients employing FES locomotion daily for more than five years in their household environment, the presented methodology may be considered still as a feasibility demonstration and the first step toward future commercial rehabilitative systems. The potential and impact of FES on the treatment and rehabilitation of paraplegic patients are hard to be predicted. However, it is already evident today that with chronic implants, proprioceptive feedback and smart stimulator controller, improved safety, function, cosmesis, and permanent availability will be attained introducing FES as an important rehabilitation modality. Because technological changes are gradually influencing the FES field, there is no need for this book to concentrate on technological issues, but rather on principles, fundamentals, and rules which compose the basic essentials of the FES methodology and will remain unchanged regardless of applied technology. The basic knowledge considered in the next paragraphs was developed while utilizing open-loop FES systems and is built upon our experience gained during more than 15 years of multichannel FES use in stroke patients, and more than 8 years of utilization of surface FES in SCI patients.

The patients selection for FES treatment was described in Chapter 4, Section III. The selection starts by examining the injury level, its status, and type of lesion. It is carried out according to the results of neurological and physiological status verification and outcomes of the physical evaluation concentrated on biomechanical issues. The physiological evaluation should include also the elements of general patients suitability for FES therapy in regard to cooperation, motivation, etc. Here, we will broaden and emphasize some elements of the patient selection aspects explained in Chapter 4, Section III according to the specific needs important for gait restoration. It is evident that reliable and effortless standing is a prerequisite for successful gait. In this regard, evaluation of joints integrity, range of motion (ROM), and contractures are essential. Any limitations preventing adequate standing posture are penalized with increased muscular effort and higher energy required during standing and additional increased effort during walking. Limited range of motion in ankle joint provides satisfactory standing, but will be found insufficient for enabling effective gait. Ankle joint mobility for at least 3 to 5° of dorsiflexion is essential. Slight flexion spasticity or tightness in hips are not contraindications for FES-assisted gait, because after several minutes of standing or walking, hip flexion spasticity, usually associated with abdominal spasticity, diminishes and does not represent a serious problem. The biomechanical evaluation must search also for bone integrity. Patients displaying osteoporosis and unstable spine must be excluded from the program to prevent unexpected pathological developments. Obesity is also a temporal contraindication as well as pressure sores. The ability to change the position of the upper body while standing, sense of balance, and the ability of transferring body weight between the legs are important elements for later gait training and should be checked during the FES standing sessions. A substantial difference in the FES-induced knee extensors force between the left and right side is also a contraindication because of preventing reliable single-leg support on the weak extremity and thus preventing reciprocal gait pattern. For obtaining sufficient knee extensor torques, relatively high stimulation currents must be delivered. Large electrodes are to be employed for ensuring low current density and hence, preventing skin damage. In this regard, skin tolerance is an important element in surface stimulation and needs to be carefully evaluated. It is logical and there are many fundamental reasons why it is recommended to train and evaluate patients capabilities, performance, and acceptability of FES-assisted reciprocal gait by means of surface stimulation first and not immediately by implanted stimulators. At the present state of knowledge and experience, the prediction of outcomes and achievements is not adequate. Taking into account ethical aspects, it appears to be, for the time being, appropriate to evaluate and train the patient by surface FES. When the patient remains motivated and demonstrates capabilities of using the FES-enabled locomotion functions in daily activities, the consideration should be made for implanting the orthotic system. We are in an early period of developing knowledge about FES locomotion restoration in SCI patients. Therefore, the patient selection is narrow and should be carried out very strictly until more experience and better prediction criteria will be gained. In this regard, it is rational to expect better results from younger patients. The current FES-assisted locomotion requires higher efforts than wheelchair propulsion. If a patient is not ready to accept this fact, he will sooner or later remain confined to the wheelchair. The most experienced patients with the longest use of FES for standing and walking can not be considered as representatives because so far we only have 2 to 4 years experience gained. It can be speculated that even if some of these patients will give up FES in the near future, they may probably remain permanent users in case of the availability of advanced implanted system.

II. FUNDAMENTALS OF FES GAIT RESTORATION

Nature invented different types of locomotion. The type selected was adapted to the surrounding media or terrain. The need for locomotion originates from search for food, shelter, or a safer location. Therefore, locomotion is primarily a transportation mean for carrying, in a most efficient way, the body mass from one location to another. It was perfected by the evolution process taking into account terrain characteristics, specific body construction, material used, and available energy resources. Therefore, while evolution was shaping the locomotor system and construction of body and extremities, it had to obey the physical laws of gravity, friction, construction, material characteristics, etc. This we must keep in mind permanently while discussing gait restoration in disabled persons. Equipotential mass transport in a gravitational field is most efficient and is similar to flying. In flying, only air resistance has to be overcome, while in ground transport, the losses occurring because of acceleration and deceleration of masses also must be considered and minimized. In biped gait, important body parts and heavier masses are stored well above ground for safety reasons, better avoidance of obstacles, and improved surveillance of the environment. Thus, a solid supportive structure is necessary. To enable efficient locomotion over rough terrain and adequate functionality, nature selected the segmented design of extremities. Such a segmented supportive and propelling structure is by no means moving equipotentially, but travels according to the terrain irregularities against the gravitational field, thus consumes energy. Some part of energy is stored as potential energy into the lifted leg masses. For providing support to the body by the muscle power, the lifted extremity has to be descended to the surface, thus the potential energy is converted into the kinetic energy. At the instance of touching the ground, to prevent impact damage of the extremity, the velocity of the ground approaching leg must be zero and the surplus energy dissipated. The latter may cost muscle power again. For ensuring recuperation of energy, the excessive kinetic energy is best utilized and retrieved in transportation of body masses. Indeed, nature applied in legged locomotion systems for energy conservation and optimization of energy cost-effectiveness the principle of converting potential into kinetic and kinetic into potential energy. For

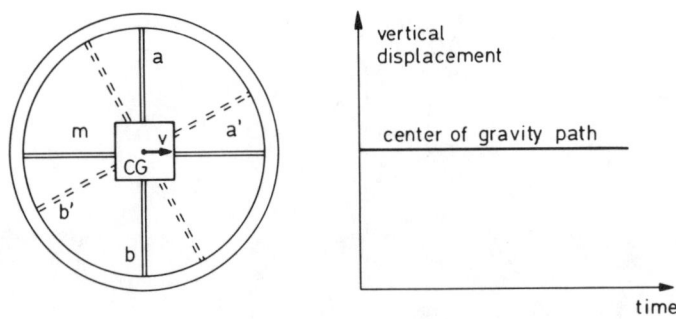

FIGURE 1. Wheeled transport and equipotential path of the center of gravity.

obtaining efficiency of the legged locomotion, first, the heavy body masses have to be carried as close as possible equipotentially or with only small oscillations. Here, the small oscillations represent kinetic to potential energy conversion among the heavier body masses and swinging limb masses. To better understand energy conversion during biped locomotion, let us compare a wheeled transport to a mass transported by the legs represented by two simple sticks. We are not going to discuss the stability problem. Obviously, the center of the gravity path in wheeled transport is equipotential and the energy is expended only because of friction. The wheel can be considered as composed of endless series of spokes serving as legs. Obviously, the spokes in Figure 1 also are moving vertically in the gravitational field, nevertheless, the resulting mass transport is optimal. The reason is the exchange of potential into kinetic energy which takes place among the spokes. Observing spoke "a" in Figure 1, it has the highest potential energy while moving toward the momentary place of spoke "b", where the potential energy is converted into the kinetic energy. Velocity in the vertical and horizontal directions of the spoke "a" is increasing until the horizontal position is reached. Equal amount of energy is consumed by the spoke "b" rotating upward to "b'" position. Further rolling of wheel is bringing "a" into the lowest position and "b" up to the maximal potential energy position. The same amount of energy as lost in descending spoke "a" was required for rising of spoke "b". The exchange of energy took place by converting potential energy of spoke "a" into kinetic and back to potential energy of spoke "b". The energy loss occurred because of air friction and load bearing friction in the axle which can be neglected if compared to the ground friction of the wheel. Note, that an increase of transported mass (m) will not substantially increase the energy required for transport. Wheeled transport is in principle efficient because of two essential characteristic properties: (1) mass is transported equipotentially in the gravitational field and (2) because of energy conversion among the wheel spokes, the wheeled transport requires only friction overcoming energy to be added for maintaining rotation. The main drawback of the wheeled transport is its unsuitability for uneven terrain. Irregularities and obstacles on the terrain result in lifting of the wheel and also change position of the transported mass. At the instance when the wheel returns to the lower path level, the majority of potential energy of mass m is not recuperated and is lost in the impact. Anyone driving a car knows the results of these impacts dissipating the energy into destructing both the vehicle and the road. It is obvious that the wheeled transport was not selected by nature because the natural terrain configuration is predominantly uneven. However, the principles of wheeled transport represent an optimal locomotion and therefore, nature adopted them by inventing the legged system construction obeying the two important principles of wheeled transport. The physical construction of the locomotor system should, as close as possible, ensure the equipotential mass transport. For the masses which are not equipotentially transferred, the potential to kinetic and vice versa conversion of energy must be very efficiently utilized. For better understanding of the legged system construction

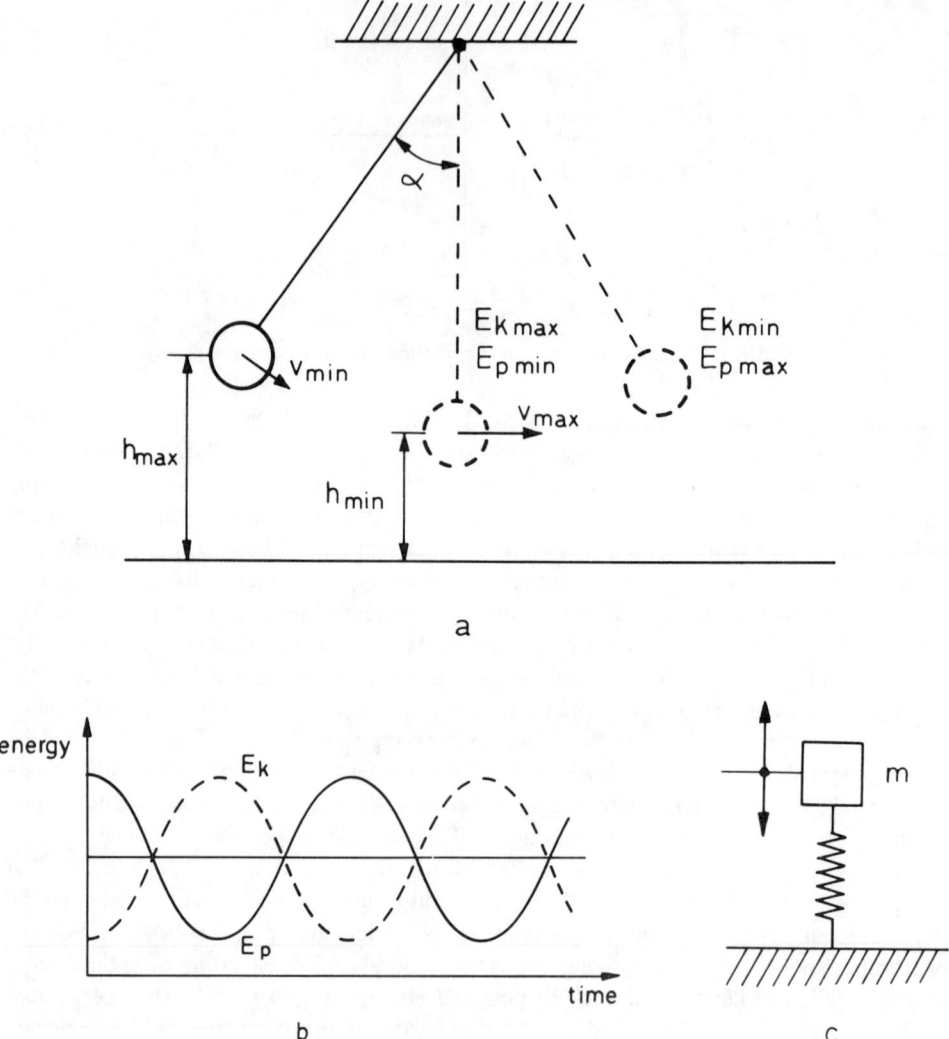

FIGURE 2. Mathematical pendulum (a), energy conversion during swinging of a pendulum (b), and a system of mass and spring (c).

principles and fundamentals of functioning, let us first consider the pendulum oscillatory movements in Figure 2. Here, the conversion of potential into kinetic energy and variations of both energies during swinging of an ideal mathematical pendulum is important (Figure 2b). Observing the shape of the curves belonging to potential and kinetic energy vs. time, one can see that they are smooth and 180° out of phase. Mathematically expressed, these are the sinusoidal curves. Here, we learned that in principle, oscillatory movements are nearly ideal for energy exchange and conversion. The latter is enabled by the specific physical system construction. There are also other arrangements providing oscillatory motion. Consider, for example, a spring and a load as presented in Figure 2c, where energy is exchanged among potential, kinetic, and spring energy. For a physical pendulum, the only energy is dissipated because of bearing friction and air friction. For good bearing of the grandfather's clock pendulum, the energy, required to keep the pendulum moving and oscillating for a week, is obtained from a weight of approximately 10 N which must be lifted 1 m higher during the clock winding. This energy is about 10 J (1 J = 1 Nm) and is sufficient for 600,000 pendulum swings covered in 7 d. Indeed, the system dissipates very little energy.

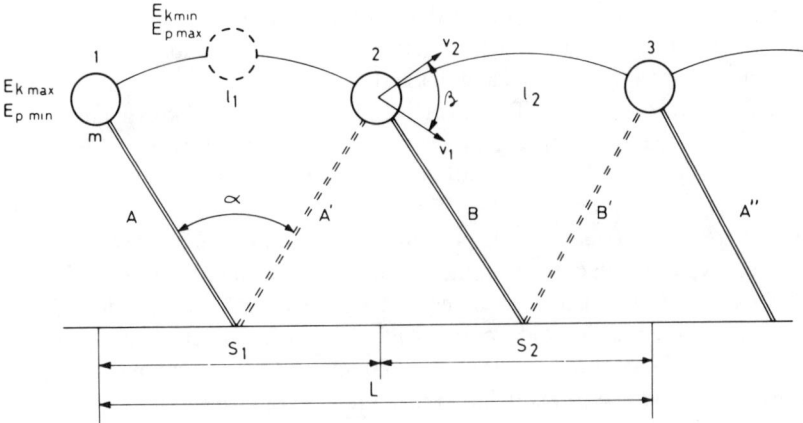

FIGURE 3. Representation of a human walking by a simple inverted pendulum model.

Similar to the pendulum is the inverted pendulum such as presented in Figure 3. Here, the mass is supported by a stick carrying the load, while the bearing is placed in the bottom. Here, the starting energy is represented by a given initial kinetic energy. A swing from position 1 into position 2 has the same energy conversion characteristics as observed with the noninverted pendulum. Because of specific system construction and its layout, position 2 is not stable, therefore, the mass is accelerated toward the ground and no oscillations occur. Let us suppose that we are able to exchange the supportive stick in position A′ instantly by stick in position B and, at the same time, change the velocity direction of mass m in position 2. With the support in the position B and proper direction of velocity, the mass m is ready to make another swing toward position 3. With the two swings l_1 and l_2, the mass m has moved for two swing distances, S_1 and S_2, or for the length L. To continue the motion and progression of mass m into position 3, again the supporting stick B′ has to be instantly exchanged by the A″. At each instance of the supporting stick exchange, the kinetic energy must be modified and the energy dissipated because friction in bearing must be added. The air friction losses can be neglected, particularly at velocities being similar to regular gait. It seems that the motion of the inverted pendulum can rather closely fulfill both criteria: (1) nearly equipotential mass trajectory and (2) exchange of potential into kinetic energy. The representation in Figure 3 also clearly points out the problem of inadequate velocity direction at the instance of supporting stick exchange. The sticks will be in further text called legs. For a smaller swing distance S_1, also the swing angle α is smaller. Even more important to observe is the β angle between the velocity vectors. With shorter swing distance, β decreases as well. According to the representation from Figure 3, nature selected smaller swing or step distances, and for ensuring proper velocity direction alignment, several additional measures were employed. The underlayed leg is not solid, but behaves like the spring-mass system such as presented in Figure 2c. In addition, at the instance of leg exchange (position 2, 3, etc.) across the trailing leg (A′, B′, . . .), a pushing force is generated to assist the velocity changing and, at the same time, adds some of the energy dissipated during the previous step. There are also other instances in gait cycle when energy is added:

1. During the acceleration phase of the swinging leg A′ (the leg B is supporting the mass m), kinetic energy is provided, which later during the braking phase, when starting supportive phase A″, is added to the kinetic energy of mass m.
2. Potential energy is added across the leg during the supportive phase by extending the extremity beyond the point of "spring" retracting action.

So far, it seems that our findings provided by the simple inverted pendulum model correlate well with the human locomotor system because ankle plantar flexor and extensor muscles of knee and hip are large when compared to the flexors of ankle and hip, but also comparable to the knee flexors. The reason will be explained in further text. For explaining it, we have to observe closely the swinging leg function like the movement from A' to A". At the instance of the underlaying leg B in position 2, the transported mass is at its minimal height and both legs are supporting the mass. This time period is called double support phase. During this phase, the trailing limb is pushing the mass m out of the low potential energy position. Also, we can observe that in the middle of the swing phase, the mass reaches its peak of the mass vertical displacement trajectory. The curve of the mass vertical displacement during human walking is a sinusoidal curve, having for each oscillation across the supportive leg or swinging of the contralateral leg, one minimum and one maximum. For two steps, i.e., for one stride, the mass m is twice in maximum and twice in minimum position. One stride is measured from an event belonging to one foot to the subsequent occurrence of the same event for the ipsilateral foot. In Figure 3, it is, for example, the time from the initial contact in instance A to that of A". Stride length can be measured with regard to any specific point of the system, for example, with regard to body mass position or with regard to the foot position as displayed in Figure 3.

When observing two minima and two maxima, the swinging leg mass must be because of clearance from the ground and because of uneven terrain moved up and down in the gravitational field. To conserve energy, nature has segmented the leg and, at approximately half of the length of the extremity, the knee joint was added. Because of necessary lifting of the foot and shank masses, the knee flexors have to be powerful. The potential energy of the lifted shank and foot is, during swinging and extending of the leg, to a great extent converted into kinetic energy. Because of braking of the swinging leg performed by hip and trunk muscles, the energy is then transferred as propulsion in the forward direction to the mass m. In such a way, nature has again employed the principle of energy conversion for recuperating the energy introduced into the swinging leg. Note, that the distal parts of the segmented leg which travel over the largest vertical distances have the smallest masses, again with the aim to conserve energy and gain other benefits such as low moment of inertia and hence, possible larger acceleration at the same muscular power. The locomotion activities explained raised thinking that the locomotor system functions as a coupled system of regular and inverted pendulum combined with springs providing smoother function and energy recuperation. One may say the human locomotion system acts like a coupled pendulum system, which oscillates near the resonant system frequency. When a man is walking, all the described coupled pendulum oscillations and springs actions are orchestrated by the neural control, while active propulsion power is added by the muscles. The muscles generate, maintain, and absorb forces as required for efficient mass transfer. All these muscle functions have to be kept in mind together with the principles of gait and orchestrated pendulum oscillations when considering gait restoration in general. The phenomena of mass-spring system and inverted pendulum oscillations are taking place also in the frontal plane providing effective body weight shifting between the extremities. The couple of forces[1,2] created by the heel-striking left leg (negative shear backward force) and pushing-off right leg (positive forward shear force) is causing trunk rotation in a positive direction (when right leg is pushing), which is synchronized with the hip extensors and abductors activity, utilizing the tractus iliotibialis[3] as a bandage and spring for frontal load shifting on the leading leg. At the heel strike, part of the inertial moment in the direction towards the push-off leg is damped, and the energy is stored by the tractus iliotibialis acting as a spring which constant is adjusted by the hip extensors of the heel-striking leg. Also, energy is stored in the foot arch acting as a spring. Later, this energy is rebounded. The energy stored is returned during the phase of starting the medial-lateral trunk movement in order to transfer the whole trunk

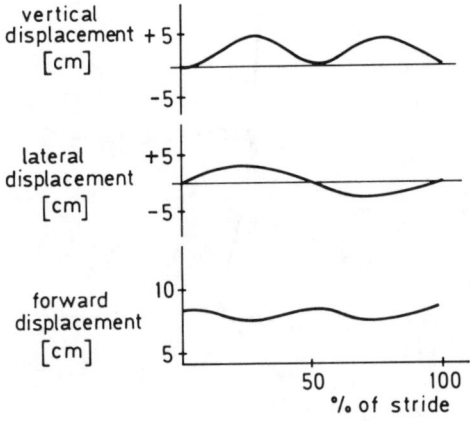

FIGURE 4. Vertical, lateral, and forward trajectories of the head and neck during normal walking (redrawn after Winter[5]).

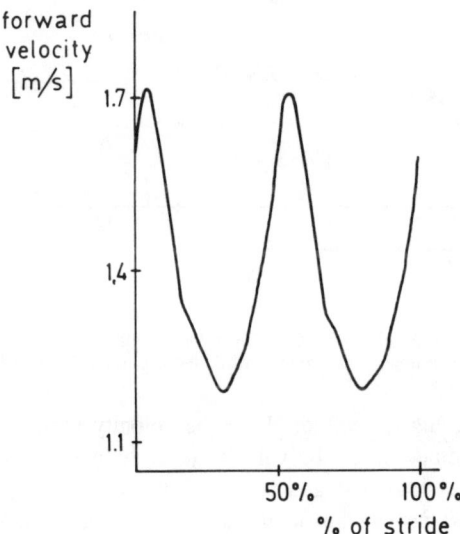

FIGURE 5. Forward velocity of head, arms, and trunk, as assessed during normal walking.

load onto the leg entering the single-limb support phase. The movement of head and neck in the vertical, lateral-medial, and forward direction[4] is shown in Figure 4. The medial-lateral displacement in the frontal plane and vertical displacement in the sagittal plane, when combined, result in smooth low frequency oscillations. Vertical displacement of the mass m in the sagittal plane as presented in Figure 3 (in particular for small steps) strikes for similarity when compared to the data obtained in a normal man (Figure 4). Also, the progression velocity[5] is oscillating as can be seen from the data measured[5] in Figure 5. Here, the velocity for head, arms, and trunk is given. Figures 4 and 5 are indicating that the energy dissipation is very small. It seems that most of energy is consumed because of the leg movements. In the case that small steps are made, the instantaneous inverted pendulum mass velocity is similar to the instantaneous progression velocity. The latter can be determined by employing the principle presented in Figure 3 and applying it in the midswing where the

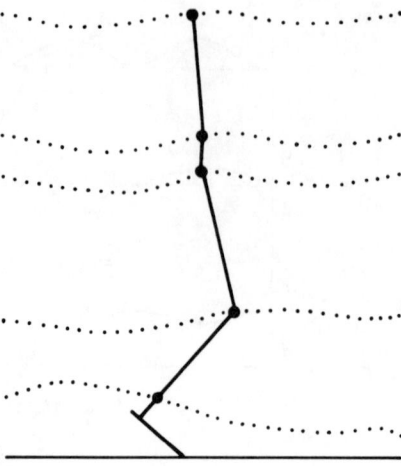

FIGURE 6. Displacements of different anatomic points during normal walking.

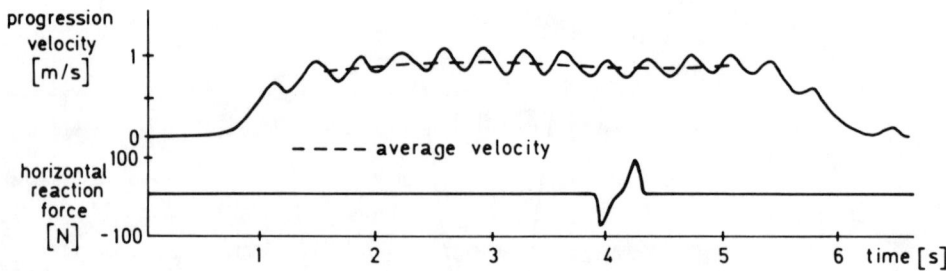

FIGURE 7. Instantaneous progression velocity of the trunk during normal walking. During steady state gait positive and negative shear force impulses are equal, while the average velocity is constant.

potential energy has the highest value. Here, the velocity is minimal. At the positions of average vertical displacement also, the velocity takes its average value, while for minimal displacement, velocity is maximal and so is the kinetic energy. Therefore, the forward progression velocity must have a sinusoidal shape. And indeed, the measurements published[5] confirm our deduction (Figure 5). For a sine wave progression, velocity and also the progression displacement will be sine-wave shaped (Figure 4). Combining the lateral and sagittal displacement curves for the head, we obtain a spiraling curve in the space. The vertical peak displacement of head, arms, and trunk (HAT), representing about $2/3$ of the body mass, is for normal gait cadence in order of 2.5 cm[4,5] or 3% for slow, 3.5% for normal, and 4.5% for fast cadence if normalized to the average value of the stride length. Regardless of the amplitude of head displacement in the vertical or horizontal plane, the important quality of energy conservation is the smooth shape of curves. Similar to HAT displacements are also rather small displacements of different anatomic points[6] as displayed in Figure 6.

The progression velocity of the center of body vs. time is presented in Figure 7. Our discussion was concentrated on the rhythmic phases of gait and not to the accelerating and decelerating phases. The main contributions of the forces required for maintaining forward progression are occurring during push-off phase when the following power can be assessed in different joints: about 10 W at the knee, 2.5 W in hip, and 35 W at the ankle joint. Most of the power is contributed by the ankle joint, while in the knee joint, there is mainly dissipated energy.[6] Inman et al.[6] also determined that there is a necessary increase of body weight above the umbilicus for 8 to 10 kg for increasing the locomotion energy requirements for more than 16%. This is evidence that considerable weight can be carried without considerably increasing the energy demand. In his studies, Inman[7] finally concluded that about 50% of the total energy of a moving subject is conserved because of energy transfer between legs and trunk with arms, while the remaining 50% of energy is required to accelerate and decelerate the lower extremities. This energy is lost and must be generated by muscles (see also Figure 39). He also stated that nature does not care very much how an individual walks because the important goal of walking appears to be transport of body mass in a most efficient way with the least expenditure of energy. If anything disturbs the mechanisms of energy conservation displayed by sinusoidally shaped smooth curves of displacement, an increase of energy expenditure will result.

From this brief presentation of the fundamentals of human walking, let us summarize some conclusions in regard to the dilemmas and recommendations for FES gait restoration. Average and normal man gait patterns cannot be copied for FES gait restoration, because low energy expenditure and efficiency are more important than appearance and cosmesis. Each individual is using locomotor apparatus, which nature gave to him, attempting to function with the least expenditure of energy.[6] This is valid also for a SCI patient. With FES, we are trying to increase his capabilities of performing locomotor functions with minimal expenditure of energy and not with regard to his aesthetic appearance. FES muscles should be, therefore, added only and only if the function is improved and thus reduced energy expenditure is obtained. Normal subject is not an adequate reference model for a SCI patients gait restoration. In SCI, there is always missing FES control over some muscles due to lower motor neuron lesion (LMNL). Restoring a simpler gait pattern is more adequate and may ensure reasonable efficiency. Also, the dilemma of walking with large or small steps is clear. For the time being, small steps are preferable, particularly when balance is a problem and plantar flexors are not activated to provide necessary propulsion. In such cases, the propulsion forces must be generated predominantly by arm pushing. Periodicity and smoothness of walking are of utmost importance for ensuring energy conversion and recuperation. If the latter cannot be achieved, small steps ensuring minimal vertical displacement and hence, minimized loss of energy are preferable. FES can efficiently provide vertical body support, but for generating proper propulsion forces and desired energy conversion, FES requires adequate control. From this point of view, feedback control systems must be considered as advantageous if applied in FES systems. Feedback control systems can also take into account important properties of bone, joint, tendon, ligaments, and muscle in order to prevent secondary pathology developments.

III. PRINCIPLES OF GAIT SYNTHESIS AND CONTROL

Our goal in gait synthesis is complex restoration of walking abilities in completely paralyzed paraplegic patients. Therefore, a comparison of the existing rehabilitative aids and FES means for gait restoration can provide interesting insight and conclusions. In Figure 8, a long leg braces equipped patient is compared to an FES system user. The main questions to be answered are what advantages FES is providing when compared to the classical mechanical bracing, and what are the development perspectives in both orthotic approaches. The most widely utilized mode of paraplegic patients locomotion is wheelchair. The latter has several important advantages such as high energy efficiency and relatively low cost. It is also very safe and simple to use. The following are the drawbacks of the wheelchair transportation: inadequate cosmesis, unnatural way of mobility being confined to even terrain, inappropriate for stair climbing, etc. The energy requirement for wheelchair propulsion at 70 to 80% of normal walking speed (80 m/min) is nearly equal to normal walking (oxygen rate 11.5 ± 3 mℓ/kg/min or oxygen cost 0.16 ± 0.3 mℓ/kg/m).[8] Crutch walking is char-

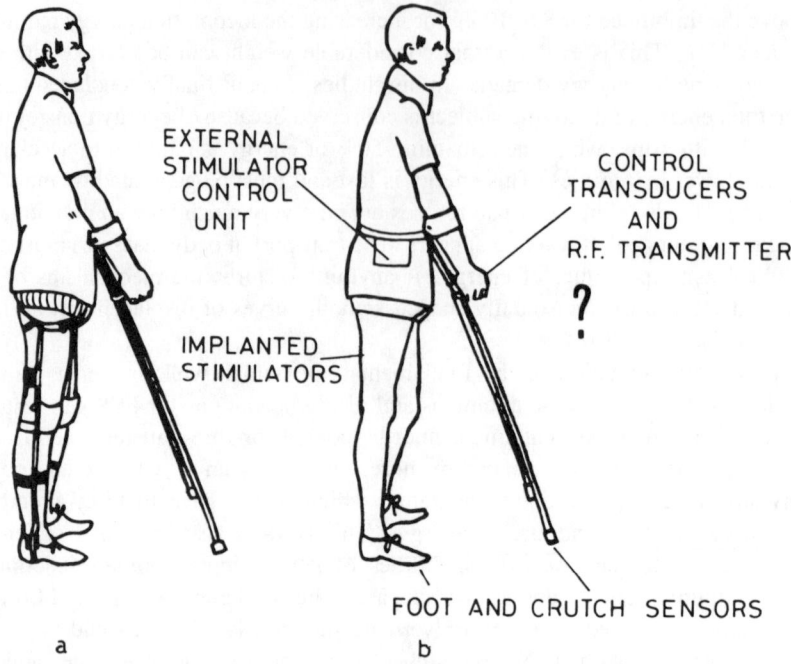

FIGURE 8. Patient standing with the help of long leg braces and maintaining balance with crutches (a), and patient with implanted FES orthotic system (b).

acterized by lower walking speeds. The average speed is 27 ± 17 m/min. It is 64% slower than normal walking (80 m/min compared to 27 m/min). The heart rate during crutch walking is increased 46%, oxygen uptake is raised 38%, and the oxygen cost is 49% higher. The energy increase is the main reason why paraplegic patients often abandon crutch walking. The energy consumption and physiologic stress are too high. It is known that work rates of up to 50% of maximum aerobic capacity can be sustained in an untrained subject for 8 h or more, but for higher work rates, the maximal working time is rapidly decreasing.[9] For FES-assisted reciprocal walking in paraplegic patients, the most important aspect is the issue of low energy consumption.

According to our discussion in Section I, the human locomotor system can be considered as composed of coupled inverted and noninverted pendula oscillating close to resonant frequency. If this hypothesis is valid, there must be an optimal walking speed characterized by minimal energy expenditure and related to the resonant oscillating frequency and magnitude of the system. Indeed, the measurements have confirmed this statement.[10-12] Any slower or faster oscillating of the subject's "coupled pendulum system" may require higher driving energy. This observation was further confirmed with the gait energy expenditure measurements in man.[12,13] Zarrugh et al.[12] developed an empirical equation for energy expenditure determination as a function of speed. It is valid for moderate speeds of walking. It was also shown that for a given step length within the normal range of walking speeds there is a determined and prescribed step rate which leads to minimal energy expenditure per unit of distance walked. Any other combination of step length and step rate results in greater energy demand. This indicates that the coupled pendula, representing the human locomotor system, must oscillate in coupled resonant mode to ensure minimal energy expenditure. Therefore, the step length is associated to the step rate as well. As Zarrugh et al.[12] pointed out, the energy optimality condition reflects a subject's dependent proportionality constant determining the step length to step rate ratio. Consequently, for a given subject's

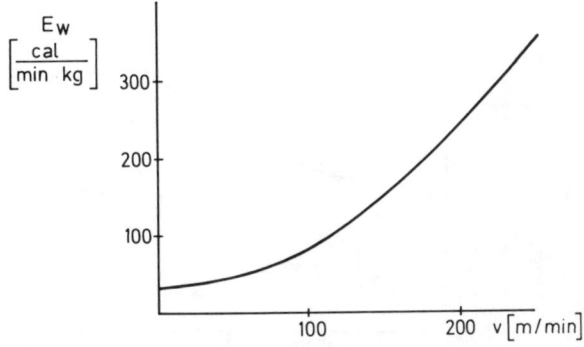

FIGURE 9. Relation between energy expenditure E_w and walking speed v for b = 32 and a = 0.0050, as found in group of normal subjects (1 cal = 4.186 J).

antropometric data, there exists an optimal step length and step rate as well as corresponding proportionality constant. Therefore, each subject possesses his optimal step length and step rate. Energy expenditure is expressed in calories required during locomotion per time unit (cal/min, 1 cal = 4.186 J). As the minimal energy expenditure differs from subject to subject, we shall introduce E_w — energy expenditure per unit of body mass (cal/min/kg). The energy expenditure can be normalized also to distance traveled measured in meters and denoted as E_m. It is obtained by dividing E_w by velocity v: $E_m = \dfrac{E_w}{v}$ ($\dfrac{cal}{m\,kg}$). As Ralston[11] pointed out, the energy expenditure E_w is linearly proportional to the kinetic energy, i.e., to the squared velocity:

$$E_w = b + a v^2 \qquad (1)$$

where E_w represents energy expenditure in cal/min/kg, b is the energy value at zero velocity v = 0 and a determines the slope of the quadratic curve in Figure 9. Zarrugh et al.[12] have found that b has a value of 32 and a of 0.0050 in a group of normal subjects.

Even more interesting is the presentation of energy expenditure curve with regard to the walking velocity itself. For this reason, Equation 1 is to be divided by velocity v:

$$\dfrac{E_w}{v} = \dfrac{b}{v} + a v = E_m \qquad (2)$$

The energy expenditure E_m as a function of velocity is presented in Figure 10.

From Equation 2, the minimal value of E_m can be found. Minimal and hence, optimal energy expenditure occurs at the velocity $v_{opt} = \dfrac{b}{a}$. The value for $E_{m\,min}$ can be calculated by the help of Equation 2 and v_{opt} and has the value of $E_{m\,min} = 2\sqrt{ba}$. By inserting the experimental values for a and b, we obtain v_{opt} = 80 m/min and $E_{m\,min}$ = 0.8 cal/m/kg. Another interesting locomotion parameter is the ratio of step length, S, and the number of steps per minute, n. For optimal energy expenditure, this relation is expressed by Equation 3:

$$S = 0.0068\,n \qquad (3)$$

For a selected speed, the energy expenditure can be calculated by the help of Equation 4:

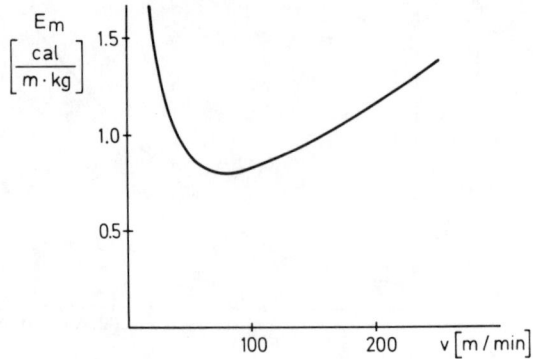

FIGURE 10. Energy expenditure E_m expressed per unit distance (1 cal = 4.186 J).

$$E_w = \frac{E_0}{(1 - \frac{v}{v_n})^2} \quad (4)$$

By using the experimental values for energy expenditure and velocity and by solving the Equations 1 and 4 simultaneously, we obtain E_0 = 28.3 cal/min/kg and the upper velocity limit v_n = 240 m/min. By the help of Equation 4, one can calculate the energy expenditure for a normal walking speed in the range of 25 to 145 m/min. The presented matter is important because the question arises of how we are going to control the walking velocity in FES orthotic systems.

It is necessary to find a method to control the stimulation pattern for obtaining walking rate dependent stimulation[30] sequences ensuring minimal energy expenditure. It is further open to discussion whether the rules given in Equations 1 to 4 apply also to pathologic gait when asymmetric walking is present and some muscles are not functional. It is also questionable as to how do these rules change if the restored gait is simplified with regard to normal walking. Our aim is to develop at least some guide rules and criteria for decision making in practical problems of FES gait synthesis. Also, we would like to have criteria for the FES gait sequences synthesis which will ensure adequate biomechanical and physical solutions and also provide efficient energy expenditure. At the same time, we would like to prevent secondary pathological system degradation or damage.

A. Patient Model

Before any planning of gait restoration utilizing FES can be started, it is important to understand in detail the impairment, preserved functions, and anatomical limitations being consequences of the spinal cord lesion. For FES restoration of gait in SCI patients, the global body mechanics must be first considered. In Figure 11, a SCI patient with thoracic lesion is presented in order to display how the lower paralyzed body part is related to the upper normally innervated body. The two body regions are tied together by the long body muscles such as erector spinae and abdominal muscles. Regardless of the lesion level, some parts of these muscles are preserved and function normally because they are innervated from many spinal cord levels as can be redrawn from Figure 12. From Figure 13, it is evident that any SCI lesion at the T-12 level or below will result predominantly in lower motor neuron lesion (LMNL) because of the spinal cord shift with regard to the vertebrae. This is even more stressed in reality because spinal lesions involve, to some extent, also the neighboring segments due to hematoma and edema development. Therefore, in practice, there are not

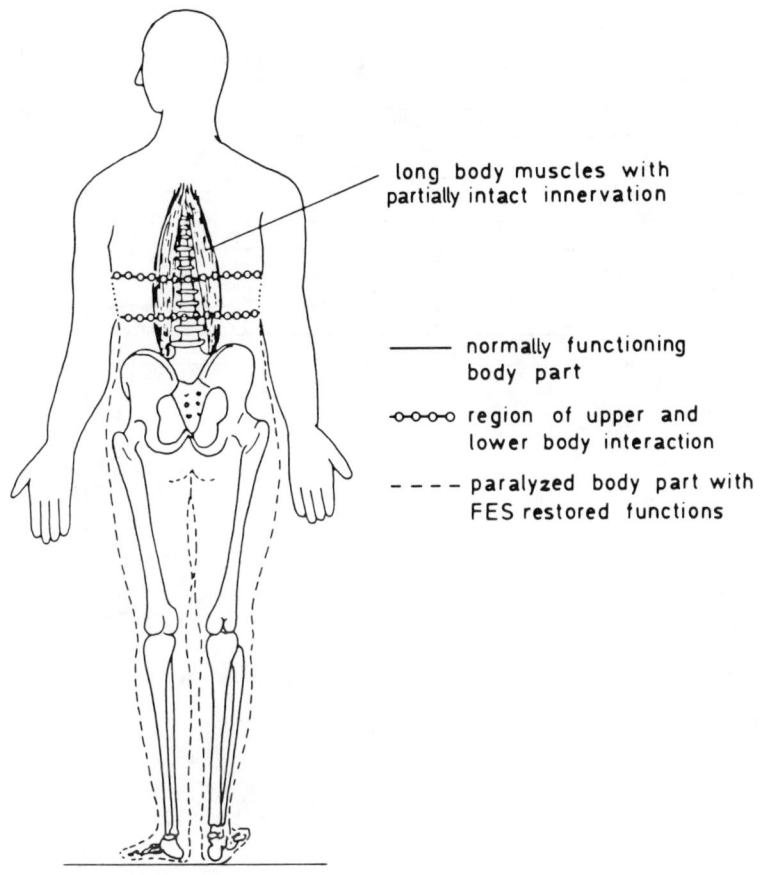

FIGURE 11. Functional body regions in thoracic SCI subject.

many patients with lesions at or below T-11,12 candidates for FES gait restoration. These patients, having LMNL of the main extensors of hip and knee, are suitable candidates for classical or hybrid (FES and mechanical) bracing. Considering the biomechanical structure in Figure 11, FES can only provide the control over the paralyzed lower part of the upper body. The coordination, control, and function of the lower body must be adjusted according to the requirements imposed by the upper body. The patient must be provided with means for conscious or subconscious control of the FES activation of his pelvis and lower extremities. The upper body part is attached through the long body muscles to the lower part of the trunk. If this connection is inadequate and very weak, it can substantially influence the ability of the patient to balance his upper body. In such cases, the stimulation of the trunk muscles is a necessity. Fortunately, nature innervated many of the muscles which are attached between the lumbar regions with the pelvis and higher trunk sites in such a way that in case of a T-4 or lower lesion, these muscles remain, to large extent, normal. In this way, the patients are able to sit and balance the trunk. They are also in a position to move and rotate the trunk in different directions while standing by braces or FES. Important to note are the following muscles: m. rectus abdominis, m. quadratus lumborum, m. erector spinae, m. spinalis, m. transversospinalis, mm. interspinales, mm. intertransversarii, m. latissimus dorsi, etc. (Figure 12). Important to distinguish is the function of these muscles in the case of firm leg support and support provided by the legs and arms with crutches. In the case of FES ambulation, the trunk movements, pelvis function, and progression forces are, to a large extent, generated by arms, while weight bearing is provided by FES. Only if the ankle

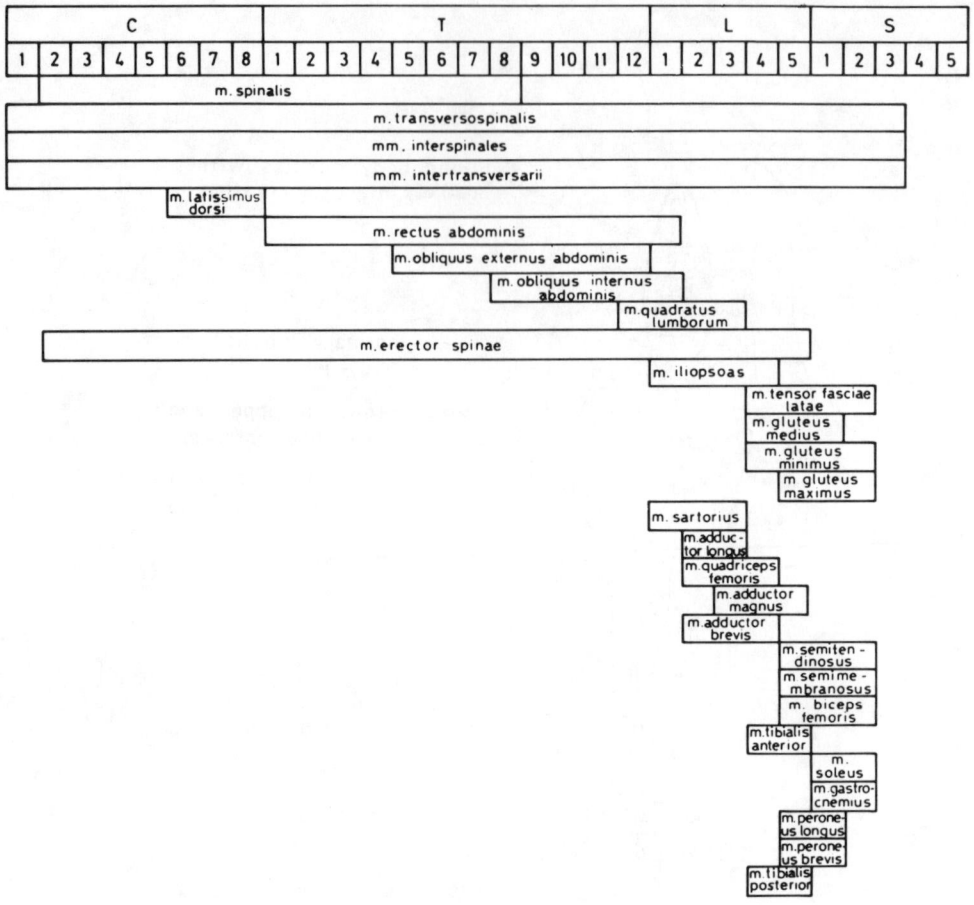

FIGURE 12. Innervation of skeletal muscles related to spinal cord level.

plantar flexors, knee and hip extensors are stimulated in a proper way, will propulsion be FES delivered also.

The long body muscles listed are important not only because they provide voluntary activity, but also due to the preserved sensation and proprioception. Natural feedback information is transferred also because of tension developed across the tissue or skin, and sometimes through existing rudimentary sensation neural channels which may be still preserved in some patients. Such sensation is important for providing at least some feeling about pelvis position in space. One may recall here the analogy with children walking with stilts. A paraplegic patient while standing and walking by means of FES is like he is walking on stilts applied at the hips. He can have some minimal information about the pelvis, but has nearly none about the events occurring in his hips, knees, and ankles. The preserved trunk muscles are very important in the locomotion restoration and therefore, it is important to restrengthen them to the maximal extent and to make the patient aware of them. This is important for improved upper body-lower body coordination and for better control during FES ambulation. For control, coordination, and FES sequences composition, understanding of Figure 14 is helpful. The movement control in man is accomplished by three main levels: cortical, supraspinal, and spinal control. Peripheral electrical excitation of muscles and nerves triggers action potentials in both afferent and efferent nerve paths. Therefore, FES is causing inflow also to higher nervous system levels. In this way, spasticity and reflexes can be triggered or inhibited by electrical excitation of peripheral neural structures. In a complete

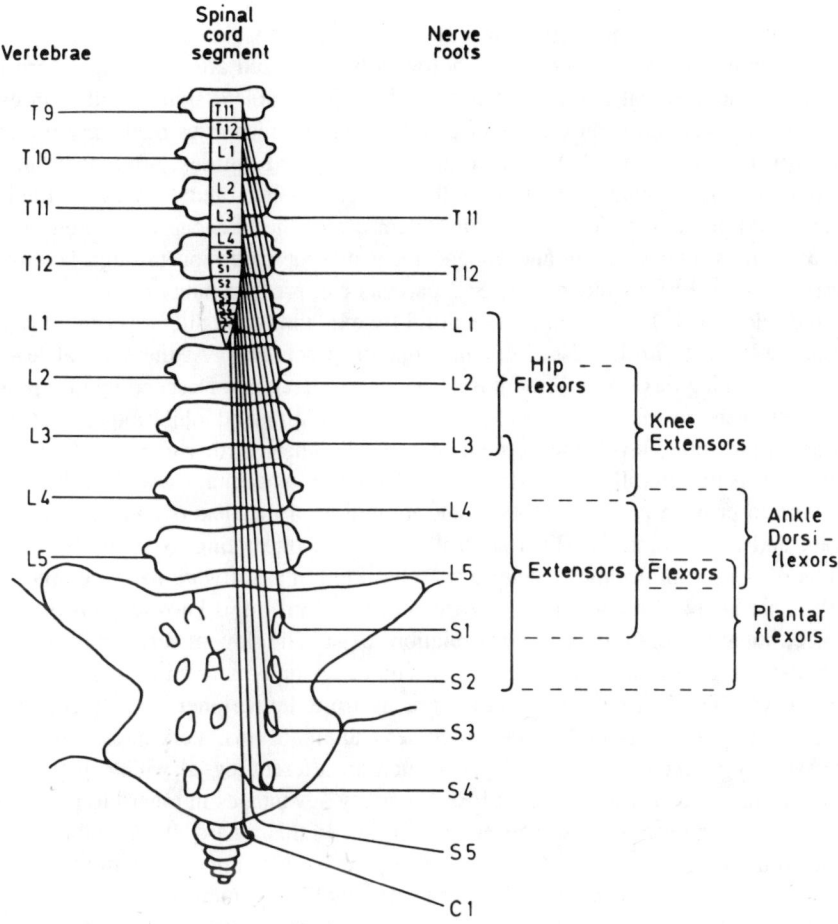

FIGURE 13. Innervation of muscle groups in lower extremity.

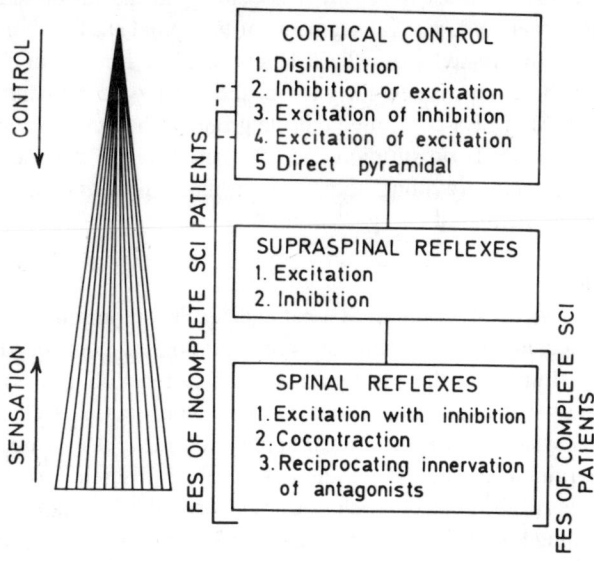

FIGURE 14. Schematic representation of neural control in man.

spinal cord injury, the spinal cord below the lesion site is isolated, but possesses neural control over spinal reflexes which are pathologically organized after the spinal cord injury due to missing supraspinal control. Therefore, FES in complete spinal cord injuries may cause efferent activation of muscles or afferently triggered responses mediated through the dissected spinal cord (Figure 14). In incomplete spinal cord injuries, afferent influence of FES also may reach higher structures of the nervous system and thus cause inhibition, excitation, and release of reflexes. Very important use of the FES-caused afferent inflow is sensory awareness augmentation and enhancement of proprioception through learning and therapy modalities. FES of incomplete SCI patients can provide many effects, particularly if delivered selectively. Figure 14 also is helpful for explaining the dilemmas and difficulties of natural feedback control and sensory information processing. At the cortical level, the intention to start a leg flexion movement is a "go no go" decision. Descending to supraspinal reflexes level, many neural structures require proper excitation and inhibition control signals, and lower on the spinal level, the number of control signals further expands. The number of control signals has literally a triangular shape from top to bottom, expanding dramatically with the aim to provide proper activation and inhibition of the flexors and extensors of the hip, knee, and ankle joint. For FES control, it may be interesting to know the rules and algorithms of neural information expansion. What kind of a software nature employs, and how is the "hardware" functioning? For efficient FES control, this knowledge is of a crucial importance, but at present only vague speculations exist. The flow of sensation signals from periphery to the higher CNS levels displays the characteristic of neural information compression (Figure 14). The extensive information arising from the periphery is filtered, selected, and compressed by not fully understood processes and algorithms. Very interesting, indeed, is the possibility to send from the periphery such an afferent signal which may elicit the desired reflex movement. Such afferent FES has many advantages in regard to more natural muscle activation and use of preserved neural control. In this regard, the spinal reflexes are of primary importance as well as the structural principles depictured in Figure 15.[65] Particularly, the combination provided by afferent and efferent FES is suitable for broad application and functional restoration of walking in SCI patients. It seems, therefore, valuable to include the afferent FES modality into the FES sequences synthesis. Patient evaluation, in regard to preserved reflexes, is of utmost importance.

Considering Figure 13, we must realize that according to the lesion site and extent of damage caused to the spinal cord, several segments of the spinal cord will display peripheral lesion and the muscles innervated from these levels are lost for use of FES. These lost functions will have to be compensated for and substituted by the remaining normally innervated muscle functions or FES-controlled muscle groups. The exact restoration of normal gait is therefore not possible. If substitution and compensation are not adequate, a simpler gait pattern is to be selected providing some compromises resulting in a somewhat less effective gait, displaying increased energy consumption.

B. Control Principles

The control issues of gait restoration in SCI patients by FES represent a complex problem from a fundamental, technological, functional, and pathological point of view. Therefore, our discussion will be limited to the practical approach to the FES gait control problems. In principle, the control system can be either an open loop or a closed loop. Almost all currently utilized FES systems for FES clinical application make use of open-loop control. Further, the control principles can be continuous[14,15,19] or discrete[16] or can use logical algorithms.[17] Regardless of the control type or principle used, basic control schemes provide a means for understanding problems involved and solutions proposed. First, we shall consider open-loop control schemes. In Figure 16, the interaction of patient and FES orthosis is presented. The FES system is bypassing the spinal cord lesion. Block 1 represents the CNS

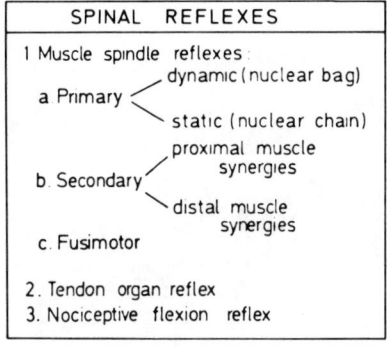

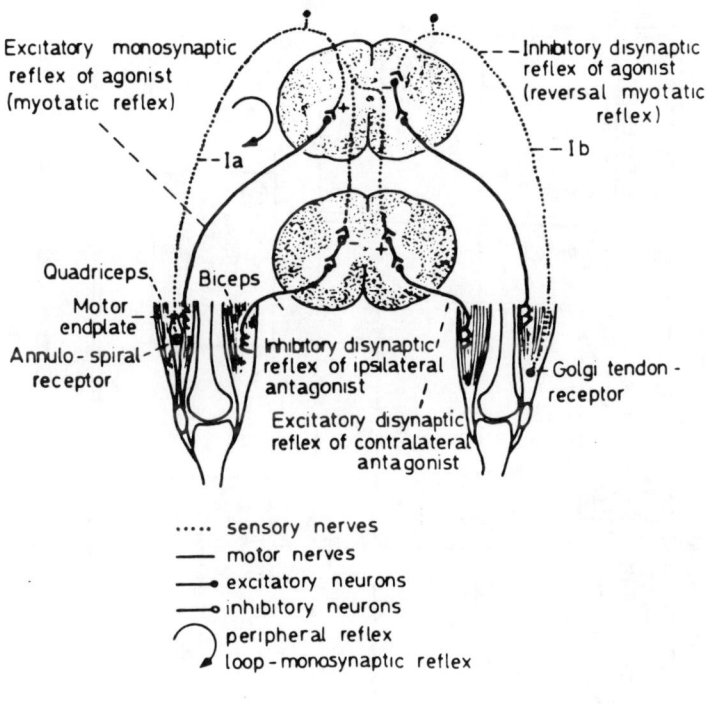

FIGURE 15. The spinal reflexes (a) and the ipsilateral and contralateral innervation (b).

function together with the part of the intact spinal cord above the lesion. Block 2 belongs to the preserved spinal cord which is disconnected from the CNS according to the lesion extent. In complete SCI, there is no functional neural connection between blocks 1 and 2. Block 3 appertains to the musculoskeletal system which is partly normally innervated and partly paralyzed. The bypass across the damaged spinal cord functionally consists of a control signal processing block 4 and a FES stimulator delivering the desired stimulation sequences and represented by block 5. The control information is picked up from a normally innervated body site. The body function, which can serve as the control source, can be muscle force, joint torque, pressure, EMG signal, or joint angle. A very common control signal is obtained by fingers activating switches, adjusting potentiometers, or manipulating

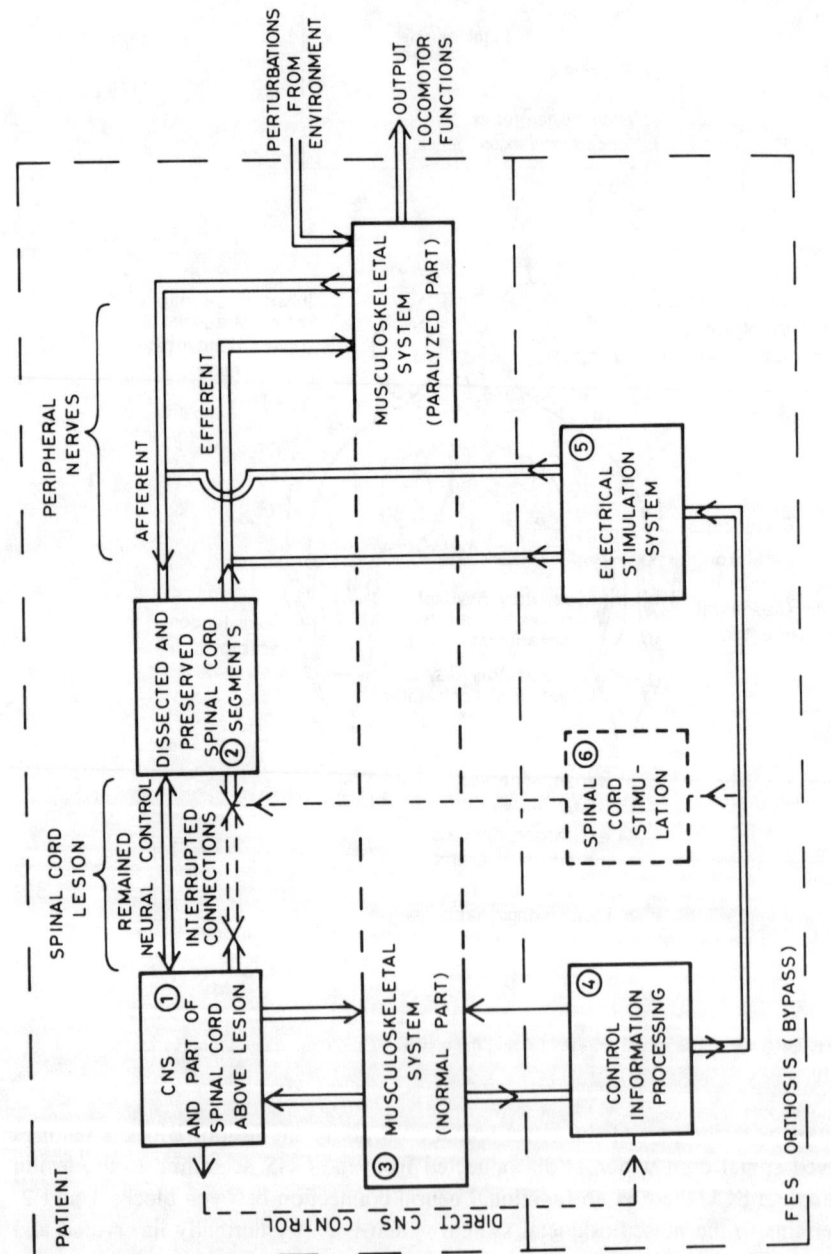

FIGURE 16. Interaction of patient and FES orthotic system.

some other device such as joy stick. In all these examples, the control signal is picked up by a transducer which is consciously controlled by the patient.[18-23] A whole different set of control signals belongs to the subconscious control. In the conscious control, a body site function is artificially selected in order to control the function lost due to paralysis. In most cases, this also means that the control body site has no natural relation with the lost function. A subconscious control signal is obtained from an intact body site which is functionally and naturally connected to the involved paralyzed body site. Obtaining such subconscious control signals is difficult, especially with regard to the design of pick-up hardware and information processing necessary for the extraction of the control signal. The common problem encountered is the separation of the control from regular functions. Control signals must be reliable and independent of noise, interference, and any other functions not being correlated with the control activity. Control signals can be continuous and/or discrete in regard to amplitude and time. In Figure 16, the control bypass is represented by the blocks 4 and 5. Electrical stimulation can be delivered to the peripheral nervous system as motoric-efferent or sensory-afferent. The latter causes the required output movement through the reflex functioning of the dissected spinal cord. In Figure 16, there is a feedback presented between blocks 4 and 3 caused by retrofunction of the control device, e.g., when controlling the force required to activate a joy stick. The futuristic control approach envisages the possibilities of placing pick-up electrodes directly in the CNS.[24] There is also a possibility to deliver FES directly to the spinal cord as represented by block 6 in Figure 16.[64]

For the open-loop control principle, it is characteristic that the FES sequences are independent of the output locomotor functions. The locomotor functions may change because of many reasons such as fatigue of stimulated muscles, cocontraction of muscles caused by pathological neural control of the dissected spinal cord, or because of external reasons such as perturbations from the environment. The FES orthotic system has no information about these undesirable events and cannot prevent or correct them. The same is true for the patient's conscious control. The patient is not aware of the events occurring in the paralyzed part of his body and cannot readjust the control of stimulator because he has no proprioceptive or exteroceptive feedback. For improving these disadvantages, feedback or a closed-loop control system is to be introduced. In regard to the type of feedback information, we can distinguish information derived from the locomotor system output and denoted as exteroceptive and information obtained by monitoring, functioning of the musculoskeletal system itself, denoted as proprioceptive information. In Figure 17, three types of feedback signals are presented: local exteroceptive and proprioceptive feedback to the FES system, feedback to the control information processing unit, and sensory feedback augmentation providing sensory information about locomotor performance to the patient. As future possibilities, dashed lines are plotted, representing the feedback signals to the spinal cord stimulator and to the CNS directly. The feedback information measured must be properly processed and extracted in block 7 before it can be efficiently used. For output or exteroceptive information assessment, there are various transducers available, yet they are, in most cases, clumsy and cumbersome for daily use. For proprioceptive or internal musculoskeletal system monitoring, there are presently numerous unsolved problems like where to place the sensors, what type of transducers to use, etc. It seems that an important complementary solution to the artificial implanted sensors is the idea to use the already present natural sensors as proposed by DeLuca[66] and Hoffer and Sinkjaer.[25]

The feedback control system can be employed for local adjusting of a muscle force[16] or a joint angle.[15] The feedback controller is therefore forcing the locomotor output according to the desired input reference signal. In this way, often more muscle power may be used[23,26] than during normal walking. Such control is therefore opposing the requirements for low energy consumption. Here, the term strategy of the control comes into importance. Instead of forcing, for example, a given joint into a desired reference angle, it may be less costly

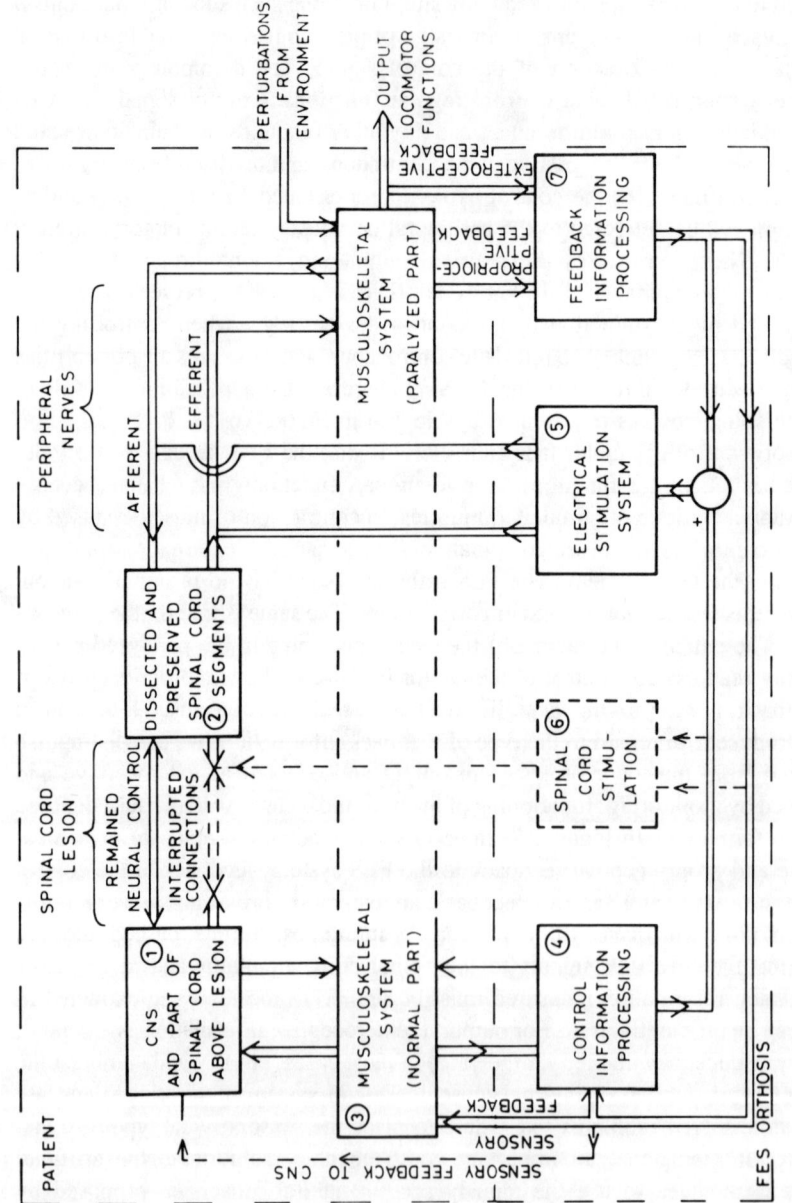

FIGURE 17. Introduction of feedback signals into the FES orthotic system for locomotion assistance.

to readjust another joint and obtain an acceptable position in the first joint by less energy. It might be appropriate also to change globally the body posture and solve the control problem at a very low cost and conserve even more energy. In such a context, the global control strategy appears to be more important as compared to a local joint control, because more energy can be saved at only slight change of locomotion pattern. Hierarchical control strategy might be an appropriate solution for the problems mentioned. On the higher control levels, joint trajectories providing low energy consumption are chosen with respect to momentary body posture and desired movement. On the lower levels regular closed-loop control of joint motions can be implemented.

C. Expansion of Control Information

In the previous Sections III.A and III.B, the need for control information expansion was presented. It is obvious that there must be found some rules or criteria for expansion of control information traveling from higher nervous levels to lower structures of the locomotor system.

It is necessary to determine the algorithms for simultaneous control of a given set of stimulated muscles. The next question is how this algorithm has to be changed in regard to exteroceptive proprioceptive feedback signals. After knowing the control algorithm, the stimulation sequences can be generated easily by only knowing the properties of stimulated muscle. The stimulation sequence prescribes the amplitude and the time period of activity for each muscle selected in the gait restoration task. The action of muscles must be orchestrated to enable biped reciprocal gait, while gait stability will not be considered in this presentation. One possibility of stimulation sequences composition is to copy and mimic the activity of muscle function as assessed by the help of an EMG recording during normal gait. In Figure 18, it is shown how the stimulation sequence for ankle dorsiflexors is determined in gait restoration of hemiplegic patients using an EMG recording of normal subject's walking. The EMG can be rectified and averaged and the envelope obtained. The stimulation sequence of fixed preset amplitude and time duration is obtained by rather crude approximation (A-case). The stimulation sequence is determined with respect to the trigger signal obtained from the heel-off shoe insole switch. It is delivered to the ankle dorsiflexors after a delay d_1, while the duration of activity is d_2. It means that for each muscle stimulated by such a mode, three parameters have to be selected with respect to a specified control signal trigger: amplitude, delay d_1, and duration d_2. Such a mode was, for instance, utilized in multichannel FES for stroke patients.[27-29] Because of selected delay d_1 and stimulation duration d_2, this sequence is suited for a given walking speed, and the patient has to adapt his walking to the FES orthotic system. To avoid this imperfection, walking rate controlled timing of the stimulation sequences was proposed.[30] For obtaining the corrective signal, the cadence time or swing time of the patient's walking are measured and, according to the patient's speed of walking, the delay d_1 and duration d_2 are adjusted. These simple principles were utilized for six-channel FES for gait restoration in hemiplegic patients.[27,29] The control principle can be even further expanded by utilizing more trigger signals in a single stride.[31] In principle, with changes in walking speed also the stimulation amplitude can be adjusted. Such an FES device was to our knowledge not yet applied. In Figure 18, the B mode of stimulation sequences utilizes discrete approximation of the FES amplitudes according to the EMG signal envelope.[32] Such a stimulation sequence results in smoother, less jerky, and more natural movements in isolated joints. Technical realization of gradually modulated stimulation envelope demands considerably more complex hardware. The most sophisticated stimulation sequence is presented by the C mode in the Figure 18. It resembles the rectified and integrated EMG activity as assessed during walking of a healthy subject. It can be obtained also mathematically from the desired joint trajectory (joint torque and angle) and musculoskeletal model.[33] Continuous stimulation sequence can be efficiently found also by

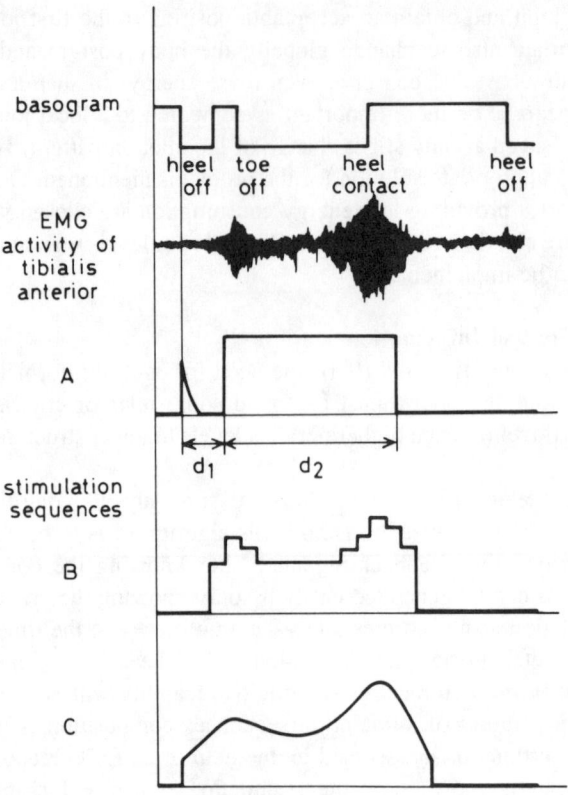

FIGURE 18. Three modes for stimulation sequence determination based on normal EMG pattern: constant stimulation amplitude (A), gradually modulated stimulation sequence (B), continuous modulated electrical stimulation (C).

an iterative trial-and-error procedure.[34] Utilizing the principles presented in Figure 18 for stimulation sequence composition, practical gait restoration system for SCI patients was most successfully developed by Marsolais et al.[23,35,36] For triggering, there was a variety of possibilities proposed, such as hand and shoe switches,[23,37,38] mercury tilt switch placed at sternum,[39] force sensors,[38,40] accelerometers,[38,41] proportional two fingers control,[22] and EMG signature discrimination of trunk movement.[38,42] Some of the transducers enumerated provide continuous control signals while only on-off information can be obtained from others. Continuous analog control signals, such as those derived from accelerometers or EMG muscle activity, need considerable preprocessing, resulting in more complex control hardware.

For each locomotor function, such as standing-up, sitting-down, stair climbing, etc., the stimulation sequences are to be stored in a memory of a microprocessor-based stimulator and selected like "menues" by the patient. This gait control mode can be called "menue mode" of the locomotor functions selection. Here, stimulation sequences composition is very flexible when including additional muscles, but requires that the patient adapts himself to the sequences selected. These FES sequences are predetermined and have poor or no adaptation possibility for changed walking conditions like obstacles in the environment. In this regard, important advantages are provided by the control mode where the patient himself is composing stimulation sequences timing. In this way, a patient can more efficiently coordinate the locomotor events and adapt his performance to his visual feedback and other feedback information he may utilize. The gait is triggered and synthesized on-line via hand switches.

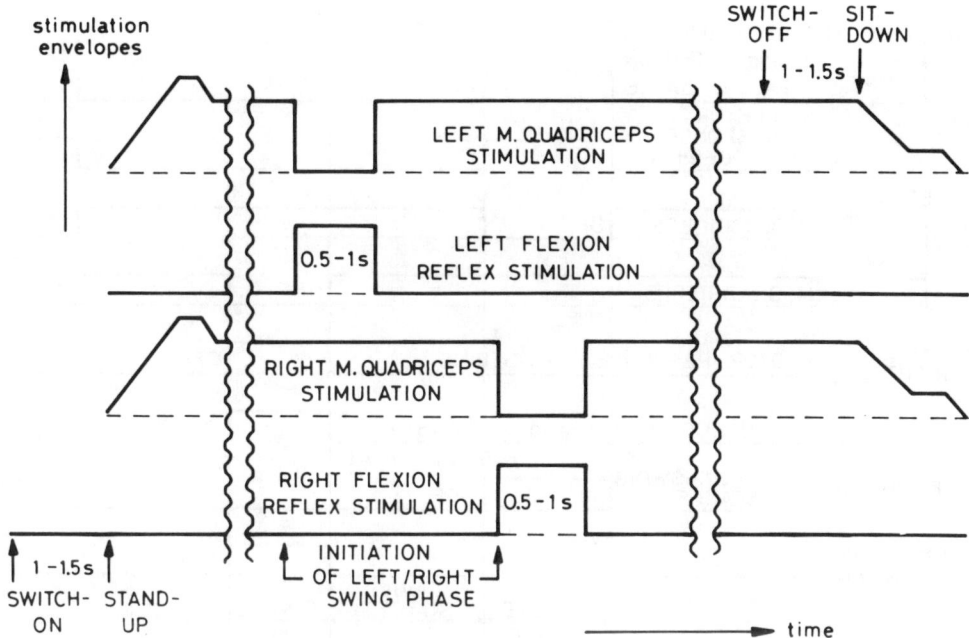

FIGURE 19. Four-channel stimulation sequences providing standing-up, standing, simple reciprocal walking, and sitting-down of a completely paralyzed paraplegic subject.

This approach was used to control simple four-channel reciprocal gait pattern. In further text, the patient composed gait synthesis will be described in detail. The characteristic gait events are double stance phase and single stance with contralateral swing phase. If no hand switch is activated, double stance is present and by pressing a switch the swing phase starts. The intensity of flexion in the leg being in the swing phase is proportional to the duration of the hand switch pressing. Release of the switch stops the flexion response and brings stimulation again to the knee extensors. The activation of switches and transitions between phases are controlled by fingers. The arm support provides stability and required progression forces. Typical four-channel stimulation sequences are given in Figure 19. The amplitude setting for each channel is available to the patient, and he can adjust the intensity of movement according to his needs and, at the same time, also compensate increasing fatigue of stimulated muscles. Additional muscles can be added easily if their activation is related to the occurrence of the stance or swing phase. Addition of the muscles which require a delayed start according to the hand switches is performed by the help of logical circuitry containing the activation algorithm ensuring adaptability to changed rhythm of gait. Figure 20 displays an example of a six-channel gait sequence. There is a dilemma present in regard to the selected number of channels, complexity of the system, reliability, and improved function. In case the addition of a stimulated muscle/channel does not improve the locomotor function adequately, the particular muscle is not used properly or it is not relevant in restored function and is therefore obsolete. The information for each stimulation channel must contain also the algorithm or some simple logic ensuring safety in case wrong or illogical triggering occurs. Such a situation may occur when both the left and right swing phase are requested at once while the patient is walking. Such a command is prohibited and must not be executed. Therefore, if such a request is obtained, the logical circuitry will neglect the command. Another complication arises when a swing phase is requested by a leg which is still bearing body weight. In the four-channel patient's-controlled gait pattern, the patient must transfer his body weight and ensure proper stability before triggering the swing phase event. In this respect, it is interesting

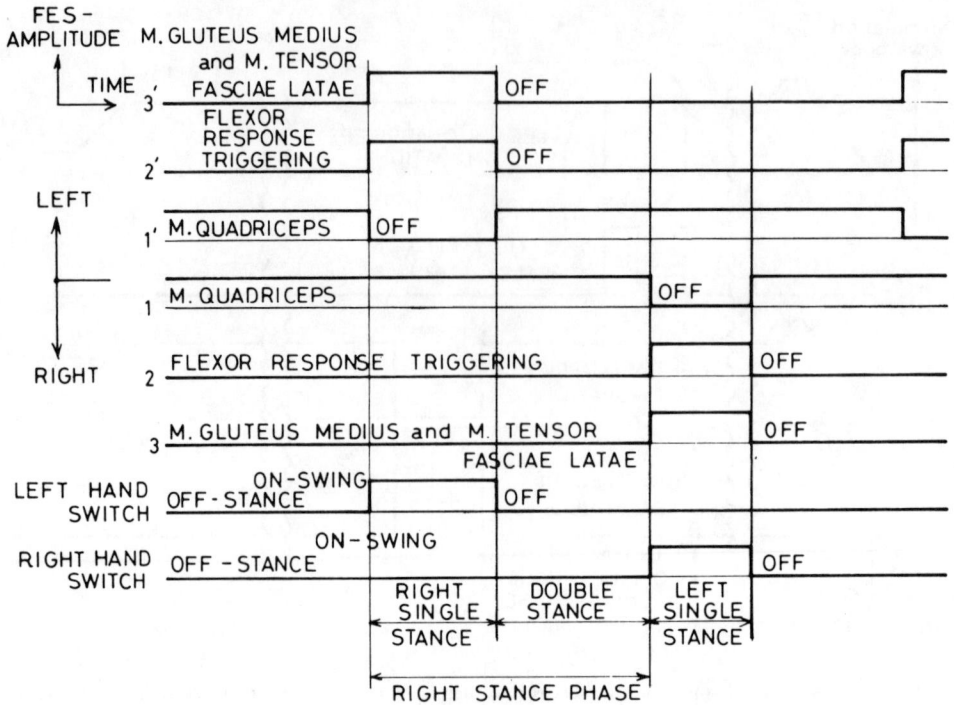

FIGURE 20. Six-channel gait pattern.

to discuss Figure 21. Quiet bilateral standing is stable if the body center ground reaction force is passing within the support area encircled by foot prints. Usually, we adjust because of comfort and safety the resulting reaction force in front of the ankle joint and in the center line, such as points 1, 2, 3, and 6 of Figure 21. If surface electrical stimulation is applied to abductor muscles, for instance, to the tensor fasciae latae or to the gluteus medius, weight shifting to the stimulated site takes place (points 4 and 5 or 7, 8, and 9). In the case that adequate stimulation is applied, the origin of the ground reaction vector will be moved into the footprint, resulting in single stance phase. Now, the contralateral leg is not providing support and therefore, swing phase flexion movements can be started. In the simple four-channel gait mode described, the body weight shifting is not assisted by electrical stimulation. Therefore, the patient has to shift the body weight from double leg support into a single leg support by trunk movement and by pushing with arms and hands on the supportive device. By introducing exteroceptive sensation and applying feedback signals from crutch or shoe attached sensors, important improvement in function and safety may be gained. Functional improvements may be substantial according to the results obtained by Kobetič et al.[43] By adding hip abduction muscles and plantar flexors for providing push-off forces, the stride length can be doubled and four times higher speed of walking achieved.[43] Again, this is suggesting that by proper addition and FES control of muscles, substantial functional improvements are possible.

Regarding propulsion of the body mass in the forward direction, Figure 22 is explaining how the plantar flexors function is dominant, while exerting propulsion for forward displacement of the center of gravity across a long moment lever. For providing forward momentum the hip and knee joints of the trailing leg must be adequately locked. Pushing is accomplished during a short period at 40 to 60% of the stride time. During this time, the plantar flexors are highly active. During that time, the opposite leg is in the late swing phase and enters the initial contact (heel strike) phase lasting up to 15% of the stance phase. In

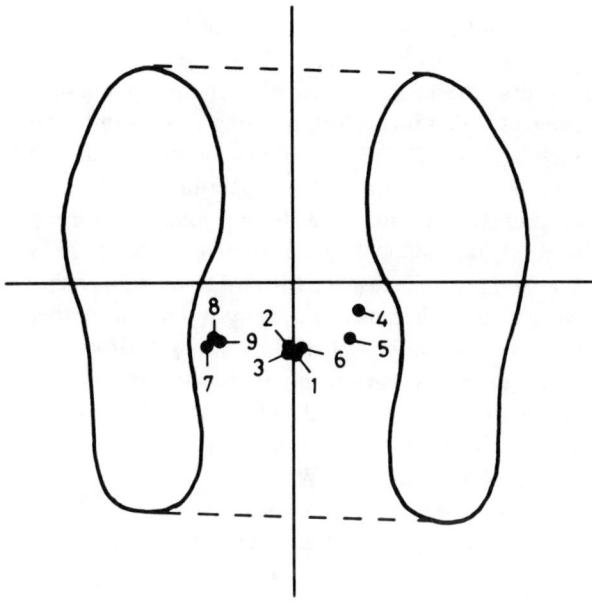

FIGURE 21. Relation of body center reaction force and supporting area during standing.

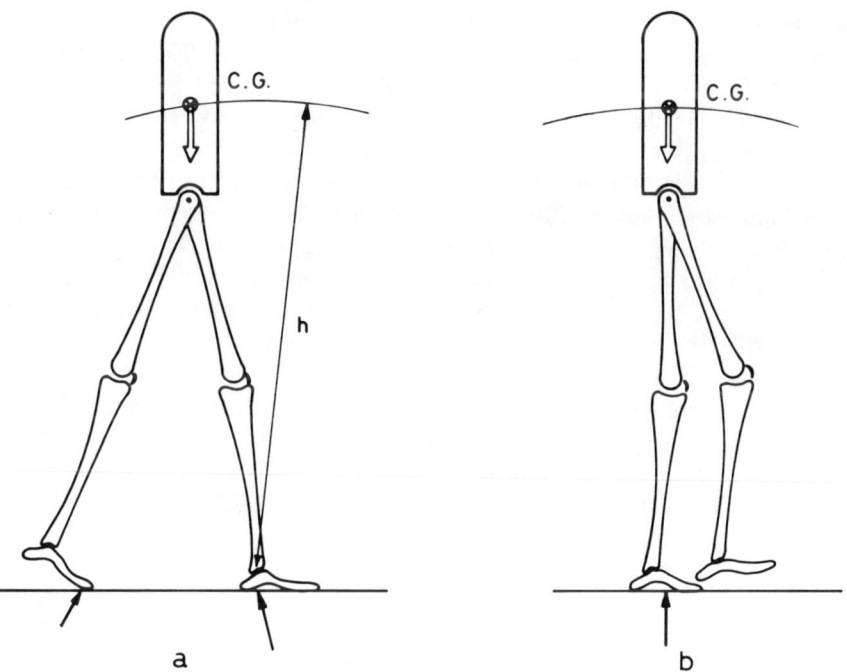

FIGURE 22. Body posture during the late stance (a) and early swing phase (b) of walking.

this phase, energy is absorbed at the knee joint of the leading leg. The trailing leg must control balance and contribute energy for rolling over the ankle joint of the leading leg. The long lever h is favourable for that reason (Figure 22a). During the late push-off phase (Figure 22b), the hip joint is powerfully flexed and produces positive work for accelerating the swing phase entering leg masses. Note, that sufficient acceleration in this phase can contribute to the step length and forward propulsion during the braking phase of the swinging leg. In case of missing hip flexors activity or because by surface FES we are not able to stimulate adequately the hip flexors, the swinging leg acceleration is missing. Knee flexors and extensors muscle action can be utilized for providing some substitution. Suppose, that in Figure 22b the swinging leg is sufficiently flexed in knee and dorsiflexed for clearance while the center of gravity is rotating forward on the supporting leg. The swinging leg will start because of pendulum properties to swing in the hip joint when the paraplegic subject is leaned forward. The pendulum action is not sufficient to bring the leg forward enough. Therefore, some physiotherapists increase the forward leaning for improving the step length. This is not a satisfactory solution because more body weight has in this way to be borne by the arms. Improved step length can be obtained by strong activation of the knee extensor, producing a sudden knee extension movement. Its braking momentum is pulling forward, substituting the missing active hip flexion and adding to the forward propulsion. The weight transfer in paraplegic four-channel walking is not easy for the patient to control.

An interesting observation was made by Winter[44] proposing the principle of lower limb support during stance phase of gait. The inconsistency of moments in the lower extremity joints during gait, if compared to kinematic data, gave rise to the principle that all leg joint moments contribute to the net supporting moment during stance phase, M_s, which prevents collapse in the lower extremity:

$$M_S = M_K - M_H - M_A \qquad (5)$$

Moment acting in a counterclockwise direction at the proximal end of any segment is positive. Owing to such notation in normal stance phase, knee joint moment, M_K, is positive, while hip joint moment, M_H, and ankle moment, M_A, are negative. The principle of the net supporting moment is saying that as long as M_S is positive and greater than moments provoking collapse in the lower extremity, the tendency of support remains. This also implicitly includes cases when a single joint moment action is missing or is even negative. As long as the net sum of moments is positive, the support is active. From the FES point of view and possible substitution for missing or inadequate extensor muscle force at a joint, the former finding is important. It indicates that by an appropriate activation of muscles at other joints, positive net supporting moment can be obtained. The latter conclusion is important and must be included into the synthesis of the stimulation sequences for gait restoration particularly in patients with LMNL of some extensor muscles. In this regard, consider also the posture switching aspects[45] described in Chapter 4.IV.C.

At the end of this paragraph, it should be noted that the present results of research directed to introduce closed-loop FES systems in paraplegic walking have not yet produced practical improvements in regard to function, duration, or reduced energy expenditure.[40,46,47] The already obtained benefits of closed-loop application were mainly observed in safety improvement, functional robustness of the performance in regard to external perturbations, and cosmesis reflected in smoother movement trajectories. Important research of applied closed-loop FES control in standing is directed toward achieving stability of standing free of hand support.[48] It is expected that in the coming decade, FES closed-loop systems will improve substantially all the locomotor functions. Main problems resistant to the immediate clinical application of closed-loop control FES systems are lack of adequate sensors and questionable cosmesis and complexity of such systems.

IV. GAIT TRAINING

Gait training can be started after the patient has accomplished independent safe and secure standing for at least 3 to 5 min. Before first gait trial, it is recommended to reevaluate the patient from a biomechanical point of view. Here, the most relevant selection criteria appear to be the presence of limited ROM, osteoporosis, or skeletal system instability. Any of these factors may exclude the patient from gait training. In principle, if a patient can be recognized to be a candidate for long leg braces locomotion, he is also suitable for FES gait training, of course, if the main lower limb muscle groups display UMNL syndrome. Before gait training, it must be assured that no sudden pathological change may occur. Therefore, bone integrity, spine stability, and joint integrity must be checked.

Patients able to stand for at least 3 to 5 min start the gait training with the help of multichannel electrical stimulation. The established minimal number of channels is four.[37,49] This gait mode includes the utilization of flexion reflex withdrawal movement for substituting efferently elicited flexion in leg joints. In further text, we are going to describe the gait training using the four-channel gait mode based on afferent and efferent FES. Two stimulation channels are assigned to each body site. Each set of two channels is controlled by a hand switch. If pressed, it will switch off the ipsilateral knee extensors stimulation and switch on the flexion reflex triggering. When left and right hand switches are not pressed, both m. quadriceps muscle groups are stimulated and the patient is able to stand in a bilateral stance with the C-posture and to maintain stability by using the hands. For hand support and stability, different devices can be utilized, such as parallel bars, special supporting frames, walkers, or, in a more advanced phase, crutches. In the early stage of gait training, the hand switches are activated by the physiotherapist. First, the patient has to learn to use the four-channel stimulator for standing-up and sitting-down. Before standing-up, he must assume the correct posture, adjust the hands on the support, and then switch on the stimulator. The built-in slow start of stimulation sequences appertaining to the knee extensors provide sufficient time for repositioning the hand used for switching on the stimulator back to the supportive aid. At this early stage, it is important to insist on good and proper posture during the standing-up maneuver. It is also a good practice to teach the patient to first switch off the stimulator before proceeding with sitting-down. The built-in delay is sufficient for providing adequate time to the patient (1.5 s) for correct placing of hands and assuming posture for sitting-down before stimulation starts to decay. Parallel bars were used in the early days of FES gait training.[50] Special supporting frames with the wheels allow longer walking runs and easier wheelchair accessibility. A four-channel stimulator is shown in Figure 23a, displaying the unit, large m. quadriceps electrodes, small electrodes for afferent stimulation, and the pair of hand switches. With walking frames, walkers, or crutches, another set of switches is foreseen. These switches are usually built into the handles of the walking frame or crutches or are suitable for attachment to different supporting devices. Figure 23b presents the switch built into the crutch handle, and Figure 23c presents a control module suitable for walking frame or crutch attachment. Different designs of stimulators were presented and described for enabling walking in SCI patients.[49-52] By observing the four-channel stimulation sequence (Figure 19), it can be recognized that at the same time for each site only one stimulation channel is active. Therefore, in principle, the four-channel unit can be replaced by a two-channel stimulator connected with the hand switches in such a way that the switch, if pressed, is switching the stimulation from m. quadriceps to the flexor reflex triggering and vice versa. Such a realization does not allow a separate amplitude setting for each stimulation channel, but a potentiometer connected serially to one of the stimulation electrodes can solve the problem. We are not going to describe further the details of different technological solutions, but rather, we shall concentrate on fundamental issues. It is our aim that the reader will be able to start and conduct the gait training and also to specify or adapt a commercially available stimulator for this purpose. The aim of gait training is to ensure safe, efficient, and functional walking. In regard to safety, it is important that the patient is aware and able to master sudden collapse or jack knifing occurring at malfunctioning of hardware or unexpected external perturbation in such a way that no hazard

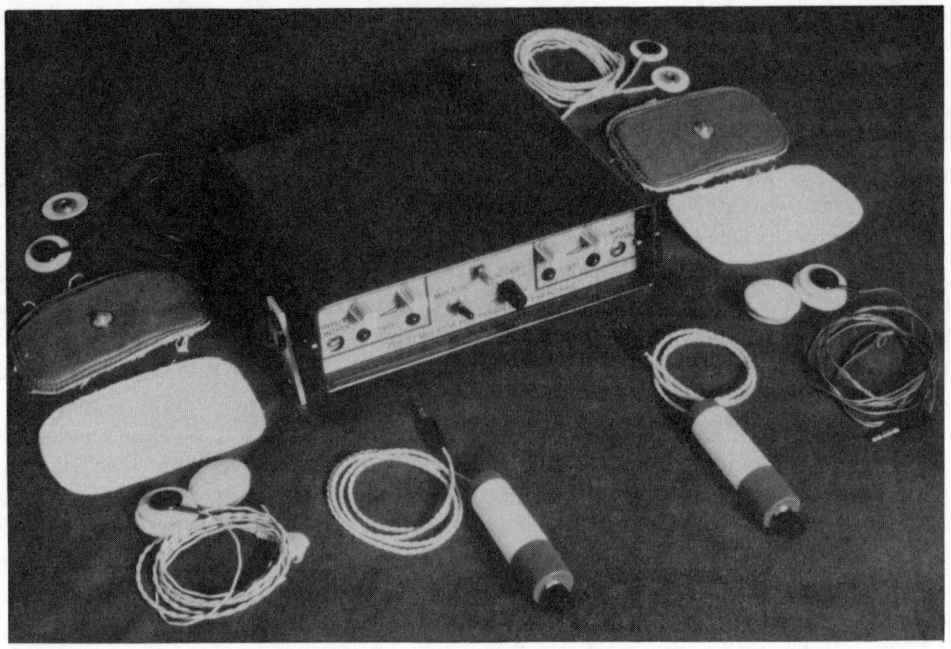

a

FIGURE 23. Four-channel electrical stimulator with electrodes (a), hand switch built into the crutch handle (b), and hand control module (c).

or harm will result. Therefore, special attention must be paid also to maneuvers necessary in cases when one electrode is detached, the electrode wire is pulled from the connector, or the stimulator does not function properly. It is also recommended that falling is practiced in the time when transfer from walker to crutches is introduced. Already, during frame- or walker-assisted walking, the patient must be made aware early of possible catching on hands and to one leg support standing. The latter is a regular part of gait training. Body weight shifting and transfer from bilateral standing is first practiced. Following body weight shifting, a single step forward is trained. The step length is kept short in the beginning, while with training time, it is increased and practiced for left and right leg. The weight shifting must be accomplished by associated trunk posture changes and helped by hand pushing and not pulling. Parallel bars and walkers are permitting not only pushing with the arms, but, to a limited extent, also pulling and are therefore easier for the patient when starting gait training. Because of later crutch walking, efforts must be made so that patient will predominantly exert pressure onto the balancing aid and that in the beginning, small steps will be made. A suitable step length is the distance of the shoe. Even shorter step length is adequate in the very beginning, but must be soon prolonged. Large step length is not recommended, particularly, in patients with higher thoracic lesions because of impaired trunk stabilizing musculature and difficult balancing. Because of large steps, knee buckling may take place. It occurs frequently when stimulated knee extensor muscles are fatiguing. Typical supporting frames used for walking training are shown in Figure 24a and b. After the patient has completed the weight shifting exercise and transfer in mediolateral and sagittal plane, he is ready to begin stepping. For safety reasons, the paraplegic subject can be secured against falling by leather straps. In this way, the physiotherapist can concentrate on the patient's locomotor functions while the patient is safe and relaxed. In the early stage of gait training, the physiotherapist is triggering the stimulator through hand switches. At the beginning,

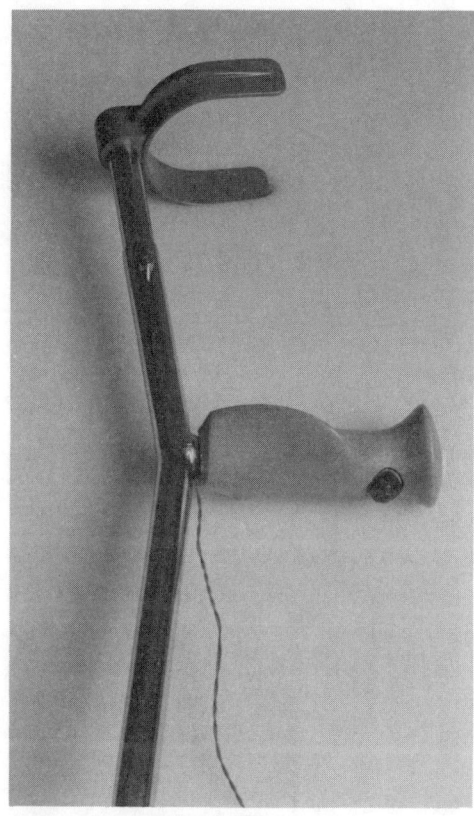 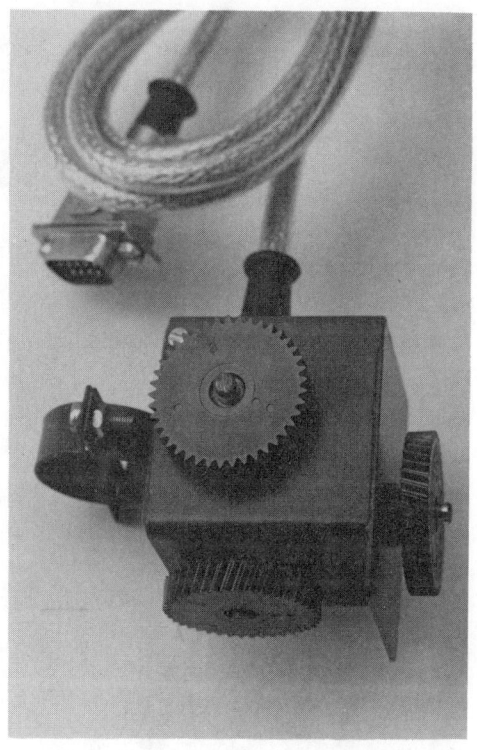

FIGURE 23b.   FIGURE 23c.

slow walking speeds are practiced. In such a way, the patient has enough time to coordinate his trunk and hand functions with locomotor activities of the lower limbs. It is important that already at the very beginning the patient is taught to walk with minimal energy expenditure and not to use his hands and arms for weight bearing, but only for progression and balance. Walking with upright C-posture is ensuring the required locomotion conditions. Large steps and prolonged patient's visual observation of the legs function are not permitted. If the patient is looking down at his legs, posture is disturbed, leaning strongly forward, and consequently, resulting in high forces carried by the arms. The patient should watch his performance in the mirror placed in front of the walking direction. Such mirror feedback is, of course, not sufficiently functional and patients prefer to look down at their legs. They should be encouraged to do this in short intervals only as a safety check and for easier coordination of triggering steps and trunk function. Later in the gait training phase, once the patient is by himself triggering the stimulator, the short time visual feedback of the legs performance is very important and helpful. At the beginning of gait training, the patient has no experience of how to select and adjust the walking speed. In this regard, it is helpful if the walking frame is on wheels and the physiotherapist is adjusting the walking speed and accelerating or slowing down the progression exerted by the patient. For minimal weight transfer experience, as required for starting the gait training, usually 3 to 5 sessions for 10 to 15 min are sufficient. The sessions should not last too long because fatiguing of electrically stimulated muscles is limiting the standing time. It is recommended to make several short time sessions per day. The latter is advantageous for faster learning. At the beginning of gait training, the walking distance and number of steps per run should be kept low, usually

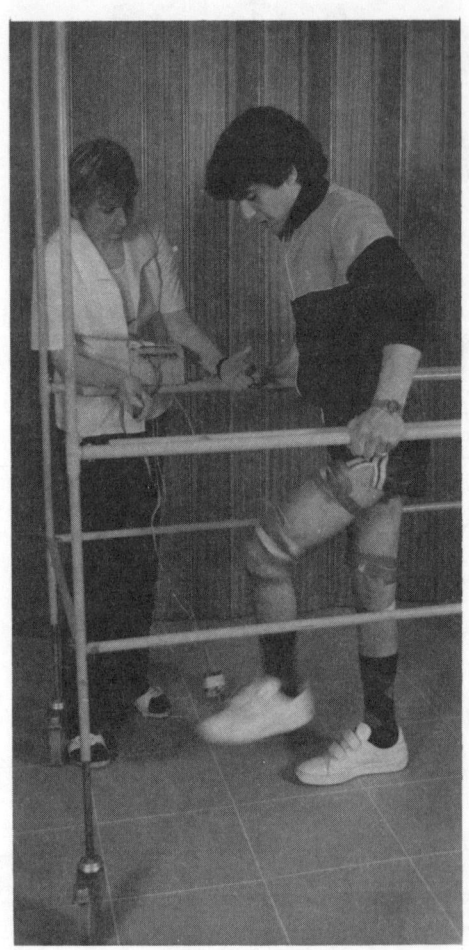 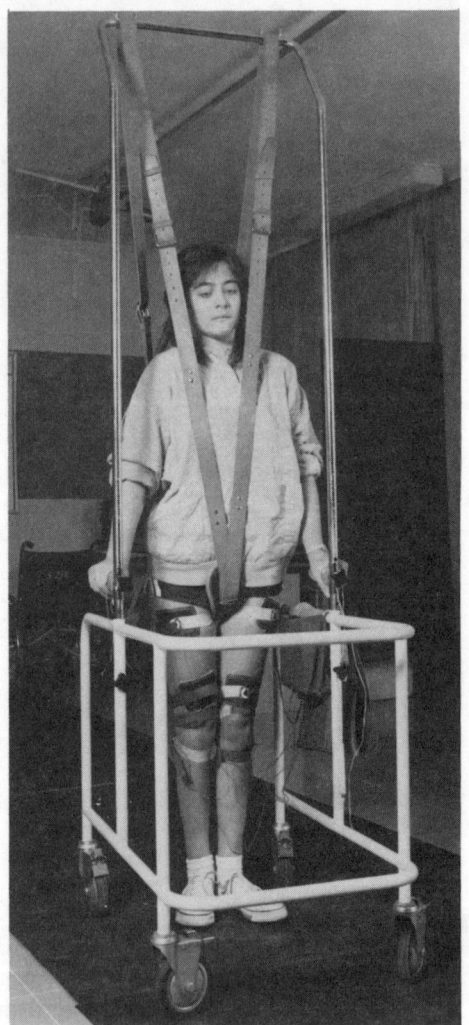

a b

FIGURE 24. Two types of supporting frames intended for initial training of walking in complete paraplegic subjects.

from only a few up to 6 to 10 steps. After each walking run, the patient must stop in a bilateral standing mode and stand independently until the physiotherapist brings the wheelchair to a new position. While the patient is sitting in the wheelchair, he gets some rest, while comments and preparations are made for the next run. Usually, if the patient is not tired, the next run can be performed after a few minutes. In case the patient is tired, he shall be allowed to rest for a longer period. It is recommended that the physiotherapist is, at the same time, exercising walking with several patients. This gives the patients time to think about their walking performance, to rest, and what is the most important, to observe the function of other patients. It is advisable that two training sessions are conducted per day.

Patients are taught at the same time to position the electrodes and to don and doff the FES system independently. At the very first trials, donning and doffing of electrodes and wires is carried out by physiotherapist, while later it is only supervised until the patient is taking care of the FES orthotic system by himself. In about a week, the patient must be able to don and doff the system independently. The physiotherapist must correct the mistakes made by patient and teach him how to select the most adequate electrode position and proper amplitude setting for all stimulation channels. After the physiotherapist decides that the patient is safe and secure enough in walking, the use of straps can be eliminated. During initial gait training, the stimulator is, conveniently for the physiotherapist, attached to the walking frame. Care must be taken for correct electrode wires location to prevent tangling and pulling out from connectors.

In patients with weak back muscles, it is recommended to introduce also FES restrengthening of long body muscles. Particularly, erector spinae and latissimus dorsi muscles should be exercised. Such electrical stimulation exercise has, according to our experience in most cases, beneficial effects with regard to improved trunk control, while also more regular defecations and bladder emptying occur together with decreased abdominal spasms. It is quite frequent that during standing-up and during the first several steps, patients will have troubles with abdominal spasms interferring with the gait. In this regard, while standing by means of FES, hyperextension stretching in hips is beneficial. In many patients, lower trunk musculature is not under voluntary control due to the spinal cord lesion, but may be synergically coactivated at upper trunk movements. In such cases, restrengthening by proprioceptive muscle facilitation also occurs.[53] Another possibility is to add stimulation of hip extensors and abductors. The latter is stabilizing the trunk and at the same time, increasing gait efficiency. Hip extensors (gluteus medius and minimus) with abductors (tensor fasciae latae) may be stimulated by a single set of correctly placed electrodes being active synchronously with the m. quadriceps stimulation.

A. Training of Walker Ambulation

When walkers are used for balance, the stimulator can be carried by the patient (Figure 25a and b) or it can be attached to the walker (Figure 25c). Walking frame or even parallel bars assistance is easier for the patient because it allows arm forces to work in the direction of pulling. Therefore, before transferring the patient to walker, it is important to ensure that he utilizes only pushing arm forces. The latter requires instrumented walking frames for evaluation of supportive forces. The alternative is to start gait training immediately with the help of a walker which requires, at the beginning, increased safety measures, stability awareness, and assistance provided by the physiotherapist. Walkers are, in general, not the most functional and best suitable supporting devices. Walker ambulation is jerky and body weight transfer is not fluent. From the other side, walkers are preferred by the patients because they provide good stability and safety. Parallelogram walkers are suitable for home ambulation, allowing sharp turning and access to furniture. Roller walkers are more difficult to turn, require somewhat more space, but they are appropriate for faster gait. An important difference is also that with the roller walker, there should be almost no body weight support when the walker is to be pushed forward. At that time, double leg stance phase is in progress. The consequence is that the patient must learn to execute the double stance phase in well-aligned "C" posture or hip extensors with plantar flexor muscles must be activated. Usually a 2- to 3-week gait training is sufficient for an average skillful patient to be able to walk with a walker. An additional 2 to 3 weeks are necessary for mastering independent and reasonably safe walker ambulation. Regarding folding and storage, parallelogram walkers are easier to handle. For outdoor walking, roller walkers appear to be more appropriate.

B. Training of Crutch Ambulation

The transfer and learning of skills necessary for changing the walking frame for a walker are easy and simple. But, the transfer to crutches is tedious and requires substantial practicing

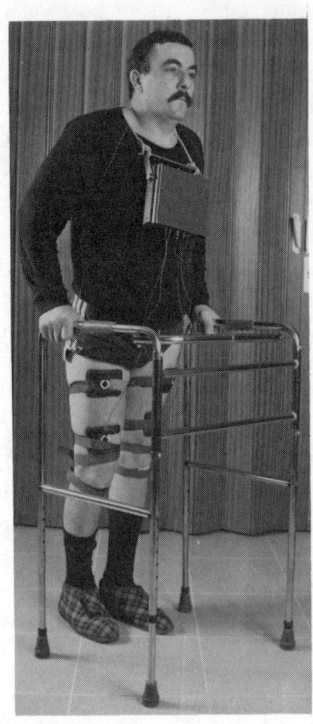 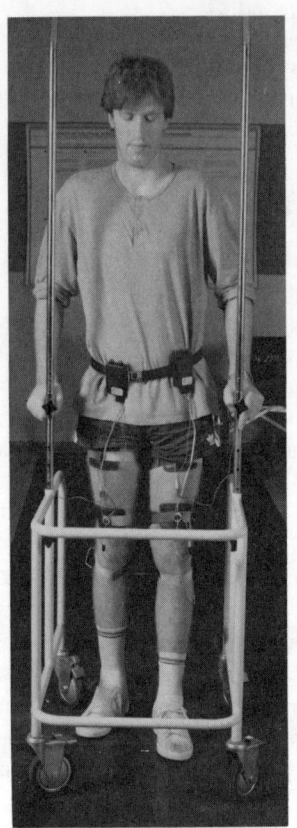

a b

FIGURE 25. Training of FES walking by the help of walker. The stimulator can be carried by the patient (a and b) or attached to the walker (c).

time. The walkers provide, for most of the time, four-point support and, for a brief time, only two-point ground support. Therefore, walkers are rather stable and allow the patients the torques around the horizontal handles of the walker in both sagittal and transverse planes. Crutches permit, in general, pushing forces and, to a much lesser extent, also torques to be transmitted in the plane defined by the horizontal longitudinal and the crutch handle axis.

Many patients are not able to master crutch-assisted FES walking. The reason is that crutch walking requires biomechanically well-aligned posture and rather strong arms, hands, and back muscles together with adequate shoulder and trunk mobility. Some patients give up because of insufficient feeling of balance and fear from falling. In particular, standing-up by the help of crutches is difficult to learn because of limited balancing possibilities. Therefore, much of time is to be devoted to practicing independent and unassisted standing-up.

Figures 26a, b, c, and d are displaying different modes of crutch-assisted standing-up. So far, the safest way of the unassisted standing-up maneuver is presented in Figure 26d. If any accident takes place during rising, the patient is falling back in to his wheelchair. The most difficult and dangerous phase occurs after the rising phase is completed and lasts until the patient is standing quietly leaned forward on his crutches. During the end period of the rising phase, the patient has to create a momentum by pushing on crutches in such a way that dynamic forces will swing the patient forward, while being in the erect position

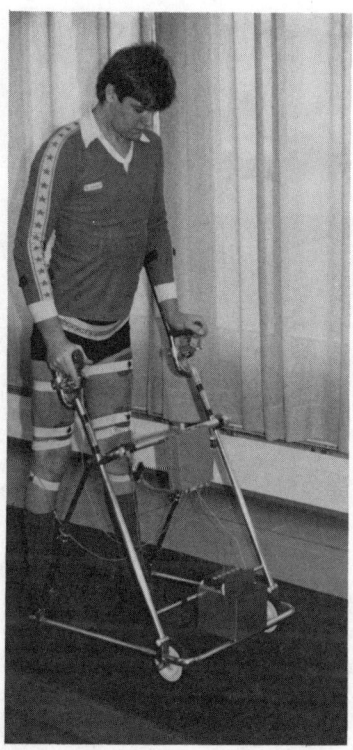

FIGURE 25c.

and standing on his legs only. At this instance, the patient must bring the crutches forward, in front of the body, and place them in a position permitting safe accepting and braking of the forward swinging body momentum. Thereafter, the patient remains standing in a posture leaning forward on the crutches. After the dynamic events have ceased, he can assume proper "C" posture. Note, that during the rising and momentum generation phase, hand, shoulder, and later, also trunk muscles are maximally utilized and knee extensors do not assist in spite of being stimulated to provide standing at the end of the rising maneuver. Therefore, only patients with strong upper body musculature and arms are capable for employing the described standing-up mode. Different is the standing-up modality presented in Figure 26c, where knee extensors are used to perform most of the lifting work. Here, the arms are also active for lifting part of the body weight and align the trunk. This standing-up mode seems to be more natural, but provides very poor means for controlling the balance. For better weight distribution of stimulator and batteries, the stimulator can be worn in special small bags as can be seen in Figure 26c. Some patients themselves like to modify the way of carrying the stimulator. Note, that additional FES-controlled muscles of the lower extremities and trunk may considerably improve the standing-up maneuver.

After the patient is taught how to stand by crutches, shift the body weight between his legs, and be confident in his feeling of balance, training for taking steps starts. Again, short steps are to be used in the beginning. For crutch-assisted walking, different gait modes are possible. Within the four-channel gait pattern, crutches have to accept the forces exerted by hands and provide progression pushing. Crutches are also used to maintain balance and must be adequately placed for braking the forward momentum produced by hands after each step of reciprocal biped gait. Such gait pattern is not smooth, namely, after each step the progression velocity drops to almost zero. During the single-leg support, while the swinging

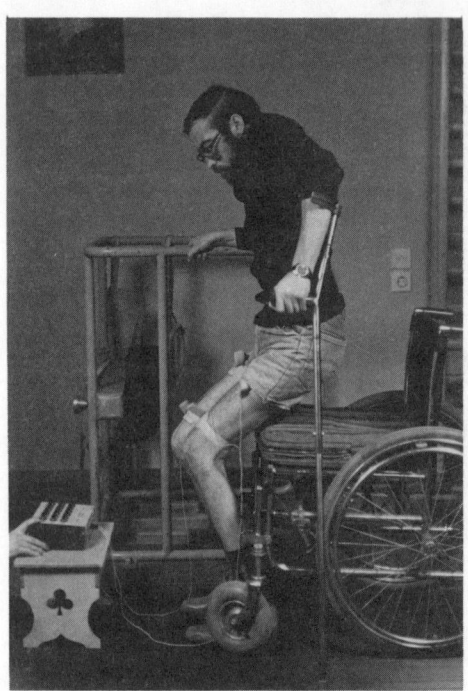
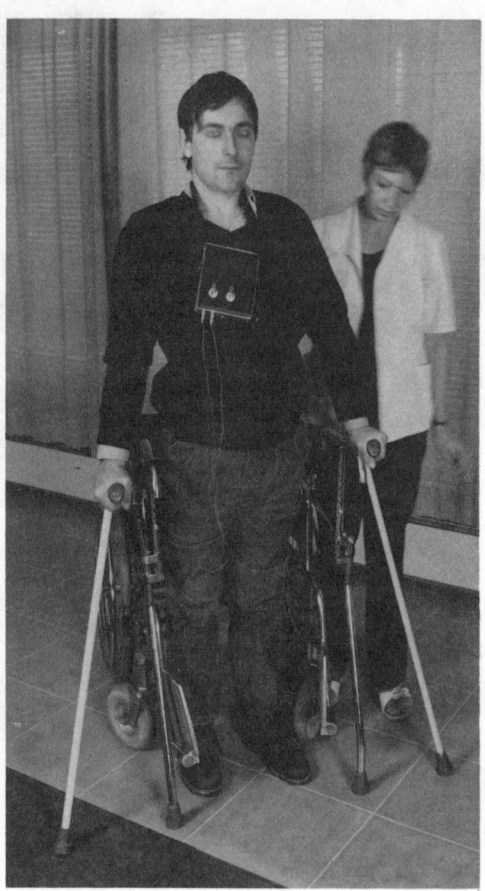

a   b

FIGURE 26. Four modes of rising from sitting to the standing position by the help of crutches: standing-up by the help of one crutch and solid support (a), standing-up maneuver using wheelchair-attached supporting frame (b), standing-up with two crutches (c), and standing-up with both lower extremities extended (d).

leg is progressing, the body stops to progress. After initial contact of the leading leg, the double stance phase starts and also, the body progression velocity increases due to hand pushing at the side of the trailing leg. After the body weight is transferred to the leading leg, the contralateral crutch is moved forward and another swing phase initiated. Figure 27 is in a diagram form presenting the events of gait and crutch transfer. The most usual order of the important gait events is the following: right crutch transfer, left step, left crutch transfer, right step, etc. With well trained patients, crutch transfer and step of the opposite leg may occur simultaneously. Different pattern of gait events is observed in incomplete SCI patients where one leg is noticeably stronger than the contralateral leg. Here, first both crutches are transferred simultaneously, and followed by the weak leg step and finally, the strong leg step. We have trained more than 20 patients for crutch walking in the last several years, but only about $1/3$ remained crutch walkers after a year post discharge. This is indicating that independent FES crutch walking is a rather tedious way of locomotion. From experiences obtained by adding stimulation of hip extensors, abductors, trunk extensors, or even plantar flexors synchronously with four-channel gait events, substantial improvements in safety, patient's feeling, and function were obtained. Let us here mention also the function of

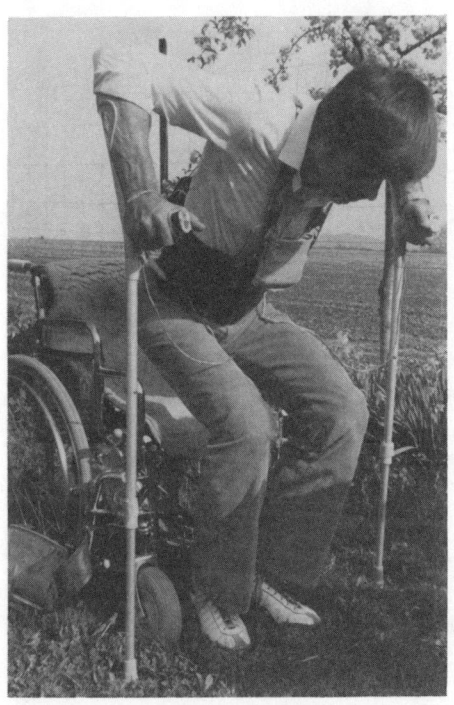 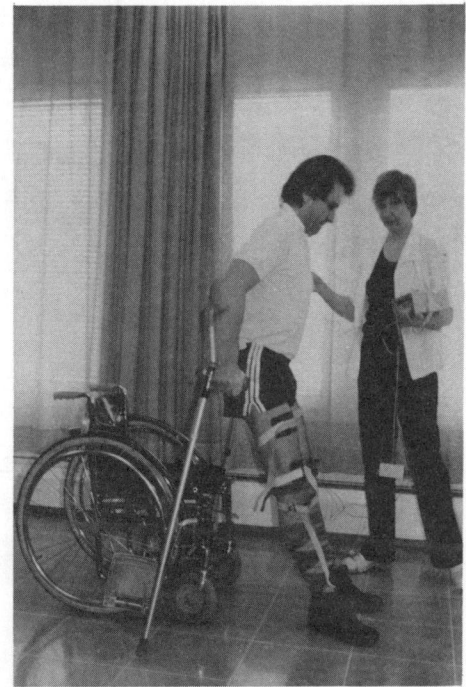

FIGURE 26c. FIGURE 26d.

ascending stairs achieved in some patients using the four-channel gait pattern, one hand rail support, and a crutch. Stair climbing was considerably improved by adding stimulation of plantar flexors and hip extensors. Patients who were not able to walk on the stairs with only four-channel FES could after addition of hip extensors and ankle plantar flexors stimulation ascend stairs. Because of practical reasons, being the consequence of surface electrodes utilization, we have not equipped patients for home independent use with more than four channels of FES. Note, that ascending stairs by utilizing two crutches and FES was not yet accomplished. A serious problem is also carrying of the unused crutch together with difficult control of balance while ascending stairs. Swing-to gait pattern with both knees locked by FES appears to be at present the appropriate way of descending stairs.

V. APPLICATIONS AND RESULTS

The achievements in FES-restored walking of complete SCI patients will be systematically presented. Since 1979, when in Ljubljana, Yugoslavia the experiments of biped reciprocal gait restoration in paraplegic patients by means of FES were started, a series of improvements were made within stimulators and control design, methodology of patients selection, training, and prescription of required balancing aids. Parallel to these accomplishments, the patients performance and achievements also advanced. In regard to different stimulators and balancing aid selection, there are several combinations possible.

First, we are going to describe some of the frequently utilized solutions for application of stimulator and balancing aid. Thereafter, the accomplishments and results with the involved patient population review are presented. In the conclusion, a discussion is presented highlighting the trends and expectations for future developments in the FES gait restoration field.

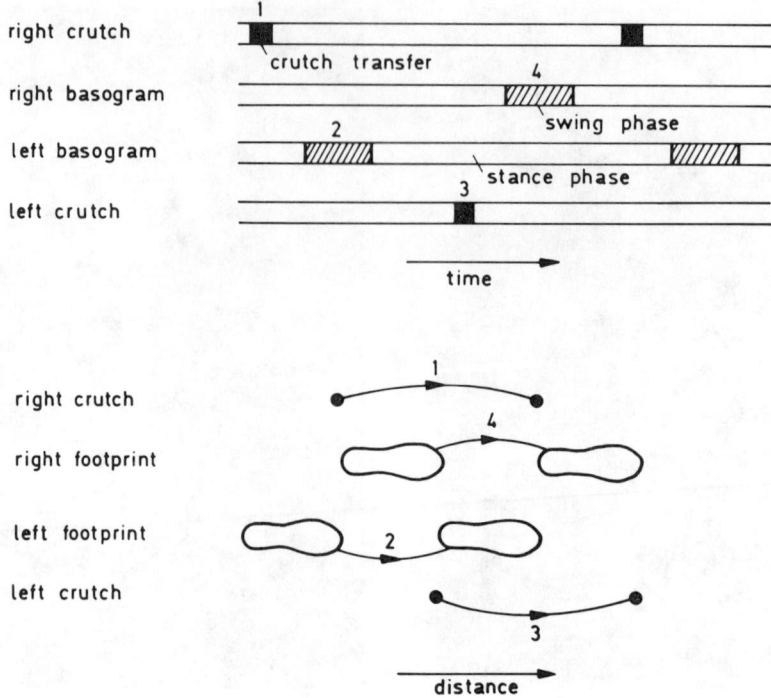

FIGURE 27. Occurrence of important gait events with respect to time and distance for crutch walking.

A. Review of Stimulators and Balancing Aids

In the early days of FES orthotic systems, self-contained stimulators and parallel bars for balancing and support were used.[50] The development of stimulators was for many years bound to the concept of a self-contained stimulator design and only in the last several years was this concept changed by the distributed stimulator design.[54] In this arrangement, some vital controls of the stimulator are arranged with respect to patient's convenience and improved functionality. Because the parallel bars are stationary, a need for mobile balancing aids soon appeared. These needs started the construction of different training frames and also the utilization of different walkers for home use. A roller walker proved to be an adequate solution for providing good functionality, reasonable speed of walking, and reliable support. Its use is favored also for outside walking in patients who achieve relatively good mobility. In Figure 28, a paraplegic patient using a roller walker is shown. In regard to stimulator placement, two solutions are important: first, the stimulator is attached to the walker to unencumber the patient, or second, the stimulator is worn by the patient. For training, the first solution appears to be more practical, allowing the physiotherapist to readjust the stimulation amplitude settings during walking. From the patient's functionality and practicality view point, the second solution is favored. Because of cosmesis and future miniaturization of stimulator hardware, the second solution is recommended. Regardless of stimulator attachment, the control transducers are connected to the FES system by wires. Solutions with wireless communications are feasible, but were not yet applied. For home use and improved mobility in small space, the parallelogram walker is a practical solution. In Figure 29, the same patient is walking, while using a stimulator with controls for swing/stance phase and amplitude setting for left/right stimulation channels dislocated to the walker handles. The standing-up and sitting-down maneuvers can be performed without using the controls attached to the walker. The on-off switch, being part of stimulator, is serving for this purpose.

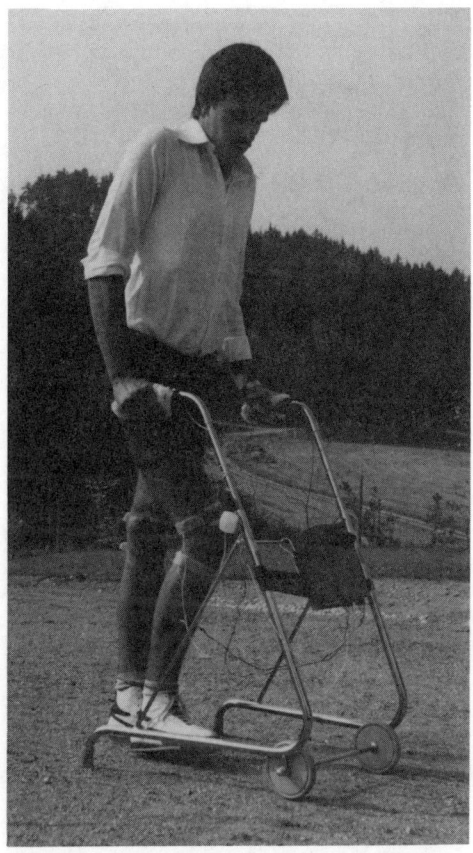

FIGURE 28. Completely paralyzed paraplegic patient using a roller walker outside of his home.

An interesting arrangement of stimulator and walker is presented in Figure 30. Here, the patient is able to adjust the m. quadriceps amplitudes at the stimulator worn on the belt. The batteries are inserted in special pockets all around the belt. This patient has a peroneal implant on each side. This one-channel radio frequency (R.F.) powered stimulator serves for flexion reflex triggering.[55] As the functioning of the implants is relatively constant in time, often readjustments are not necessary. The push buttons for the swing/stance control are attached to the walker. The position of the electrodes for m. quadriceps stimulation is clearly shown below the knee. The elastic velcro-fastened strap is carrying the output stage and the R.F. antenna of the implanted stimulator. The black knob serves for amplitude adjustment. The utilization of separate, left, and right side, two-channel stimulators worn on the belt is shown in Figure 31. Also, here the hand switches for the swing/stance control are mounted on the walker and connected to both units by wires. The amplitude controls are conveniently located on the upper side of the stimulators.

For crutch-assisted FES walking, the controls are built into the crutch handles for patient accessibility. There are two possible arrangements for carrying the stimulator: at the waist or placed higher on the chest in a special bag. For convenient load distribution, the stimulator can be attached like a backpack. Figure 32a displays a close view of the crutch-attached controls, while Figure 32b displays the outlook of a patient fitted with the backpack type of stimulator while walking. The cables for the controls are connected by means of easily detachable connectors to the crutches and stimulator. For convenience and fast assembly,

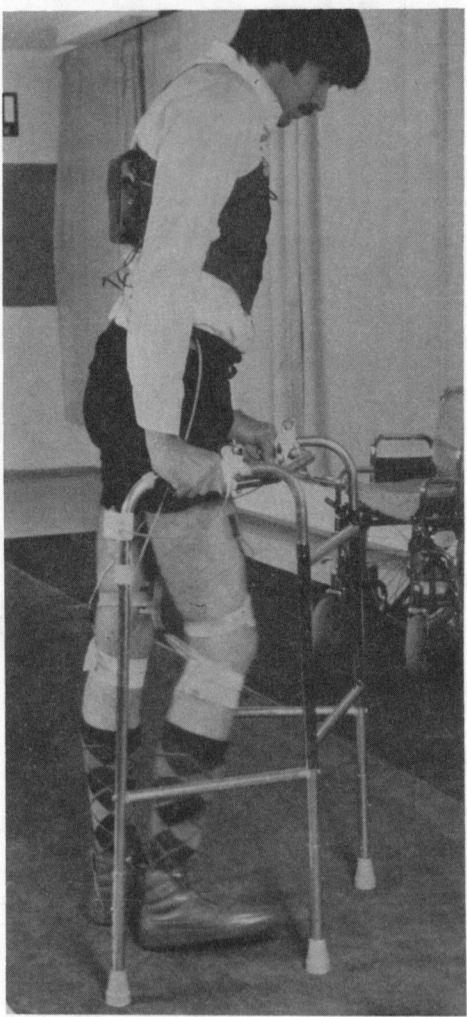

FIGURE 29. Paraplegic patient walking by the help of a parallelogram walker.

the cables can be color coded. Therefore, donning and doffing times are short and in the range of 5 min for an average patient. The belt-attached stimulator must be lightweight. Also, for the shoulder pouch carrying of the stimulator, care must be taken for preventing bouncing during stepping. For this, a trunk strap is foreseen. In Figure 33a, a patient wearing the stimulator on a belt is shown. This patient has an ankle-foot orthosis for better stabilization of ankle and to a certain extent, also for the knee joint during stance phase of walking. In Figure 33b, a paraplegic patient is walking outside of his home. A self-contained stimulator is conveniently located and attached to shoulder straps so that also the light signals can be observed for control and safety purposes. Because of high lesion (T-5) the patient wears, for improving trunk stability, also a wide elastic pelvis belt. At this point, it should be noted that different kinds of stimulators were designed for research purposes to gain knowledge, improve the methodology, and study feasibility concepts of FES-assisted gait. None of the systems displayed were designed for commercial reasons. It is not difficult to realize that with minor changes and redesigns, stimulators intended for chronic patients home use can be developed in near future.

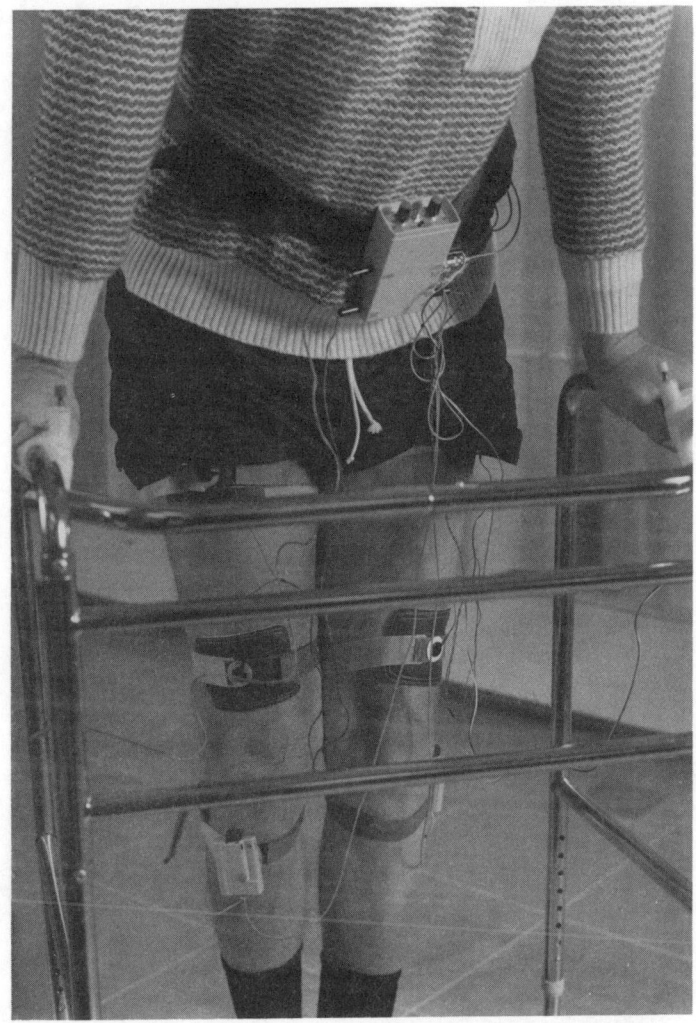

FIGURE 30. Paraplegic patient with surface electrical stimulation of knee extensors and implanted stimulation for flexion reflex triggering.

B. Accomplishments and Results

Gait restoration is indicated particularly in SCI patients with thoracic lesions between T-4 and T-12 displaying UMNL of the main lower extremities muscle groups. The patients selection criteria were described in detail in Chapter 4, Section III. With the increase of knowledge and methodology development, also the patients with higher lesions were gradually admitted to the program. In cases with injuries above T-4, the autonomic dysreflexia may be also triggered by FES. Therefore, care must be taken particularly during the first few FES sessions. Also, patients with incomplete cervical lesions are candidates if the hand function is adequately preserved for using the balancing aids. Here, we have in mind incomplete SCI patients with almost no voluntary motor functions of the lower extremities. In such patients, many times also the lower back muscles are functional and some sensation preserved. Some of these patients are also presented in our patient population review. In spite of that, we may state that these patients cannot be considered as typical cases.

Since 1978, approximately 500 patients have been treated in the spinal cord injury department of the University Rehabilitation Institute in Ljubljana, Yugoslavia. Annually, 50

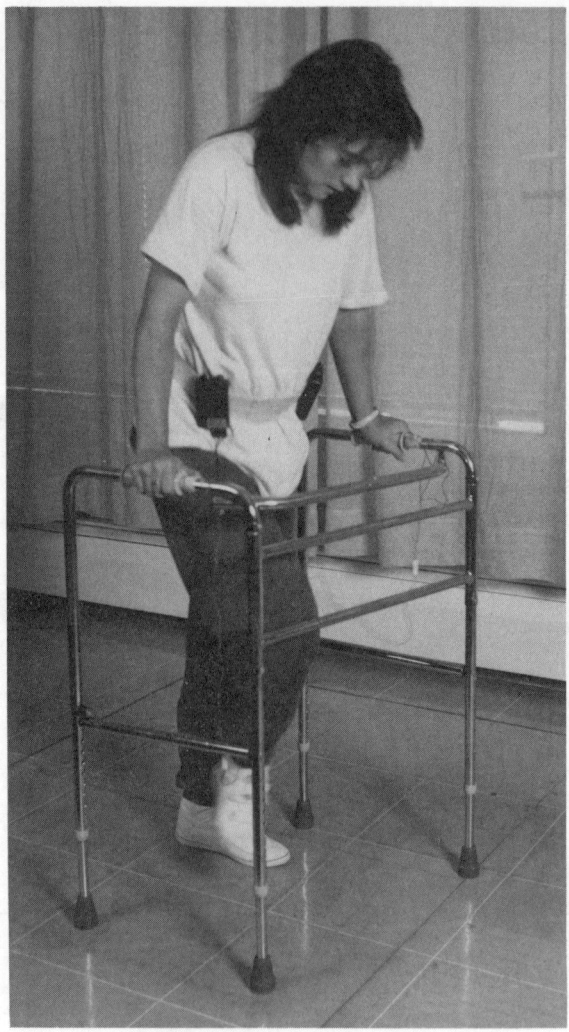

FIGURE 31. Paraplegic patient's walking restored by the help of two two-channel stimulators.

to 60 new cases have been admitted to the spinal unit. During the early years of the FES research program, in the period of 1977 to 1980, only several patients were included each year into the FES program. After 1980, more and more patients were treated annually by FES. Already in 1983, nearly all admitted and suitable patients were included into the FES rehabilitation treatment in addition to their regular rehabilitation treatment. The larger numbers of patients admitted were also the consequences of adequately elaborated FES methodology of patient selection, FES restrengthening, and standing with gait training. In 1980, the first stimulators for home use were available, such a two-channel device suitable for standing and muscle exercising and also the wheelchair-attached folding frame for standing was introduced.[56] Later, a four-channel unit intended for gait restoration was introduced[37,49] together with different walkers and crutches with built-in control transducers. In the following years and in particular after 1983, due to increased interest for FES both in SCI patients and clinicians, the number of patients started to increase because of patients being admitted to the program from other regions and countries. The patient population in our review is therefore not a typical sample of our region. Also, to note, is that patients from other regions

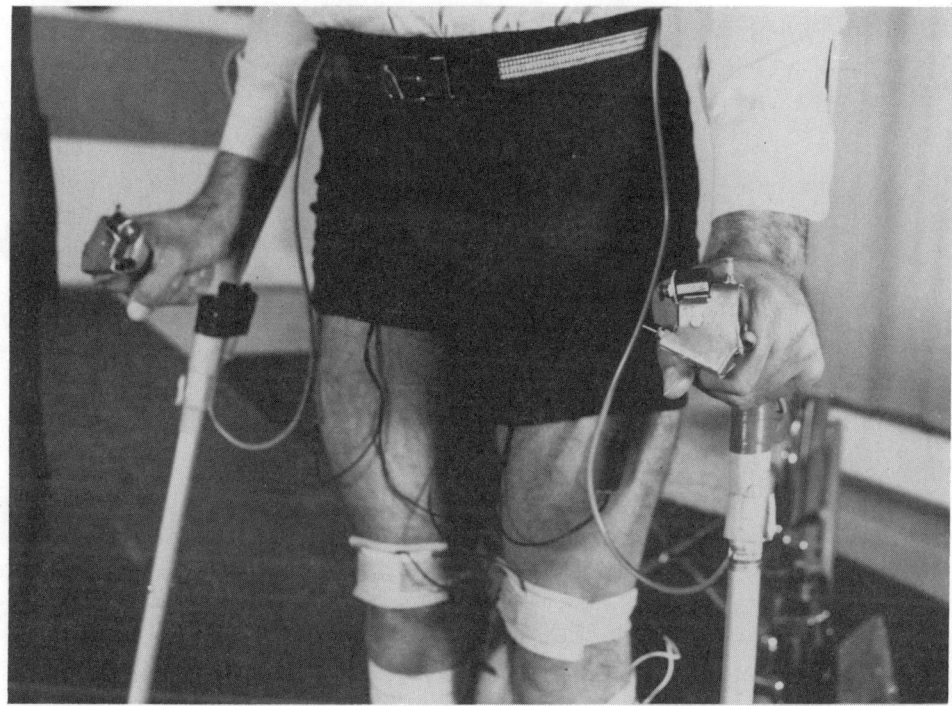

a

FIGURE 32. Gait control transducers attached to the handles of the crutches (a), and paraplegic subject with backpack type carrying of the stimulator (b).

who were included in the program were to a certain extent preselected for FES use.[17,57] Being rigorous, statistical validation and conclusions from the data on all FES-treated patients in Ljubljana are not statistically representative and must be considered as a rough preliminary estimation. This is particularly valid if we consider the fact that during the early years of the FES program, only few patients were included in spite of many suitable candidates, due to our insufficient knowledge, equipment, and personnel shortage. Because of rapidly changing FES methodology as well as hardware and training procedures, the accomplishments of patients admitted to the program during first years cannot be compared to the achievements of the patients treated in the last years. In many patients, the functional status reached at the completion of the clinical treatment was satisfactory, but for home use, they were given only the two-channel standing stimulator and frame, because four-channel units were not yet available. If the FES stimulator required for gait restoration was provided at the discharge, the functional status of the patients would be better. In some patients, due to various reasons, the in-hospital FES training time was too short or divided into intervals with long periods of inactivity.

In some cases, the home use of FES was terminated many times because of hardware failure, lack of time to continue exercising, or sometimes also due to problems not related with FES. In spite of these typical problems, the number of patients who functionally and daily use FES for standing and walking is reasonable. It is expected that the FES approach of locomotion restoration will improve also in the future and therefore, the number of patients being candidates for FES treatment will be increasing also. Taking into account all the problems mentioned, a review of the patients treated is illustrative and provides some new insights.

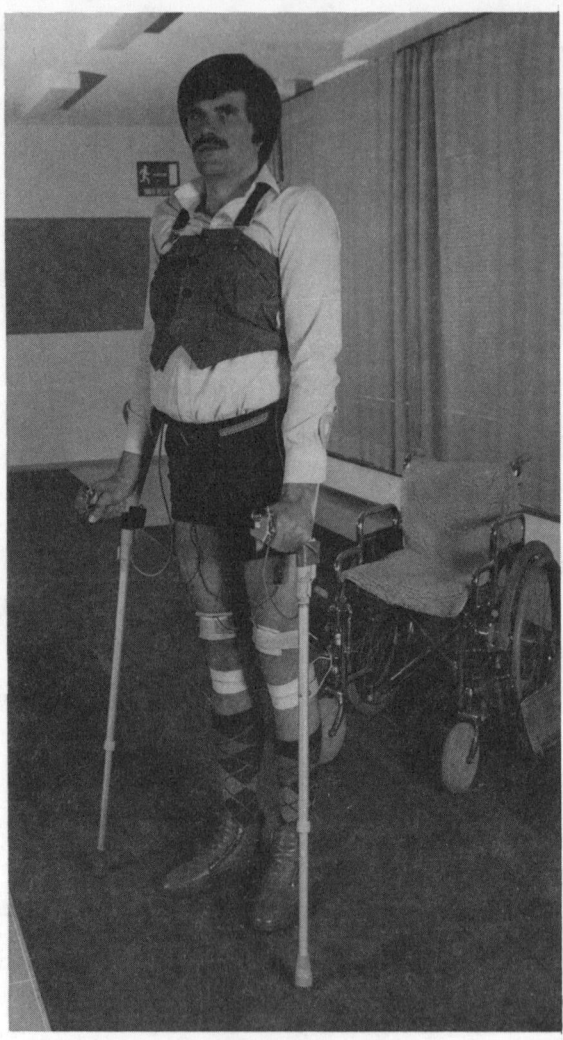

FIGURE 32b.

During the last 9 years, 54 complete SCI patients were admitted to the FES program. Four patients left the program because of reasons not related to FES. The summarized data on the 50 patients who completed the program are displayed in Table 1. During the last several years, there were also 26 cases of incomplete lesion treated by FES. These patients are not included in the table. Totally, 54 complete SCI and 26 incomplete patients were selected from the entire population of 500 patients which represents 16% of all patients. The 26 incomplete SCI patients represent 5.2% of all patients which is a rather low number due to the fact that the clinical FES program for incomplete lesions started in 1984. It is hard to estimate the number of possible candidates for the FES incomplete injury program from the previous years.

The 50 complete SCI patients, who completed the FES program, represent 10% of the whole patient population. All of these patients were treated according to the methodology described in the previous sections. It is important to note that differences exist among patients with regard to hardware applied and also treatment differences caused by knowledge and methodology development. In Table 1, the general data on 40 male and 10 female patients

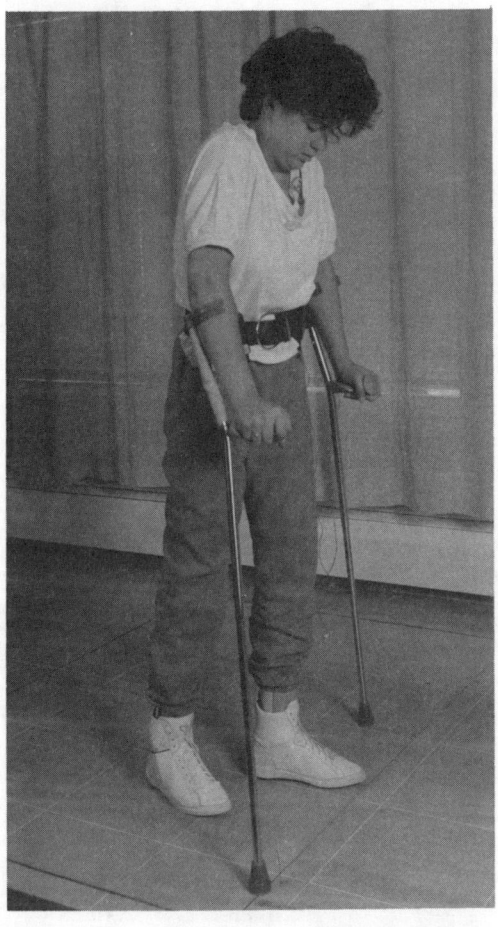 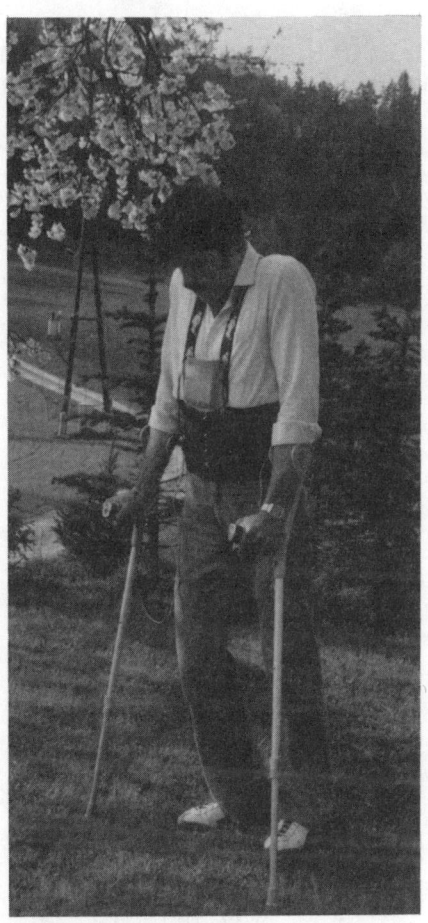

FIGURE 33. Paraplegic subject with a belt-attached stimulator and ankle-foot orthosis (a), and paraplegic subject walking outside of his home (b).

are presented. In the FES program, there were 80% males and 20% females. The level of injury distribution and the time postinjury with regard to the date, when the patients were admitted to the FES treatment, are displayed in Figure 34a and b. The majority, 33 patients or 66%, started the FES program earlier than 24 months after their injury. Regarding age, most of the patients (41 or 82%) were younger than 30 years. The spinal cord injury was in 38 (76%) patients caused by traffic accident and in 5 patients (10%) resulted from falling. In the population of the patients treated, there were 38 patients (76%) with lesions between T-4 to T-11. The age distribution for the patients treated is displayed in Figure 35.

The functional level achieved after the completion of the FES program is presented in Figure 36. Here, also the home use of FES, such as recorded 3 or more months after the discharge, is given by the dashed lines. Note, the dashes in column "FES home use" in Table 1. In these patients, we were not able to check their functional status for the last 3 months. In Figure 36, when comparing the two-channel stimulator users column with the four-channel ambulating patients, we learn that nearly half of the patients with lesions from T-4 to T-11 did not accomplish the four-channel walking level. This is, in most cases, the consequence of damage to other neural structures and caused by partial peripheral denervation

Table 1
GENERAL DATA ON 50 COMPLETELY PARALYZED PARAPLEGIC PATIENTS ADMITTED TO THE FES PROGRAM

No.	Sex	Level injury and cause	Injury date (month/year)	Age	Start of FES	FES function trained	FES home use
1	M	T-5,6, TR	X/77	30	XII/77	4CH, PB	—
2	M	T-6, TR	XII/79	27	I/85	2CH, SF	SF
3	M	T-2,3,4, TR	X/81	26	II/84	4CH, WA	4CH, WA
4	M	T-10, TR	VII/85	17	X/85	4CH, CR	4CH, CR
5	M	T-4,5, TR	I/85	33	X/83	2CH, SF	2CH, EX
6	M	C-7, TR	VI/83	21	III/86	2CH, SF	2CH, SF
7	M	T-11,12, TR	V/83	20	VIII/85	4CH, B, CR	4CH, B, CR
8	M	T-5,6, TR	VIII/79	22	I/86	4CH, WA	4CH, WA
9	M	T-10,11, TR	IX/80	25	III/81	2CH, SF	—
10	M	T-8, TR	XII/76	16	V/83	2CH, SF	2CH, SW
11	M	T-4,5, TR	X/84	25	VI/85	4CH, PB	4CH, PB
12	M	T-9,10, OT	V/64	25	VI/80	2CH, EX	2CH, EX
13	M	T-12, FA	V/83	19	VIII/85	2CH, EX	—
14	M	T-12, FA	XII/84	14	V/85	4CH, B, CR	4CH, B, CR
15	M	T-5, SH	IX/79	46	III/83	2CH, SF	2CH, SF, EX
16	M	T-7, TR	VIII/80	14	VIII/85	2CH, SF	2CH, SW
17	M	T-6, TR	III/79	20	IX/80	4CH, CR	4CH, CR
18	M	T-6, FA	VII/85	26	XI/85	4CH, WA	4CH, WA
19	M	T-10, TR	VII/78	24	II/79	4CH, PB	—
20	M	T-9, TR	XI/83	20	V/84	2CH, SF	—
21	M	T-6, TR	IV/83	26	II/84	2CH, SW	2CH, SW
22	M	T-7,8, TR	XII/83	25	IV/84	2CH, SW	2CH, SW
23	M	T-8, TR	IV/83	15	III/85	2CH, SF	2CH, SF
24	M	T-10,12, TR	I/85	22	II/86	2CH, WA	4CH, WA
25	M	T-11, TR	V/72	20	IX/82	2CH, SF	—
26	F	T-9, FA	V/81	18	X/81	4CH, PB	Lost
27	M	T-5,6, TR	V/81	18	X/81	4CH, PB	2CH, EX
28	F	C-7, OT	II/82	11	IX/83	4CH, CR	4CH, CR
29	M	T-4,5, TR	IV/84	22	X/85	4CH, WA	4CH, WA
30	M	OT	VI/75	33	VI/86	2CH, SF	2CH, EX
31	F	C-7,T-1, TR	VIII/83	21	III/84	2CH, EX	—
32	M	T-4,5, TR	VII/78	17	VI/85	4CH, PB	4CH, PB
33	M	T-8, FA	X/83	15	VI/85	4CH, WA	4CH, WA
34	M	T-3, TR	VIII/80	16	VIII/80	2CH, SF	—
35	F	T-5, OT	III/83	23	IX/84	4CH, CR	4CH, CR
36	M	T-3,4, TR	VI/82	30	IV/85	2CH, SW	4CH, SW
37	M	T-7, SH	VII/81	40	V/82	4CH, PB	—
38	M	T-7,8, TR	V/78	31	X/84	4CH, CR	4CH, CR
39	M	C-6,7, TR	VI/73	22	I/81	2CH, SF	—
40	M	C-7, DV	VII/82	24	IV/84	6CH, WF	6CH, WF
41	F	T-5,6, TR	V/82	26	XI/86	4CH, WA	4CH, WA
42	M	L-1, TR	IX/86	24	XI/86	4CH, WA	4CH, WA
43	F	T-5,6, TR	X/86	17	XI/86	4CH, WA	4CH, WA
44	M	T-11, TR	XI/86	21	III/87	4CH, WA	4CH, WA
45	M	T-8,9, TR	XI/85	24	IV/87	4CH, WA	4CH, WA
46	M	T-10,11, TR	III/87	36	VI/87	4CH, WA	2CH
47	M	T-9, TR	XI/86	48	VI/87	4CH, WA	2CH
48	M	T-11, TR	I/87	39	IV/87	2CH	IP
49	M	T-7,9, TR	IV/87	39	II/87	2CH	IP
50	M	T-4,9, TR	IV/87	18	VII/87	2CH	IP

Table 1 (continued)
GENERAL DATA ON 50 COMPLETELY PARALYZED PARAPLEGIC PATIENTS ADMITTED TO THE FES PROGRAM

Note: OT — other
TR — traffic accident
FA — fall
SH — gun shot
DV — diving
2 CH — two-channel FES
4 CH — four-channel FES
CR — crutches
WA — walker
WF — walking frame
SF — standing frame
PB — parallel bars
SW — standing wheelchair frame
EX — exercising
B — additional braces
IP — in program

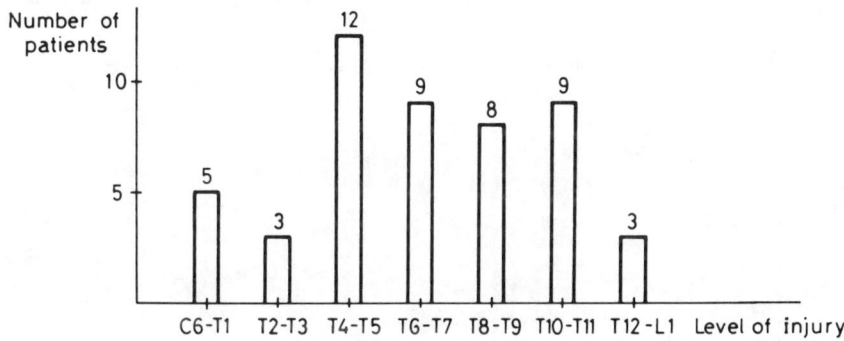

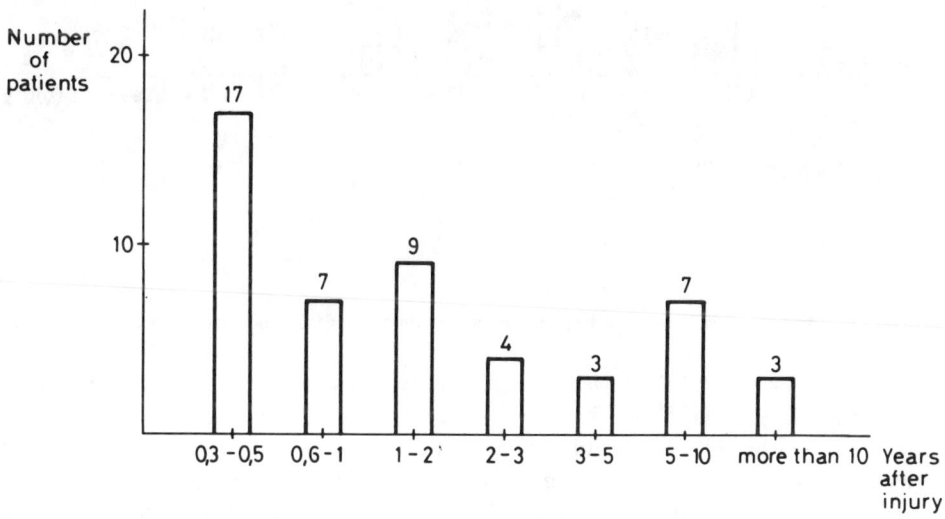

FIGURE 34. Distribution of patients with respect to the level of spinal cord injury (a) and the time after accident (b).

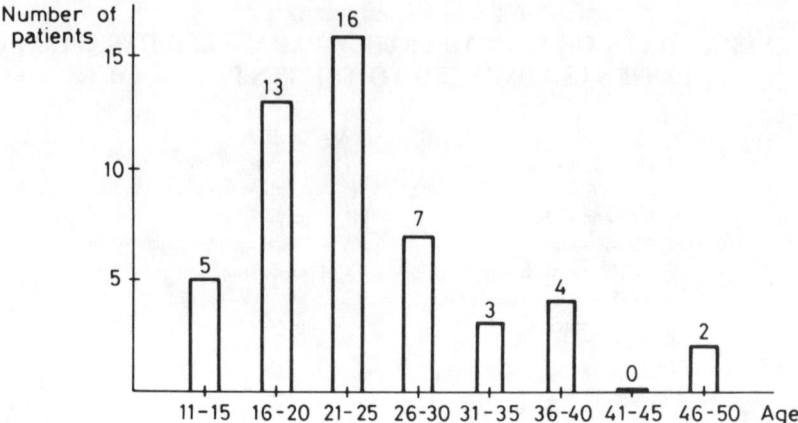

FIGURE 35. Age distribution for the patients included in FES treatment program.

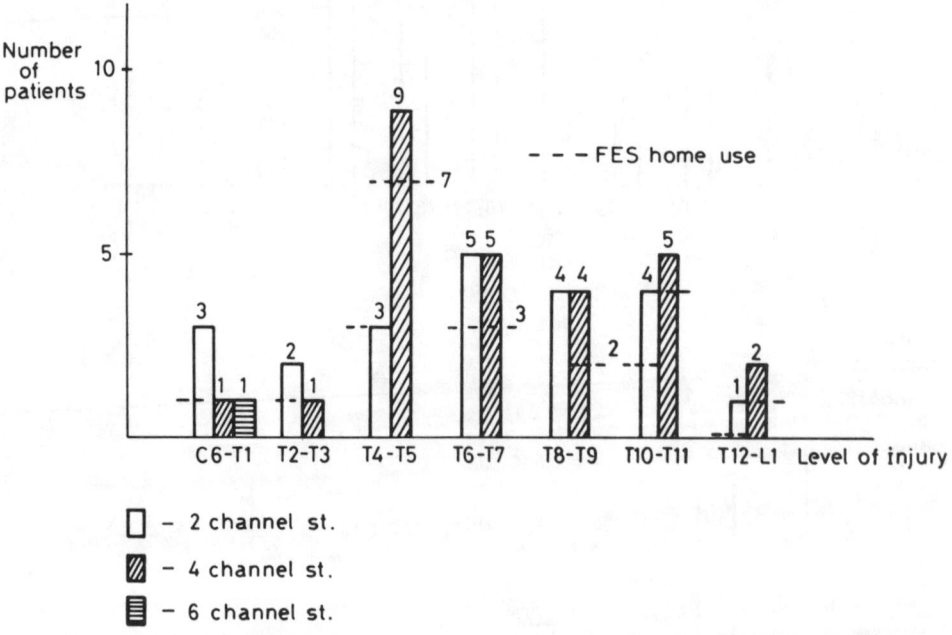

FIGURE 36. FES functional level at discharge from the rehabilitation center and later at home (dashed lines).

of some main muscles of the lower extremities. Patients with lesions T-4 to T-5 achieved four-channel walking in 75% of the cases, while those with lesion levels from T-6 to T-11 achieved four-channel walking in only 50% of all cases. All of the patients or 100% of the patients selected for FES program with lesions between T-4 to T-12 have been able to stand by means of FES. Walking, utilizing four-channel FES-assisted gait pattern, was learned by 25 patients with lesions in the range of T-4 to T-12. In regard to all the patients admitted with complete spinal cord lesion, approximately $1/2$ achieved the walking level. Of the 27 patients who learned walking, they represent 5% of the total population. After using the four-channel gait in home environment for more than 3 months, the number of patients who remained users of the four-channel stimulator dropped as can be redrawn from Figure 36. We see that ten patients gave up and only seven patients remained walkers. This represents a 37% dropout rate during first 3 months of independent FES home use. Note, that the dropout rate is very high for the first months of independent home use, while later patients do not leave FES use frequently. Among the dropout cases, there are patients who abandoned FES mainly due to the involvement required to don and doff the system. The remaining 17 patients who daily utilize four-channel FES walking systems represent, with respect to all patients admitted, 34 or 3% in regard to the total patient population. Experience indicates that patients remaining FES users for more than 1 year will use the FES orthotic system permanently for the coming years. Our oldest patients are using the four-channel gait nearly for 7 years. Most of them are walking for functional purposes or because of training only in their houses or outside. Close review of how much this locomotion mode is utilized for functional daily activities and work performance was not done.

Also in patients achieving two-channel FES-assisted standing, an interesting dropout rate can be recognized. There were 17 patients or 34% who were at the time of discharge able to stand by means of FES. After being at home for 3 or more months, only 12 patients (24%) remained FES users. The dropout rate in patients using the two-channel stimulator for standing was therefore 30%. Here, it is to note that some patients from Figure 36, indicated as two-channel stimulator users, employ the stimulator for exercising only. Many patients found the wheelchair-attached folding frame practical. While standing with the two-channel FES, they were able to free one hand and perform some task, like taking a book from a shelf or storing something in the kitchen (see also Chapter 4, Section VI). The standing time is limited due to fatiguing of the stimulated m. quadriceps muscles and is also very shortened in case of bad posture. There were attempts made for prolonging the standing time for at least three to five times by the so-called posture switching technique.[45,58] Standing times for several hours were obtained, and there are possibilities to practice the posture switching also between the left-right leg in the frontal plane to prolong the standing time even further. Among all the patients trained to walk with the four-channel gait pattern (27 patients), only 7 patients or 26% were able to master walking utilizing the elbow crutches for balance and support. All of these patients except one utilize crutch ambulation also at their homes. Experience shows that most of the patients prefer parallelogram walkers for FES locomotion at their homes. Even crutch users, due to space limitations at home, better accessibility and mobility, prefer to use parallelogram walkers at home.

Because of rather demanding electrode placement for eliciting flexion reflex withdrawal movement in one patient first on one side and after a 4-month period also on the other side, one-channel implant was surgically inserted.[55] The first implant is now functioning already for 1 year and giving great satisfaction to the patient. The second implant was displaced after being functional for nearly 2 months. The unit was removed and a new stimulator implanted. At the time of this report, both units are performing satisfactory. The patient favors the implants because they simplify and shorten his donning/doffing time while the flexion reflex function is repeatable from day to day. The implant was placed close to the caput fibulae near the common peroneal nerve. The commercially available peroneal stimulator unit aimed for correcting drop foot in hemiplegic patients was used.[59,60]

The walking speed of four-channel gait is low being from 0.2 to 0.45 m. The stance phase lasts 82% and swing phase 18% of the stride time. In normals, this ratio is 60/40%. The double stance phase lasts 27 to 32% of stride time.[37] The sagittal plane goniograms recorded with a patient walking by the help of walker and crutches and four-channel FES orthotic aid are presented in Figures 37a and 37b, respectively. The average vertical ground reaction force is displayed in Figure 38. The ground reaction forces were assessed with the help of the force shoes developed by Kljajić.[61] Such a measurement is favorable because many steps can be statistically evaluated, and average data can be obtained. In Figure 38, it is evident that patient is supporting his body weight mostly in the middle of the foot area throughout the stance phase. Unfortunately, no energy expenditure measurements were performed. The only energy data for FES-assisted paraplegic patients walking were published

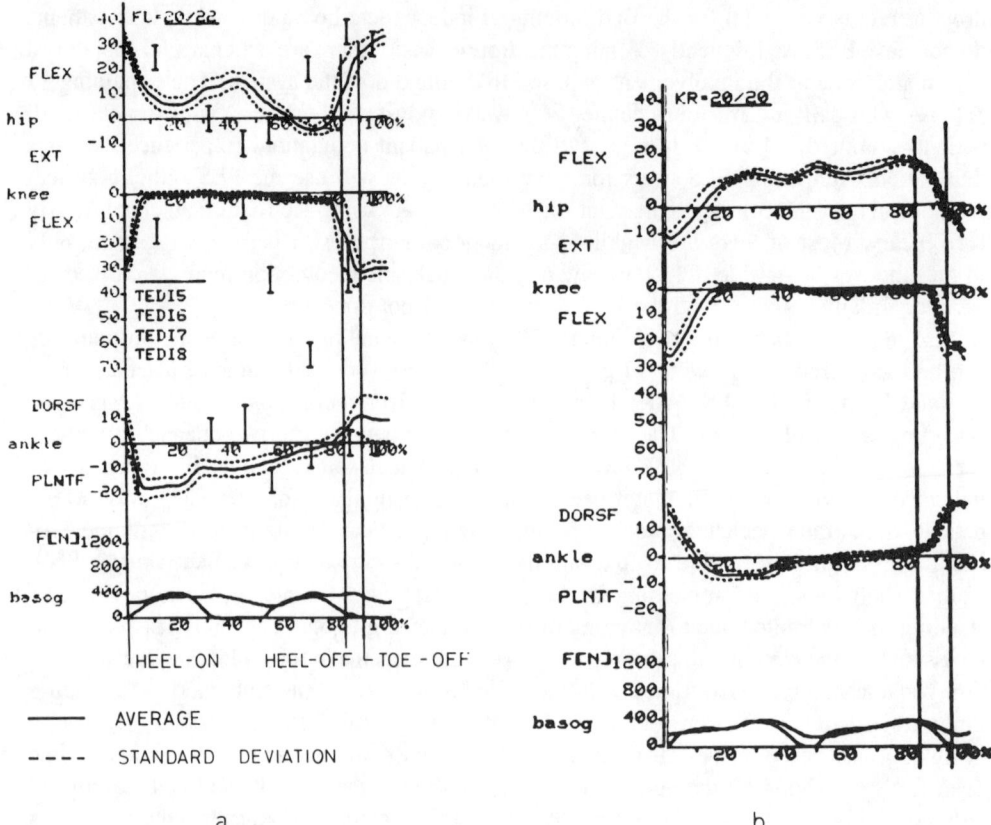

FIGURE 37. Ankle, hip, and knee goniograms during walker (a)- and crutch (b)-assisted walking of completely paralyzed paraplegic subject using a four-channel stimulator. The average duration of stride time during walker-assisted walking was 10.4 s and 4.4 s during crutch walking.

by Marsolais[36] and Edwards et al.[62] The authors are quoting that for a walking speed of 0.18 m/s, the energy expenditure is 4.2 times greater than normal, for 0.35 m/s, 2.5 times as normal, and for 0.56 m/s, 2.2 times as normal. (Energy expenditure of normal walking is about 40 cal/min/kg at low walking speed of 20 m/min.) They conclude that energy expenditure at a speed of 1 m/s will be acceptable. They also report using a 32-channel FES system providing 1 m/s walking speed in patients utilizing the FES system and a rolling walker.[36] Energy expenditure during different locomotor activities is presented in Figure 39.[6]

Walking in most of the completely paralyzed paraplegic patients, which may, when compared to a normal person's gait, be considered as stepping, is limited because of fatigue in electrically stimulated m. quadriceps muscles. In our new stimulator designs, the amplitude controls for the stimulation channels are easily accessible on the crutch handles or on the stimulator on the chest or waist. The patient can readjust the amplitude and thus, for a certain time, prolong the overall walking time. At present, attempts are made to accomplish faster and more functional gait by improved stimulation, adding stimulation of other muscles and introducing improved gait synthesis modes. Particularly, including hip and trunk musculature can provide substantial benefits. The stimulation of triceps surae muscles is also very important because they provide propulsion during gait. The introduction of new FES muscles and new stimulation control schemes will broaden the number of patients who can benefit from FES. It is also evident that in stimulation schemes, where almost normal walking

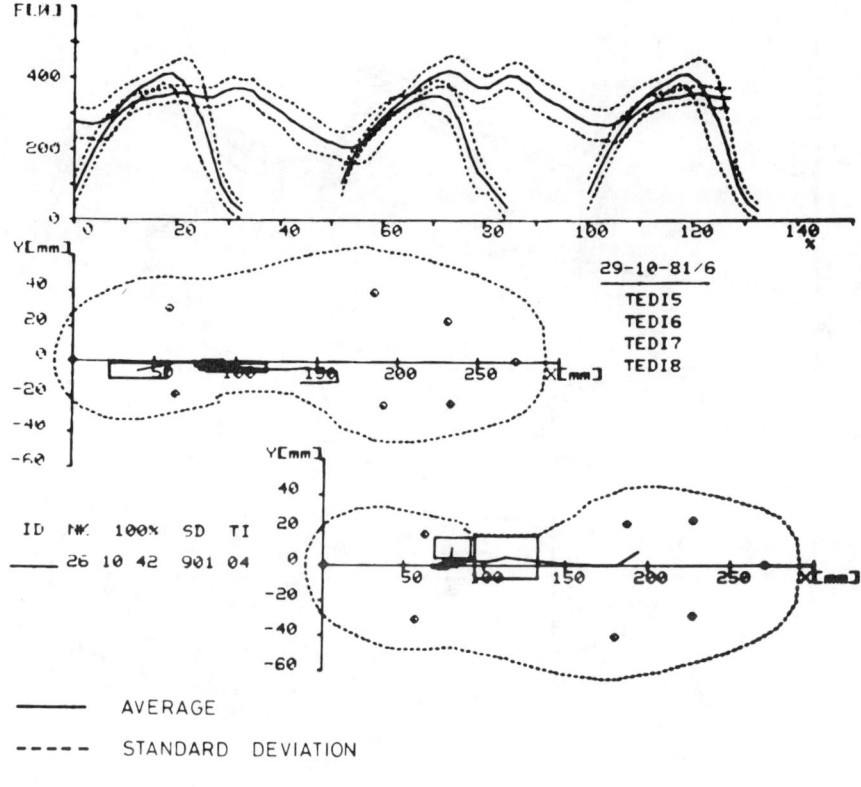

FIGURE 38. Vertical ground reaction forces and trajectory of resultant force application during paraplegic reciprocal FES gait assisted by walker (a) and crutches (b).

velocities will be achieved, bone and joint stressing must be considered in the synthesis of stimulation sequences.[63] Proper bone stressing, joint loading, prevention of ligament overstressing, and muscles overstimulation are important elements of FES gait control. In this way, protection against the development of secondary pathologies will be achieved.

All present FES control schemes are open-loop approaches. The introduction of closed-loop FES principles is of great interest and appears to be promising. However, it seems that without the incorporation of bone and joint mechanics, it is not likely to provide long-term practical and biomechanical adequate solutions. The development of sensors required for closed-loop FES systems is in an infancy stage. The cosmesis problem is very serious because patients do not like external equipment. Implanted sensors appear to be the only acceptable solution. Nevertheless, the closed-loop FES system methodology development will be an intensive research area in the coming years.

Attention should be drawn to the fact that the functional status provided by FES is higher in patients at the time of discharge than later at home. This indicates that present hardware, training, and methodology are not adequate. It further indicates that patient involvement is still too high. Regardless of these problems, it can be stated that at least 10% of complete SCI patients are candidates for FES locomotion restoration. The number of patients and statistical estimation presented in this section should be considered as a preliminary report and a very rough approximation due to the fact that during the nearly 10 years of data collection also the methodology and patient admittance were constantly changing. We consider the data presented here as an illustrative addition to the basic text presented in the

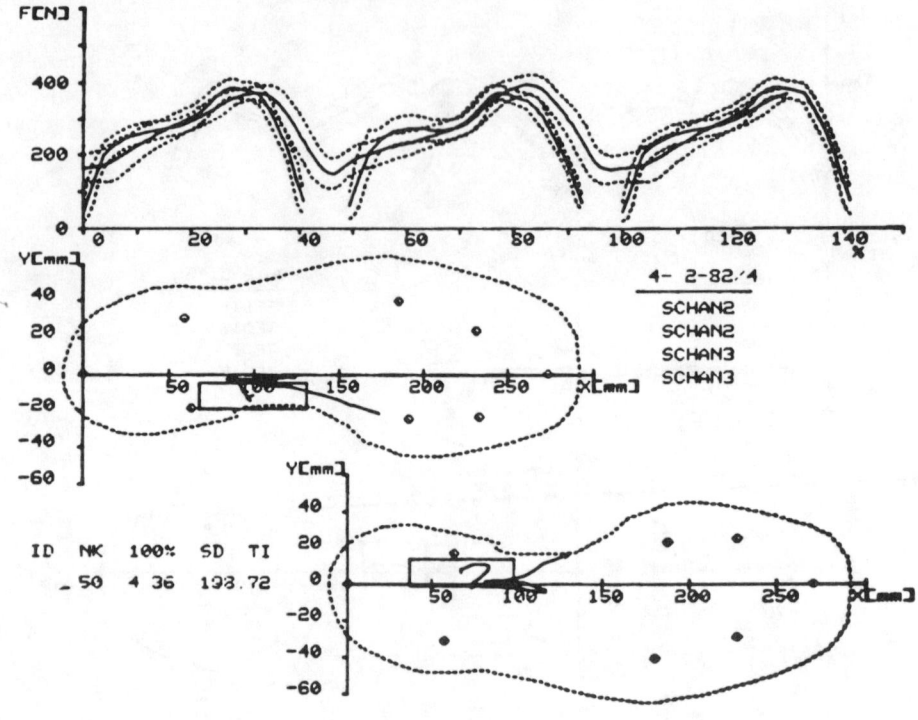

FIGURE 38b.

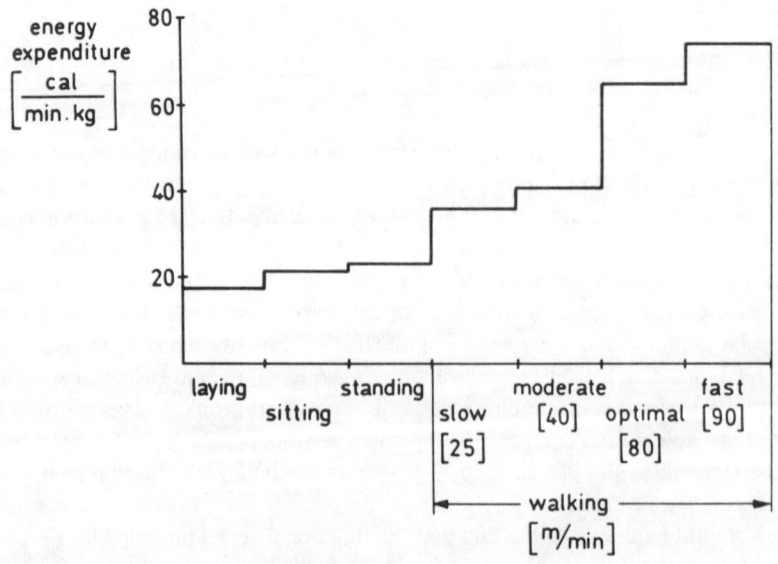

FIGURE 39. Energy expenditure during different locomotor activities assessed in male subjects. In female subjects, few percents lower values were found (1 cal = 4.186 J).

book and supportive findings important for the feasibility demonstration of locomotion restoration in spinal injury patients utilizing FES.

In discussing trends of development and expectations of the FES in SCI patients, several remarks should be made. Commercial systems developed for chronic patients independent home use will be available within the next several years. Probably, first simple FES orthotic systems will provide standing and very limited locomotor activities at the patient's home, such as assistance at transfers and the ability of making several steps. The safety elements and sensory driven logic control principles will have to be included in this new generation of practical, user-oriented orthotic systems. It is also to expect that functionality of such systems in the daily life of SCI patients needs to be closely studied. The FES system donning/doffing times, cosmesis, and instant availability of the FES-assisted functions are of prime importance. Therefore, in perspective, only implanted systems can provide satisfactory function. Surface systems can be considered as therapeutic, evaluation, and training means, important for preparing the patients selected for future implants use. We believe that FES of SCI patients is an established field which will be gaining in importance and clinical utilization in the coming years.

REFERENCES

1. **McLeish, R. D. and Charnley, J.**, Abduction forces in the one-legged stance, *J. Biomech.*, 3, 191, 1970.
2. **Capozzo, A.**, The forces and couples in the human trunk during level walking, *J. Biomech.*, 16, 265, 1983.
3. **Huggler, A. H. and Jacob, H. A. C.**, Zur funktionellen Bedeutung des Tractus iliotibialis, *Z. Orthop.*, 121, 44, 1983.
4. **Murray, M. P.**, Gait as total pattern of movement, *Am. J. Phys. Med.*, 46, 290, 1967.
5. **Winter, D. A.**, *The Biomechanics and Motor Control of Human Gait*, University of Waterloo Press, Waterloo, Ontario, 1987.
6. **Inman, V. T., Ralston, H. J., and Rodd, F.**, Human walking, Williams & Wilkins, Baltimore, 1981.
7. **Inman, V. T.**, Conservation of energy in ambulation, *Bull. Prosthet. Res.*, BPR 10-9, 26, 1968.
8. **Watters, R. L. and Lunsford, B. R.**, Energy cost of paraplegic locomotion, *J. Bone Jt. Surg.*, 67-A, 1245, 1985.
9. **Astrand, P. and Rodahl, K.**, *Textbook of Work Physiology*, McGraw-Hill, New York, 1977.
10. **Molen, N. H., Rozendal, R. H., and Boon, W.**, Graphic representation of the relationship between oxygen consumption and characteristics of normal gait of the human male, *Proc. K. Ned. Akad. Wet. Ser. C.*, 75, 305, 1972.
11. **Ralston, H. J.**, Energy-speed relation and optimal speed during level walking, *Int. Z. Angew. Physiol. Einsch. Arbeitsphysiol.*, 17, 277, 1958.
12. **Zarrugh, M. Y., Todd, F. N., and Ralston, H. J.**, Optimization of energy expenditure during level walking, *Eur. J. Appl. Physiol.*, 33, 293, 1974.
13. **Kljajić, M. and Trnkoczy, A.**, A study of adaptive control principle orthoses for lower extremities, *IEEE Trans. Syst. Man, Cybernet.*, 8, 313, 1978.
14. **Vodovnik, L., Crochetiere, W. J., and Reswick, J. B.**, Control of a skeletal joint by electrical stimulation of antagonist, *Med. Biol. Eng.*, 5, 97, 1967.
15. **Stanič, U. and Trnkoczy, A.**, Closed-loop positioning of hemiplegic patient's joint by means of functional electrical stimulation, *IEEE Trans. Biomed. Eng.*, 21, 365, 1974.
16. **Crago, P. E., Mortimer, J. T., and Peckham, P. H.**, Closed-loop control of force during electrical stimulation of muscle, *IEEE Trans. Biomed. Eng.*, BME-27, 306, 1980.
17. **Tomović, R.**, On man and machine, Norbert Wiener memorial lecture, in Proc. Int. Symp. External Control of Human Extremities, Dubrovnik, Yugoslavia, August 31 to September 5, 1987, 3.
18. **Liberson, W. T., Holmquest, H. J., Scott, D., and Dow, A.**, Functional electrotherapy: stimulation of the peroneal nerve synchronized with the swing phase of the gait in hemiplegic patients, *Arch. Phys. Med. Rehabil.*, 42, 101, 1961.
19. **Vodovnik, L., Long, C., Reswick, J. B., Lippay, A., and Starbuck, D.**, Myo-electric control of paralyzed muscles, *IEEE Trans. Biomed. Eng.*, 12, 169, 1965.
20. **Vodovnik, L. and Reberšek, S.**, Information content of mio-control signals for orthotic and prosthetic systems, *Arch. Phys. Med. Rehabil.*, 55, 52, 1974.
21. **Peckham, P. H., Marsolais, E. B., and Mortimer, J. T.**, Restoration of key grip and release in the C6 tetraplegic patient through functional electrical stimulation, *J. Hand Surg.*, 5, 462, 1980.
22. **Thoma, H., Frey, M., Holle, J., Kern, H., Reiner, E., Schwanda, G., and Stöhr, H.**, Paraplegics should learn to walk with fingers, in *Proc. Conf. IEEE Frontiers of Engineering and Computing in Health Care*, IEEE Service Center, Piscataway, NJ, 1983, 579.

23. **Marsolais, E. B., Massiello, A. L., Ko, W. H., and Spear, T.**, Finger switch for a portable microprocessor system to restore walking in paraplegics. in Proc. RESNA 8th Annu. Conf., Memphis, TN., 1985, 376.
24. **Siegfried, J. and Hood, T.**, Brain stimulation procedures in dystonic, hypertonic, dyskinetic and hyperkinetic conditions, in *Recent Achievements in Restorative Neurology, Upper Motor Neuron Functions and Dysfunctions*, Eccles, J. and Dimitrijević, Eds., S. Karger, Basel, 1985, 79.
25. **Hoffer, J. A. and Sinkjaer, T.**, A natural "force sensor" suitable for closed-loop control of functional neuromuscular stimulation, in Proc. 2nd Vienna Int. Workshop on Functional Elektrostimulation, Vienna, Austria, September 21 to 24, 1986, 47.
26. **Chizeck, H. J., Selwan, P. M., and Merat, F. L.**, A foot pressure sensor for use in lower extremity neuroprosthetic development, in *Proc. RESNA 8th Ann. Conf.*, RESNA Association for the Advancement of Rehabilitation Technology, Washington, D.C.,195, 379.
27. **Kralj, A., Trnkoczy, A., and Aćimović, R.**, Improvement of locomotion in hemiplegic patients with multichannel electrical stimulation, in *Human Locomotor Engineering*, Institution of Mechanical Engineers, London, 1971, 45.
28. **Kralj, A. and Vodovnik, L.**, Functional electrical stimulation of the extremities, *J. Med. Eng. Technol.*, 1, 12, 1977.
29. **Stanič, U., Aćimović-Janežič, R., Gros, N., Trnkoczy, A., Bajd, T., and Kljajić, M.**, Multichannel electrical stimulation for correction of hemiplegic gait, *Scand. J. Rehabil. Med.*, 10, 75, 1978.
30. **Gračanin, F., Kralj, A., and Rebersek, S.**, Advanced version of the Ljubljana functional electronic peroneal brace with walking rate controlled tetanization, in Proc. Int. Symp. External Control of Human Extremities, Dubrovnik, Yugoslavia, 1969, 487.
31. **Trnkoczy, A., Stanić, U., and Maležič, M.**, Present state and prospects in the design of multichannel FES stimulators for gait correction in paretic patients, *T.I.T.J. Life Sci.*, 8, 17, 1978.
32. **Stanič, U., Trnkoczy, A., Aćimović, R., and Gros, N.**, Effect of gradually modulated electrical stimulation on the plasticity of artificially evoked movements, *Med. Biol. Eng. Comput.*, 15, 62, 1977.
33. **Bajd, T. and Trnkoczy, A.**, Attempts to optimise functional electrical stimulation of antagonistic muscles by mathematical modelling, *J. Biomech.*, 12, 921, 1979.
34. **McNeal, D. R., Nakai, R. J., Meadows, P., and Tu, W.**, Control of the freely-swinging paralyzed leg before and after exercise, in Proc. Int. Symp. Adv. in External Control of Human Extremities, Dubrovnik, Yugoslavia, August 31 to September 5, 1987, 261.
35. **Marsolais, E. B. and Kobetic, R.**, Functional walking in paralyzed patients by means of electrical stimulation, *Clin. Orthop.*, 175, 30, 1983.
36. **Marsolais, E. B.**, Establishing and fulfilling criteria for practical FNS systems, in Proc. Int. Symp. Adv. External Control of Human Extremities, Dubrovnik, Yugoslavia, August 31 to September 5, 1987, 105.
37. **Kralj, A., Bajd, T., Turk, R., Krajnik, J., and Benko, H.**, Gait restoration in paraplegic patients: a feasibility demonstration using multichannel surface electrode FES, *J. Rehabil. Res. Dev.*, 20, 3, 1983.
38. **Symons, J., Axelgaard, J., Bellatti, J., McNeal, D. R., and Watters, R. L.**, Electromyography and acceleration of the trunk as trigger sources for implantable gait stimulation, in *Proc. RESNA 8th Annu. Conf.*, RESNA Association for the Advancement of Rehabilitation Technology, Washington, D.C., 1985, 385.
39. **Cooper, E. B., Bunch, W. H., and Campa, J. F.**, Effects of chronic human neuromuscular stimulation, *Surg. Forum*, 14, 477, 1973.
40. **Chizek, H. J., Lalonde, R., Chang, C. W., Rosenthal, J. A., and Marsolais, E. B.**, Performance of a closed-loop controller for electrically-stimulated standing in paralyzed patients, in *Proc. RESNA 8th Annu. Conf.*, RESNA Association for the Advancement of Rehabilitation Technology, Washington, D.C., 1985, 231.
41. **Willemsen, A. M. and van Alste, J. A.**, Accelerometry: a method for angle assessment of the lower extremities with the potential of implantation, in Proc. Int. Symp. Adv. External Control of Human Extremities, Dubrovnik, Yugoslavia, August 31 to September 5, 1987, 283.
42. **Graupe, D., Kohn, K. H., Kralj, A., and Basseas, S.**, Patient controlled electrical stimulation via EMG signature discrimination for providing certain paraplegics with primitive walking functions, *J. Biomed. Eng.*, 5, 220, 1983.
43. **Kobetič, R., Pereira, M., and Marsolais, E. B.**, Effect of muscle stimulation on weight shifting in paraplegics, in *Proc. RESNA 8th Annu. Conf.*, RESNA Association for the Advancement of Rehabilitation Technology, Washington, D.C., 1985, 234.
44. **Winter, D. A.**, Overall principles of lower limb support during stance phase of gait, *J. Biomech.*, 13, 923, 1980.
45. **Kralj, A., Bajd, T., Turk, R., and Benko, H.**, Posture switching for prolonging functional electrical stimulation standing in paraplegic patients, *Paraplegia*, 24, 221, 1986.
46. **Marsolais, E. B., Kobetič, R., Chizeck, H., Mansour, J., Borges, G., and Rosenthal, J.**, Standing of paraplegics using closed-loop controlled stimulation, in Proc. Int. Symp. External Control of Human Extremities, Dubrovnik, Yugoslavia, September 3 to 7, 1984, 63.

47. **McNeal, D. R. and Bekey, G. A.**, Closed-loop control of the human leg using electrical stimulation, in *Proc. Int. Symp. External Control of Human Extremities*, Dubrovnik, Yugoslavia, September 3 to 7, 1984, 113.
48. **Jaeger, R. J.**, Design and stimulation of closed-loop electrical stimulation orthoses for restoration of quiet standing in paraplegia, *J. Biomech.*, 19, 825, 1986.
49. **Bajd, T., Kralj, A., Turk, R., Benko, H., and Šega, J.**, The use of a four-channel electrical stimulator as an ambulatory aid for paraplegic patients, *Phys. Ther.*, 63, 1116, 1983.
50. **Kralj, A., Bajd, T., and Turk, R.**, Electrical stimulation providing functional use of paraplegic patient muscles, *Med. Progr. Technol.*, 1, 3, 1980.
51. **Strojnik, P., Kralj, A., and Uršič, I.**, Programmed six-channel electrical stimulator for complex stimulation of leg muscles during walking, *IEEE Trans. Biomed. Eng.*, BME-26, 112, 1979.
52. **Šega, J., Kralj, A., Rudel, D., Bajd, T., Balorda, Z., Munih, M., and Stamos, D.**, Six-channel microprocessor based electrical stimulator as an ambulatory aid for paraplegic patients, in *Prog. Rep. Electronics in Medicine and Biology*, Institution of Electronic and Radio Engineers, London, 1986, 167.
53. **Knott, M. and Voss, D. E.**, *Proprioceptive Neuromuscular Facilitation: Patterns and Techniques*, Hoeder Medical Division, Harper & Row, New York, 1968.
54. **Kralj, A., Bajd, T., Turk, R., Rudel, D., and Benko, H.**, The control of FES enabled gait in spinal cord injured patients, in *Proc. RESNA Annu. Conf. Eng.*, RESNA Association for the Advancement of Rehabilitation Technology, Washington, D.C., 1984, 545.
55. **Strojnik, P., Aćimović, R., Vavken, E., Simič, V., and Stanič, U.**, Treatment of drop foot using an implantable peroneal underknee stimulator, *Scand. J. Rehabil. Med.*, 19, 37, 1987.
56. **Bajd, T., Kralj, A., Šega, J., Turk, R., Benko, H., and Strojnik, P.**, Two channel electrical stimulator providing standing of paraplegic patients, *Phys. Ther.*, 61, 526, 1981.
57. **Kralj, A., Bajd, T., and Turk, R.**, Enhancement of gait restoration in spinal injury patient by functional electrical stimulation, *Clin. Orthop. Relat. Res.*, 233, 34, 1988.
58. **Kralj, A., Jaeger, R. J., and Bajd, T.**, Posture switching enables prolonged standing in paraplegic patients functionally electrically stimulated, in *Proc. 5th RESNA Annu. Conf.*, RESNA Association for the Advancement of Rehabilitation Technology, Washington, D.C., 1982, 60.
59. **Aćimović, R., Gros, N., Maležič, M., Strojnik, P., Kljajić, M., Stanič, U., and Simič, V.**, A comparative study of the functionality of the second generation of peroneal stimulators, in *Proc. RESNA 10th Annu. Conf.*, RESNA Association for the Advancement of Rehabilitation Technology, Washington, D.C., 1987, 621.
60. **Rozman, J., Kelih, B., and Pihlar, B.**, Potentials of platinum electrodes versus Ag/AgCl reference electrode, in Proc. 2nd Vienna Int. Workshop of Functional Electrostimulation, Vienna, Austria, September 21 to 24, 1986, 121.
61. **Kljajić, M. and Krajnik, J.**, The use of ground reaction measuring shoes in gait evaluation, *Clin. Phys. Physiol. Meas.*, 8, 133, 1987.
62. **Edwards, B. G., Lew, R. D., and Marsolais, E. B.**, Relative energy costs of long-leg-brace and FNS ambulation, in *Proc. 9th RESNA Annu. Conf.*, RESNA Association for the Advancement of Rehabilitation Technology, Washington, D.C., 1986, 322.
63. **Kralj, A., Bajd, T., Turk, R., and Munih, M.**, Mathematical synthesis of FES sequences, in Proc. Int. Symp. Adv. External Control of Human Extremities, Dubrovnik, Yugoslavia, August 31 to September 5, 1987, 249.
64. **Dimitrijević, M. R., Sherwood, A. M., and Faganel, J.**, Mechanisms of motor control augmentation using continuous epidural spinal cord stimulation, in Proc. Int. Symp. External Control of Human Extremities, Dubrovnik, Yugoslavia, August 28 to September 1, 1978, 657.
65. **Kottke, F.**, Neurophysiologic therapy in stroke, in *Stroke and Its Rehabilitation*, Light, S., Ed., Weverly Press, Baltimore, MD., 1975, 256.
66. **DeLuca, C. J.**, Considerations for using the nerve signal as a control source for above-elbow prostheses, in *Proc. Int. Symp. Adv. External Control of Human Extremeties*, Dubrovnik, Yugoslavia, August 25 to 30, 1975, 101.

INDEX

A

Acceptance problem, 111—112
Action potential, 1, 17
Acute anterior cervical cord syndrome, 129
Acute central cervicular cord syndrome, 129
Adipose tissue, 130
Aerobic metabolism, 95
Afferent influences, 7, 9
Afferent nerve, 125
Afferent nerve paths, 152
Afferent neurons, 124—125
Afferent pathways, 129
Age distribution, 181, 184
Ambulation, 38, 47
Amplitude, 4—5, 12, 18—19, 27, 125
Amuscular standing, 49, 60
Anaerobic metabolism, 95
Animal models, 25—26
Ankle-foot orthosis, 58, 176, 181
Ankle joint mobility, 139
Ankle plantar flexors, 2
Assessment of effects of exercise, 28
Atrophy, 8—9, 24, 128
Autonomic dysreflexia, 177
Autonomous nervous system, 9, 68

B

Babinski response, 37
Balancing aids, 174—177
Balancing forces, 61
Below-knee orthosis, 8
Belt-attached stimulator, 176, 181
Bending stress, 69—75
Bending torques, 68, 71
Bicycle, 3
Bicycle exercise, 23
Biofeedback, 28, 130
Biological work, 58
Blood circulation, 18
Blood pressure, 33
Blood supply, 92
Body weight, 52, 59—60, 81—82
Bone, 8
Bone density, 113
Bone functions, 67—75
Bone integrity, 139
Bone stressing, 49, 68—71, 73, 187
Brown-Sequard lesion, 129

C

Capillary density, 26
Cardiac output, 95
Cauda equina, injuries to, 129
Center of gravity, 52, 57, 67
Central nervous system (CNS), 1, 19, 38, 157
Centrally denervated muscles, 124
Cerebellar stimulation, 43—44

Cerebral ischaemia, 96
Chrondromalacia patellae, 24—25
Closed-loop concept, 7
Closed-loop control, 4, 27, 154, 157, 164, 187
CNS, see Central nervous system
Coactivation, 125
Compartmentalization activation, 72
Complete SCI patients, FES-assisted walking, 139—191, see also FES-assisted walking
Compressive stressing, 69—70
Computerized tomography, 128
Conservation of energy, 55
Conservative force, 55
Contractures, 11, 33, 61, 68, 129—130, 134—135
Contraindications, 92, 96—98
Control, 7
Control information, 155, 157, 159—164
Control source, 155
Control strategy, 157, 159
Coordination, 151—152
Cortical control, 152—153
Cosmesis problem, 187, 189
Crutch ambulation, training of, 169—173
Crutch-attached controls, 175
Crutches, 1—3, 6—8, 135, 147—148, 151, 166
Current density, 140
Currents, 1, 4, 18—19
Cutaneous reflexes, 37

D

Decubiti, 8, 11, 46, 92, 97
Defecation, 33
Denervated muscles, 127—128
Denervation hypertrophy, 26
Dermatomes, 10, 44—47
Dissected spinal cord, 154, 157
Distributed stimulator, 174
Disuse atrophied muscle, 127, 130, 132
Doffing, 111
Donning, 111
Dorsiflexion, 134
Double-support phase, 12, 144
Drop foot, 185
Duration, 18—19, 125
Duty cycle, 22—24, 32—33
Dynamics, 54
Dyspnea, 96

E

Ectopic ossification, 68
Edema, 92, 150
Efferent influences, 7
Efferent nerve paths, 152
Efferent neurons, 124
Electrical stimulators, 1—2
Electrodes, 1—8, 27, 125—126, 129—130, 134, 157, 168
Electrogoniometers, 3, 39—40

Electrogoniometric system, 136
Electromyogram (EMG), 3, 38, 40, 155, 159
EMG, see Electromyogram
Energy, 7—8, 10, 22, 53—56, 135, 139—144, 147, 159
Energy criteria related to standing, 57—63
Energy expenditure, 49, 75, 148—150, 188
Equilibrium, 57, 67, 73
Equipotential movement, 55
Ergonometry, 95
Exercise, 23, 28—33, 131
Exercise bicycle ergometer, 28
Exhaustion, 95
Extension spasticity, 37—38, 46
Extensor reflex activity, 37
Extensor spasticity, 94
Extensor tone, 124—125
Exteroceptive feedback, 157
Extrinsic stability, 49, 58, 60, 62—63

F

Facilitation, 130
Fast twitch fibers, 17—18
Fatigability, see Fatigue
Fatigue, 2, 4—5, 7—9, 11, 17—18, 20, 22—25, 27, 33, 132—133, 185—186
Fatigue index, 22, 32, 133
Fatigue resistance, 2, 4, 10, 25—26, 29—33
Fatiguing, see Fatigue
Feedback control, 154
Feedback control system, 147, 157
Feedback information, 157, 160
Femoral nerves, 2, 4
FES, see also specific topics
  advantages, 8
  barriers, 9
  candidates for, 18
  lower extremity in paraplegic subjects, 1—9
  restoration of locomotion in paraplegic patients, 9—13
  therapeutic effects, 8
  training program, 27
FES ambulation, 9
FES ambulation program, incomplete SCI patients, 123—138
FES-assisted walking
  applications, 173—189
  balancing aids, 174—177
  complete SCI patients, 139—191
  gait restoration, 140—147
  gait synthesis and control, 147—164
  gait training, 164—173
  incomplete SCI patients, 133—137
  patient selection, 139—140
  results, 173—189
  stimulators, 174—177
FES exercise, 2—3, 10, 33
FES-implanted system, 113
FES orthosis, 9
FES orthotic systems, 8—9, 150, 156—158
FES restrengthening, see Restrengthening

FES sequences, 49
FES standing, 11, 97—119
  acceptance problem, 111—112
  benefits of, 109—114
  functional uses of, 114—119
  physiological advantages of, 112
  physiological factors associated to, 113
  posture dependence of standing, performance, 102—105
  posture switching, 105—109
  prerequisites, 97
  procedure, 97—101
  supporting frames for, 101—102
FES therapeutic program, 129—133
FES training, 2—3, 5, 10, 31, 33
FES walking, 6—7
Flaccid muscle, 128
Flexion reflex, 3, 8, 11—12, 37, 124—125, 128, 135, 165, 177, 185
Flexion response, 2—3, 7, 12, 37, 126
Flexion spasticity, 37—38
Flexion synergy, 37
Flexion withdrawal reflex, 94
Flexor reflex, 38
Foot reaction force, 52
Foot switches, 17
Force, 4, 17, 27, 49—53, 131
Force plate, 52
Four-channel gait, 184
Four-channel gait mode, 165
Four-channel gait pattern, 185
Four-channel stimulation sequences, 161
Four-channel stimulator, 165—166
Frequency, 5, 18, 20, 125
Friction, 53
Friction force, 54
Frontal plane, 61
Functional electrical stimulation, see FES and related topics
Functional status of patient, 92—93
Fusion frequency, 20

G

Gait, 2—3, 5, 7—8, 11—12, 59, 130, 134—136
Gait cycle, 143
Gait restoration, 75, 139—147, 177
Gait stability, 159
Gait synthesis and control, 147—164
Gait training, 164—173
Gait velocity, 3
Gluteal nerves, 2, 4
Goniograms, 40, 80, 185—186
Ground reaction forces, 185, 187

H

Habituation, 127—128
Hand switches, 12, 17, 130, 134, 160, 166
Hat, see Hand, arms, and trunk
Head, arms, and trunk (Hat), 76, 145—146
Heart rate, 95

Heel-striking, 144
Heel switch, 1
Heel-switch control, 134
Hematoma, 92, 150
Hemorrhages, 92
Hierarchical control strategy, 159
High-frequency sinusoidal stimulation, 25
High-frequency stimulation, 26
Hip abductors, 2
Hip extensors, 2
Hip flexion contractures, 111
Hoffmann reflex, 39
Homeostatic regulation, 110
Hybrid applications, 93
Hybrid orthosis, 7—8
Hybrid orthotics, 7
Hypercalciuria, 113—114
Hyperextended knee, 61—62
Hypoventilation, 96

I

Immobilization, 23
Implanted FES, 4—5
Implanted FES orthotic system, 148
Implanted multichannel FES system, 4
Implanted sensors, 187
Implanted stimulation systems, 112
Implanted stimulators, 140
Implants, 2, 4
Incomplete SCI lesions
   general characteristics, 123—124
   neurophysiological characteristics, 124—129
   incomplete SCI patients, 11, 28, 39
   FES ambulation program, 123—138
   FES-assisted walking, 133—137
   FES therapeutic program, 129—133
Incomplete spinal cord injury, 22
incomplete tetraplegics, 123
Indications for FES, 96—98
Injury distribution, 181, 183
Innervation of muscles, 152—153
Intrinsic stability, 49, 58, 73
Inverted pendulum oscillations, 144
Isokinetic dynamometer, 28
Isokinetic modality, 28—29
Isokinetic training, 23, 27
Isometric contraction, 58
Isometric exercise, 23, 25
Isometric measurements, 10
Isometric modality, 28—29
Isometric torque, 19—23, 28, 97, 131—132
Isometric training, 27
Isotonic contractions, 26, 130
Isotonic training, 27

J

Jackknifing, 100
Jendrassik maneuver, 38
Joint angle, 155, 157
Joint compliance, 39
Joint contractures, 49
Joint loading, 187
Joint pressure, 74
Joint torque, 19, 28—31, 76, 81, 131—132, 155
Joint trajectories, 159
Joints, 8
Joy stick, 157

K

Kinetic energy, 55
Knee-ankle-foot orthoses, 4, 6—7, 58
Knee buckling, 166
Knee extensors, 3
Knee joint torque, 10—11

L

Lability, 57
Lactic acid, 95
Level of lesion, 92—94
Life expectancy, 1
Limb circumferences, 29
Locking, 7, 67, 74
Locomotion, 6—7
Locomotion restoration, 1, 9—13
Locomotor system, 12
Long leg braces, 1, 6, 8, 148, 165
Lordosis, 61
Low frequency oscillations, 145
Low-frequency stimulation, 25—26, 33, 133
Lower limb support, principle of, 164
Lower motor neuron, 1, 6
Lower motor neuron lesions, 7, 18, 26, 128, 147, 150

M

Magnetic resonance imaging (MRI), 29
Maximum aerobic capacity, 148
Menue mode, 160
Metabolic energy, 54
Mobility rehabilitation, 1—2
Moment of inertia, 144
Monoarticular muscles, 72
Monosynaptic reflexes, 39
Motoneurons, 17—18
Motor points, 5
Movements, 49—53
MRI, see Magnetic resonance imaging
Multichannel implantable FES systems, 9
Multichannel stimulator, 135
Muscle atrophy, 135
Muscle biopsy, 29
Muscle facilitation, 169
Muscle fatigue, 10, see also Fatigue
Muscle fibers, 4, 17—18, 20, 25, 29
Muscle force, 2, 31, 58, 155, 157, see also Force
Muscle restrengthening, see Restrengthening
Muscle spindle, 37, 124
Muscle-twitch, 17, 20
Muscles, 124
Muscular activation space, 67

Muscular status, 92
Musculoskeletal system, 155, 157

N

Needle electrodes, 125
Nerve fibers, 4, 19—20
Net supporting moment, principle of, 164
Neural cell, 1
Neural control, 152—153
Neurological status of patient, 94
Neurologically intact patients, 23—25
Neuromuscular fatigue, 33, see also Fatigue
Neuromuscular system, 92
Nociceptive reflexes, 125
Nonerect standing, 67
Nontubular bone, 69

O

Obesity, 97, 139
One-channel radio frequency powered stimulator, 175
One-joint muscles, 72
Open loop control system, 154, 187
Orthoses, 133
Oscillations, 141, 144
Oscillatory movements, 142
Ossification, 33, 68
Osteoporosis, 49, 68
Oxygen cost, 147
Oxygen rate, 147

P

Pacemaker, 1, 4
Pain, sensation of, 130
Parallelogram walkers, 169, 174, 185
Paraplegic patients, 1—3, 123, 129
Passive movement, 39
Passive orthoses, 6
Patient composed gait synthesis, 161
Patient selection, 92, 96—98
    FES-assisted walking, 139—140
    functional status, 92—93
    indications for FES, 96—98
    level of lesion, 92—94
    neurological status, 94
    physical evaluation, 96—97
    physical examination, 92
    physiological status, 94—96
    standing, 91—97
    status of lesion, 92—94
Pendulum test, 10, 39, 43, 45—47
Percutaneous electrodes, 5
Peripheral nerve lesions, 9
Peripheral nerves, 1
Peripheral nervous system, 157
Peripherally denervated muscles, 124, 127, 129
Peroneal implant, 175
Peroneal nerve, 1, 8, 134
Peroneal stimulation, 11

Peroneal stimulator unit, 185
Phasic motoneurons, 18
Phasic reflexes, 37—38
Phasic spasticity, 38
Physical evaluation of patient, 96—97
Physical examination, 92
Physical exercise, see Exercise or specific types of exercise
Physiological status of patient, 94—96
Plantar flexion contractures, 111
Polysynaptic reflexes, 39
Postural movements, 67—75
Postural space, 10, 49, 65—67
Postural trajectory, 91
Posture, 49, 59
Posture dependence of standing performance, 102—105
Posture selection and standing, 63—65
Posture switching, 2, 11, 49, 105—109, 185
Potential energy, 49, 54
Power, 53—56
Precision potentiometer, 3
Pressure, 155
Pressure sores, 33, 131, 135
Presynaptic inhibition, 41
Progressive resistance exercise, 23
Proprioception, 76
Proprioceptive feedback, 157
Propulsion, 93
Pulse duration, 2, 10, 20—22, 27, 33, 125—127, 130
Pulse train, 126
Pulse width, 5
Pulses, 1, 3, 5, 18—19, 125
Pushing, 162, 166

R

Range of joint motion, 58
Range of motion (ROM), 61—62, 67, 129
Reaction, 52
Reaction force, 73
Reciprocal gait pattern, 139, 161
Reciprocating-brace orthosis, 8
Reflexes, 8, 92, 152
Regeneration of spinal cord, 123
Relaxation index, 40
Resistance, 19
Resonant system frequency, 144
Restrengthening, 9—10, 17—35, 47, 169, 178
Restrengthening program, 26—28
Resultant force, 53, 73
Roller walkers, 169, 174—175
ROM, see Range of motion
Roundabout stimulation, 4
Russian technique of electrical stimulation, 24—25

S

Safety, 7, 93, 165, 189
Sagittal plane postures, 61
Sciatic nerve, 2
Segmented structures, 49, 58—63

Self-contained stimulators, 174
Sensation, 152
Sensibility, 128
Sensors, 9
Sensory augmentation, 154, 157
Sensory driven logic control principles, 189
Sensory-evoked potentials, 38
Sensory information processing, 154
Sensory nerves, 12
Sexual abilities, 33
Shear force, 53, 144
Shoe insole switch, 159
Single-limb support phase, 145
Sitting, 49
Sitting-down, 75—91, 115
Six-channel gait pattern, 162
Skeletal system, 11
Skin sensors, 125
Slow-twitch fibers, 17—18
Slow twitch muscle, 25
Solid objects, 57—58
Somatosensory-evoked potentials, 38
Spasms, 30, 38, 46, 169
Spastic muscle, 128
Spastic paraplegia, 6
Spasticity, 8—11, 33, 92, 114, 129—130, 134, 139, 152
    agonist, 41—45
    antagonist, 41—45
    biomechanical measurements, 38—39
    cerebellar stimulation, 43—44
    clinical assessment, 38—41
    dermatomes, 46
    influence of electrical stimulation, 37—48
    neurophysiological measurements, 38—39
    physical therapy, 43
    spinal cord stimulation, 43—44
    surgical treatment, 41
    treatment, 41—45
    types, 37—38
Spinal control, 152—153
Spinal cord injury, 1
Spinal cord stimulation, 43—44
Spinal reflexes, 153—155
Spinal shock, 37, 124
Spinal spasticity, see Spasticity
Stability, 57—63
Stairs, 12, 173
Stance phase, 134, 185
Stand/sit maneuvers, 79—85
Stand/sit trajectories, 49, 85—91
Standing, 2—3, 9—10, 30, 38, 47, 49—122, 189
    bone functions, 67—75
    energy, 53—56
    energy criteria, 57—63
    FES, see FES standing
    forces, 49—53
    fundamentals of, 56—57
    mechanics of, 49—91, see also other subtopics hereunder
    movements, 49—53
    patient selection, 91—97

    postural movements, 67—75
    postural space, 65—67
    posture selection, 63—65
    power, 53—56
    segmented structures, 58—63
    solid objects, 57—58
    stability, 57—63
    work, 53—56
Standing frame, 97
Standing-up, 10, 75—91, 114
Static coefficient of friction, 53
Static stability, 54
Status of lesion, 92—94
Steady balance, 50
Step length, 149, 164
Step length to step rate ratio, 148
Step rate, 148—149
Stimulated response, 131
Stimulation amplitude, 10, 126—127, 130
Stimulation envelope, 159
Stimulation frequency, 2, 4, 10, 12, 21—24, 27, 125—127, 130
Stimulation sequences, 4—5, 11, 67, 159, 160, 187
Stimulation site, 126
Stimulation trains, 130
Stimulators, 5, 27, 129, 135, 174—178, see also Electrical stimulators
Stooping, 67
Strain gauges transducer, 3
Strength, 2, 8, 25, 29—33
Strengthening, 129—132
Strengthening program, 29—33
Stretch reflex, 37—39, 124
Stride length, 3, 6, 144, 146, 162
Stride time, 185
Stroke volume, 95
Subconscious control, 151, 157
Support area, 57—58, 60
Supraspinal control, 152—153
Surface electrodes, 8—9, 125, 173
Sway, 63
Swing phase, 12, 134, 163
Swing/stance control, 175
Swing/stance phase, 174
Swing-to gait pattern, 173
Swinging, 143—144, 164
Synchronization, 76
Synergies, 67
Synergistic pattern, 94

T

Tendon, 52
Tendon reflex, 39
Tension bands, 71
Tetanic contraction, 20
Tetanic tension, 25—26, 33
Tetraplegic patients, 11, 33, 123, 129
Therapeutic effects of FES, 8
Therapeutic electrical stimulation, 11, 129
Tidal volume, 95
Tilt table, 97

Toe standing, 62—63
Tonic inhibition, 38
Tonic motoneurons, 18
Tonic reflexes, 37—38
Tonic spasticity, 38
Tonic vibration reflex, 39
Transcutaneous electrical stimulation, 44—47
Transducers, 157, 160, 174, 178—179
Tremor, 92
Tubular bone, 69, 73
Twitch contraction, 25
Twitch tension, 25
Two-channel standing stimulator and frame, 179
Two-channel stimulators, 47, 114, 134—135, 165, 178
Two-joint muscle, 71
Type I fibers, 17—18, 29
Type II fibers, 17—18, 29
Type II motors fibers, 33

U

Ultrasound, 29
Upper motor neuron, 1
Upper motor neuron lesion, 7, 9, 18, 26, 37
Upper motor neuron lesion syndrome, 165
Urine calcium, 133—114

V

Vector, 52
Velocity, 7, 37, 39, 55
Ventilation, 95
Vibration reflex, 38
Volitional movement, 17
Voltage, 18—19
Voluntary response, 131

W

Walker, 2—3, 8, 166
Walker ambulation, training of, 169
Walking, 2—4, 6, 9, 12, 30, 47, 135—136
Walking frame, 167, 169
Walking rate, 150
Walking speed, 5—6, 148, 167, 185
Weight force, 72
Weight shifting, 166
Weight vector line, 59
Wheelchair, 1, 6, 9, 11, 94, 114, 133, 147
Wheelchair-attached folding frame, 185
Wheelchair-attached supporting frame, 114—116
Wheeled transport, 141
Wire electrodes, 5
Wires, 4
Withdrawal, 37
Withdrawal reflex, 2, 12
Work, 53—56

DISCARDED
URI LIBRARY